Stabilization and Resuscitation of Newborns

Editor

Bernhard Schwaberger

MDPI • Basel • Beijing • Wuhan • Barcelona • Belgrade • Manchester • Tokyo • Cluj • Tianjin

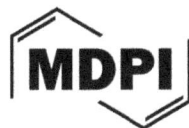

Editor
Bernhard Schwaberger
Division of Neonatology
Medical University of Graz
Graz
Austria

Editorial Office
MDPI
St. Alban-Anlage 66
4052 Basel, Switzerland

This is a reprint of articles from the Special Issue published online in the open access journal *Children* (ISSN 2227-9067) (available at: www.mdpi.com/journal/children/special_issues/Stabilization_Resuscitation_Newborns).

For citation purposes, cite each article independently as indicated on the article page online and as indicated below:

LastName, A.A.; LastName, B.B.; LastName, C.C. Article Title. *Journal Name* **Year**, *Volume Number*, Page Range.

ISBN 978-3-0365-6447-0 (Hbk)
ISBN 978-3-0365-6446-3 (PDF)

© 2023 by the authors. Articles in this book are Open Access and distributed under the Creative Commons Attribution (CC BY) license, which allows users to download, copy and build upon published articles, as long as the author and publisher are properly credited, which ensures maximum dissemination and a wider impact of our publications.

The book as a whole is distributed by MDPI under the terms and conditions of the Creative Commons license CC BY-NC-ND.

Contents

About the Editor vii

Preface to "Stabilization and Resuscitation of Newborns" ix

Bernhard Schwaberger
Stabilization and Resuscitation of Newborns
Reprinted from: *Children* **2022**, *9*, 1492, doi:10.3390/children9101492 1

Lukas Aichhorn, Erik Küng, Lisa Habrina, Tobias Werther, Angelika Berger and Berndt Urlesberger et al.
The Role of Lung Ultrasound in the Management of the Critically Ill Neonate—A Narrative Review and Practical Guide
Reprinted from: *Children* **2021**, *8*, 628, doi:10.3390/children8080628 5

Marlies Bruckner, Nicholas M. Morris, Gerhard Pichler, Christina H. Wolfsberger, Stefan Heschl and Lukas P. Mileder et al.
In Newborn Infants a New Intubation Method May Reduce the Number of Intubation Attempts: A Randomized Pilot Study
Reprinted from: *Children* **2021**, *8*, 553, doi:10.3390/children8070553 19

Hueng-Chuen Fan, Fung-Wei Chang, Ying-Ru Pan, Szu-I Yu, Kuang-Hsi Chang and Chuan-Mu Chen et al.
Approach to the Connection between Meconium Consistency and Adverse Neonatal Outcomes: A Retrospective Clinical Review and Prospective In Vitro Study
Reprinted from: *Children* **2021**, *8*, 1082, doi:10.3390/children8121082 25

Amy L. Lesneski, Payam Vali, Morgan E. Hardie, Satyan Lakshminrusimha and Deepika Sankaran
Randomized Trial of Oxygen Saturation Targets during and after Resuscitation and Reversal of Ductal Flow in an Ovine Model of Meconium Aspiration and Pulmonary Hypertension
Reprinted from: *Children* **2021**, *8*, 594, doi:10.3390/children8070594 43

Satyan Lakshminrusimha, Sylvia F. Gugino, Krishnamurthy Sekar, Stephen Wedgwood, Carmon Koenigsknecht and Jayasree Nair et al.
Inhaled Nitric Oxide at Birth Reduces Pulmonary Vascular Resistance and Improves Oxygenation in Preterm Lambs
Reprinted from: *Children* **2021**, *8*, 378, doi:10.3390/children8050378 53

Stamatios Giannakis, Maria Ruhfus, Mona Markus, Anja Stein, Thomas Hoehn and Ursula Felderhoff-Mueser et al.
Mechanical Ventilation, Partial Pressure of Carbon Dioxide, Increased Fraction of Inspired Oxygen and the Increased Risk for Adverse Short-Term Outcomes in Cooled Asphyxiated Newborns
Reprinted from: *Children* **2021**, *8*, 430, doi:10.3390/children8060430 65

Seung Yeon Kim, Gyu-Hong Shim and Georg M. Schmölzer
Is Chest Compression Superimposed with Sustained Inflation during Cardiopulmonary Resuscitation an Alternative to 3:1 Compression to Ventilation Ratio in Newborn Infants?
Reprinted from: *Children* **2021**, *8*, 97, doi:10.3390/children8020097 81

Bernhard Schwaberger, Christoph Schlatzer, Daniel Freidorfer, Marlies Bruckner, Christina H. Wolfsberger and Lukas P. Mileder et al.
The Use of a Disposable Umbilical Clamp to Secure an Umbilical Venous Catheter in Neonatal Emergencies—An Experimental Feasibility Study
Reprinted from: *Children* **2021**, *8*, 1093, doi:10.3390/children8121093 . . . . **91**

Deepika Sankaran, Payam Vali, Praveen Chandrasekharan, Peggy Chen, Sylvia F. Gugino and Carmon Koenigsknecht et al.
Effect of a Larger Flush Volume on Bioavailability and Efficacy of Umbilical Venous Epinephrine during Neonatal Resuscitation in Ovine Asphyxial Arrest
Reprinted from: *Children* **2021**, *8*, 464, doi:10.3390/children8060464 . . . . **101**

Ahmed Aboalqez, Philipp Deindl, Chinedu Ulrich Ebenebe, Dominique Singer and Martin Ernst Blohm
Iatrogenic Blood Loss in Very Low Birth Weight Infants and Transfusion of Packed Red Blood Cells in a Tertiary Care Neonatal Intensive Care Unit
Reprinted from: *Children* **2021**, *8*, 847, doi:10.3390/children8100847 . . . . **111**

Lukas Peter Mileder, Nicholas Mark Morris, Stefan Kurath-Koller, Jasmin Pansy, Gerhard Pichler and Mirjam Pocivalnik et al.
Successful Postnatal Cardiopulmonary Resuscitation Due to Defibrillation
Reprinted from: *Children* **2021**, *8*, 421, doi:10.3390/children8050421 . . . . **121**

Ena Pritišanac, Berndt Urlesberger, Bernhard Schwaberger and Gerhard Pichler
Accuracy of Pulse Oximetry in the Presence of Fetal Hemoglobin—A Systematic Review
Reprinted from: *Children* **2021**, *8*, 361, doi:10.3390/children8050361 . . . . **127**

Nariae Baik-Schneditz, Bernhard Schwaberger, Lukas Mileder, Nina Höller, Alexander Avian and Berndt Urlesberger et al.
Cardiac Output and Cerebral Oxygenation in Term Neonates during Neonatal Transition
Reprinted from: *Children* **2021**, *8*, 439, doi:10.3390/children8060439 . . . . **139**

David B. Healy, Eugene M. Dempsey, John M. O'Toole and Christoph E. Schwarz
In-Silico Evaluation of Anthropomorphic Measurement Variations on Electrical Cardiometry in Neonates
Reprinted from: *Children* **2021**, *8*, 936, doi:10.3390/children8100936 . . . . **147**

Ravindra Pawar, Vijay Gavade, Nivedita Patil, Vijay Mali, Amol Girwalkar and Vyankatesh Tarkasband et al.
Neonatal Multisystem Inflammatory Syndrome (MIS-N) Associated with Prenatal Maternal SARS-CoV-2: A Case Series
Reprinted from: *Children* **2021**, *8*, 572, doi:10.3390/children8070572 . . . . **151**

About the Editor

Bernhard Schwaberger

Bernhard Schwaberger is a neonatologist and researcher affiliated with the Division of Neonatology at the Medical University of Graz, Austria. His research interests include neonatal resuscitation, near-infrared spectroscopy, prehospital emergency medicine, neonatal transition, cerebral blood volume, vascular access in the newborn, lung ultrasonography (point-of-care ultrasonography), (non-)invasive ventilation of the neonate, and congenital diaphragmatic hernia. He has published about 80 scientific articles in the field.

Preface to "Stabilization and Resuscitation of Newborns"

The majority of newborns do not need medical interventions to manage the neonatal transition after birth. However, every year millions of newborns worldwide require respiratory support immediately after birth, and another considerable number of newborns additionally require extensive resuscitation including chest compressions and drug administration. Despite a significant increase in knowledge and development of enhanced therapy strategies over the past few years, morbidity and mortality caused by failures in neonatal transition remain an important health issue. The purpose of this book is to support or introduce novel concepts and add information in the area of the "Stabilization and Resuscitation of Newborns", aiming to improve neonatal care and, as the major objective, to enhance neuro-developmental outcomes.

I believe that this book helps to contribute to consolidating the current body of information with the hopes of enhancing and stimulating further studies on all spectra of "Stabilization and Resuscitation of Newborns".

Bernhard Schwaberger
Editor

Editorial

Stabilization and Resuscitation of Newborns

Bernhard Schwaberger

Division of Neonatology, Department of Pediatrics and Adolescent Medicine, Medical University of Graz, 8036 Graz, Austria; bernhard.schwaberger@medunigraz.at; Tel.: +43-316-385-30018

The majority of newborns do not need medical interventions to manage the neonatal transition after birth. However, every year millions of newborns worldwide require respiratory support immediately after birth, and another considerable number of newborns additionally require extensive resuscitation including chest compressions and drug administration. Despite a significant increase in knowledge and development of enhanced therapy strategies over the past few years, morbidity and mortality caused by failures in neonatal transition remain an important health issue. The purpose of this Special Issue is to support or introduce novel concepts and add information in the area of the "Stabilization and Resuscitation of Newborns", aiming to improve neonatal care and, as the major objective, to enhance neuro-developmental outcomes.

1. Respiratory Support

Most emergency situations in the newborn are respiratory conditions, often during the neonatal transition after birth. Neonatologists are confronted with the challenging task of achieving optimal care for term and preterm newborns which often requires quick and decisive action. The review by Aichhorn et al. [1] describes the neonatologist-performed lung ultrasound (NPLUS) as a point-of-care examination and its use for the stabilization and resuscitation of newborns. NPLUS immediately provides knowledge about the respiratory condition of the patient and helps to rule out pneumothorax, and visualize ventilation or atelectases, effusions, or consolidations in less than one minute. More experienced sonographers may use NPLUS for assessment of tracheal tube placement, diagnosis of congenital malformations, diaphragmatic movement, and pneumomediastinum as well as assessment of laryngeal anatomy. Thereby, NPLUS further reduces exposure to ionizing radiation.

Neonatal tracheal intubation is a life-saving procedure, but adverse events are not uncommon. A small randomized controlled trial by Bruckner et al. [2] evaluated the concept of providing continuous gas flow through the tracheal tube during neonatal intubation to prevent severe desaturation or bradycardia. This novel approach seems to be favorable compared to the standard procedure without increasing the risk for major unexpected adverse events.

Meconium aspiration syndrome remains a major contributor to neonatal morbidity and mortality. The study by Fan et al. [3] suggested that thick meconium in newborns might be associated with poorer outcomes compared with thin meconium based on chart reviews. Additionally, they presented cell survival assays following the incubation of various meconium concentrations with monolayers of certain cell lines, which were consistent with the results obtained from the chart reviews.

Lesneski et al. [4] compared time to reversal of ductal shunting in persistent pulmonary hypertension of the newborn (PPHN) between standard and high oxygen saturation (SpO2) targets during resuscitation and in the post-resuscitation period. In this term lamb model of meconium aspiration syndrome and PPHN, targeting SpO2 at a higher range (95–99%) during resuscitation and in the immediate post-resuscitation period led to a quicker transition to left-to-right shunting across the ductus arteriosus but did not result in a sustained increase in pulmonary blood flow.

Inhaled nitric oxide (iNO) is a common therapy for newborns suffering from PPHN in the neonatal intensive care unit, but the potential effects of its use during stabilization and resuscitation immediately after birth have not been investigated in detail. In their animal study, Lakshminrusimha et al. [5] studied the effects of iNO on oxygenation and pulmonary vascular resistance in preterm lambs with and without PPHN during resuscitation and stabilization at birth. They concluded that iNO at birth is effective for improving oxygenation and reducing pulmonary vascular resistance in both preterm lambs with and without PPHN without increasing inspired oxygen.

In newborns treated with therapeutic hypothermia following perinatal asphyxia, several risk factors are associated with adverse outcomes. In their retrospective study including 71 asphyxiated cooled newborns, Giannakis et al. [6] analyzed the association between ventilation status (mechanical ventilation versus spontaneously breathing newborns) and adverse short-term outcomes. The need for mechanical ventilation was significantly higher in newborns with more severe asphyxia. In ventilated newborns, higher levels of encephalopathy, lower partial pressure of carbon dioxide, and increased oxygen supplementation were associated with adverse short-term outcomes.

2. Cardio-Circulatory Support

Cardio-circulatory support after birth may include interventions such as chest compressions, the establishment of vascular access and emergent drug administration (e.g., epinephrine, volume expanders), and–in very rare cases–may also include defibrillation.

While the current neonatal resuscitation guidelines recommend a 3:1 compression to ventilation ratio, it was recently demonstrated that providing continuous chest compressions superimposed with high distending pressure or sustained inflation may reduce the time to return of spontaneous circulation and mortality in both asphyxiated piglets and newborn infants. A review by Kim et al. [7] summarizes the currently available evidence of continuous chest compressions superimposed with sustained inflation.

Drug administration during neonatal resuscitation requires immediate vascular access to the newborn. Recent guidelines recommend the umbilical venous catheter (UVC) as the optimal vascular access during neonatal resuscitation. However, the UVC securement may be challenging and time-consuming. Therefore, our study group [8] introduced a new concept of UVC securement by using a peripheral catheter and a disposable umbilical clamp. This experimental study on umbilical cord remnants was designed to test the feasibility of this concept. It may be a rewarding option for umbilical venous catheterization and securement, but the experimental data need to be confirmed in clinical trials before being introduced into clinical practice.

In case of persistent bradycardia despite effective ventilation and chest compressions, the administration of epinephrine via a UVC is recommended and should be followed by a certain amount of flush volume. The flush may be essential to push epinephrine to the right atrium in the absence of intrinsic cardiac activity during chest compression. Sankaran et al. [9] evaluated the effect of 1 mL versus 2.5 mL flush volumes of normal saline after epinephrine administration via a UVC in a near-term ovine model of perinatal asphyxia-induced cardiac arrest. Three out of seven (43%) and 12/15 (80%) lambs achieved the return of spontaneous circulation after the first dose of epinephrine with 1 mL versus 2.5 mL flush, respectively ($p = 0.08$). From this pilot study, higher flush volume after the first dose of epinephrine may be beneficial during neonatal resuscitation.

An adequate blood volume is important for neonatal resuscitation and stabilization. In their retrospective single-center study, Aboalqez et al. [10] quantified the cumulative iatrogenic blood loss in very low birth weight infants by blood sampling and the necessity of packed red cell transfusions from birth until discharge from the hospital. They concluded that iatrogenic blood loss should be limited to a minimum in the interest of patient blood management.

The case presentation by Mileder et al. [11] is the first reported case of a newborn with perinatal asphyxia, who required postnatal resuscitation and defibrillation due to ventricular fibrillation following epinephrine administration. Based on this case, the authors suggest that health care providers managing neonatal resuscitation should be aware of the possible need for defibrillation, even though it may be very rare. Therefore, they suggest providing a defibrillator with appropriately sized pediatric defibrillation pads in every delivery room, allowing for weight-adapted, gradual titration of the energy level.

3. Cardio-Respiratory Monitoring

Cardio-respiratory monitoring may assist health care providers to identify the newborn in need of medical interventions after birth and may be used for evaluating and observing the newborn's condition at the neonatal intensive care unit. For these purposes, pulse oximetry is routinely used during neonatal care. The review by Pritišanac et al. [12] compared non-invasive arterial oxygen saturation monitoring by pulse oximetry (SpO2) to oxygen saturation measurements from arterial blood samples (SaO2) in preterm and term newborns in terms of fetal hemoglobin (HbF) measurements. They found a considerable SpO2-SaO2 bias and concluded that the influence of HbF on SpO2 readings may result in an overestimation of SpO2 for the lower saturation ranges.

Advanced monitoring of the cardio-circulatory system and/or the brain provides further information during the neonatal transition after birth. Baik-Schneditz et al. [13] combined non-invasive cardiac output (CO) monitoring by electrical velocimetry and cerebral near-infrared spectroscopy in term newborns after cesarean section, in order to analyze the potential influence of CO on cerebral oxygenation during the neonatal transition. In term infants with uncomplicated neonatal transition after cesarean section, they found no correlation of CO and cerebral oxygenation.

Healy et al. [14] described in their in silico study that anthropometric measures as weight and length of the newborn affect non-invasive CO measurements. Therefore, inaccurate estimates or measurements of anthropometric values can lead to clinically relevant differences in CO measurements, which are more pronounced in preterm infants compared to term infants. This should be considered in the design of future clinical trials and in the interpretation of previous studies including non-invasive CO measurements in the newborn.

4. COVID-19

The recent coronavirus disease 2019 (COVID-19) pandemic affected all segments of health care including obstetrics and neonatology. Pawar et al. [15] published a case series of 20 newborns with features of a hyperinflammatory syndrome associated with prenatal maternal SARS-CoV-2 infection potentially caused by transplacental transfer of anti-SARS-CoV-2 antibodies. Ninety percent had cardiac involvement with prolonged QTc (corrected QT interval), 2:1 atrioventricular block, cardiogenic shock, or coronary dilatation. Other findings included respiratory failure, fever, feeding intolerance and melena. All infants had elevated inflammatory biomarkers and received immunomodulatory therapy (e.g., steroids and intravenous immunoglobulins). Two infants (10%) died. This condition was named "Neonatal Multisystem Inflammatory Syndrome" (MIS-N) in conformity with the post-infectious immune-mediated condition in children, "Multisystem inflammatory syndrome in children" (MIS-C), usually seen 3–5 weeks after COVID-19.

I believe that this Special Issue of *Children* helps to contribute to consolidating the current body of information with the hopes of enhancing and stimulating further studies on all spectra of "Stabilization and Resuscitation of Newborns".

Funding: This research received no external funding.

Institutional Review Board Statement: Not applicable.

Informed Consent Statement: Not applicable.

Acknowledgments: The author would like to thank Lukas P. Mileder and Andreas Trobisch for proofreading the Editorial manuscript.

Conflicts of Interest: The author declares no conflict of interest.

References

1. Aichhorn, L.; Küng, E.; Habrina, L.; Werther, T.; Berger, A.; Urlesberger, B.; Schwaberger, B. The Role of Lung Ultrasound in the Management of the Critically Ill Neonate—A Narrative Review and Practical Guide. *Children* **2021**, *8*, 628. [CrossRef] [PubMed]
2. Bruckner, M.; Morris, N.M.; Pichler, G.; Wolfsberger, C.H.; Heschl, S.; Mileder, L.P.; Schwaberger, B.; Schmölzer, G.M.; Urlesberger, B. In Newborn Infants a New Intubation Method May Reduce the Number of Intubation Attempts: A Randomized Pilot Study. *Children* **2021**, *8*, 553. [CrossRef] [PubMed]
3. Fan, H.-C.; Chang, F.-W.; Pan, Y.-R.; Yu, S.-I.; Chang, K.-H.; Chen, C.-M.; Liu, C.-A. Approach to the Connection between Meconium Consistency and Adverse Neonatal Outcomes: A Retrospective Clinical Review and Prospective In Vitro Study. *Children* **2021**, *8*, 1082. [CrossRef] [PubMed]
4. Lesneski, A.L.; Vali, P.; Hardie, M.E.; Lakshminrusimha, S.; Sankaran, D. Randomized Trial of Oxygen Saturation Targets during and after Resuscitation and Reversal of Ductal Flow in an Ovine Model of Meconium Aspiration and Pulmonary Hypertension. *Children* **2021**, *8*, 594. [CrossRef] [PubMed]
5. Lakshminrusimha, S.; Gugino, S.F.; Sekar, K.; Wedgwood, S.; Koenigsknecht, C.; Nair, J.; Mathew, B. Inhaled Nitric Oxide at Birth Reduces Pulmonary Vascular Resistance and Improves Oxygenation in Preterm Lambs. *Children* **2021**, *8*, 378. [CrossRef] [PubMed]
6. Giannakis, S.; Ruhfus, M.; Markus, M.; Stein, A.; Hoehn, T.; Felderhoff-Mueser, U.; Sabir, H. Mechanical Ventilation, Partial Pressure of Carbon Dioxide, Increased Fraction of Inspired Oxygen and the Increased Risk for Adverse Short-Term Outcomes in Cooled Asphyxiated Newborns. *Children* **2021**, *8*, 430. [CrossRef] [PubMed]
7. Kim, S.Y.; Shim, G.-H.; Schmölzer, G.M. Is Chest Compression Superimposed with Sustained Inflation during Cardiopulmonary Resuscitation an Alternative to 3:1 Compression to Ventilation Ratio in Newborn Infants? *Children* **2021**, *8*, 97. [CrossRef] [PubMed]
8. Schwaberger, B.; Schlatzer, C.; Freidorfer, D.; Bruckner, M.; Wolfsberger, C.H.; Mileder, L.P.; Pichler, G.; Urlesberger, B. The Use of a Disposable Umbilical Clamp to Secure an Umbilical Venous Catheter in Neonatal Emergencies—An Experimental Feasibility Study. *Children* **2021**, *8*, 1093. [CrossRef] [PubMed]
9. Sankaran, D.; Vali, P.; Chandrasekharan, P.; Chen, P.; Gugino, S.F.; Koenigsknecht, C.; Helman, J.; Nair, J.; Mathew, B.; Rawat, M.; et al. Effect of a Larger Flush Volume on Bioavailability and Efficacy of Umbilical Venous Epinephrine during Neonatal Resuscitation in Ovine Asphyxial Arrest. *Children* **2021**, *8*, 464. [CrossRef] [PubMed]
10. Aboalqez, A.; Deindl, P.; Ebenebe, C.U.; Singer, D.; Blohm, M.E. Iatrogenic Blood Loss in Very Low Birth Weight Infants and Transfusion of Packed Red Blood Cells in a Tertiary Care Neonatal Intensive Care Unit. *Children* **2021**, *8*, 847. [CrossRef] [PubMed]
11. Mileder, L.P.; Morris, N.M.; Kurath-Koller, S.; Pansy, J.; Pichler, G.; Pocivalnik, M.; Schwaberger, B.; Burmas, A.; Urlesberger, B. Successful Postnatal Cardiopulmonary Resuscitation Due to Defibrillation. *Children* **2021**, *8*, 421. [CrossRef] [PubMed]
12. Pritišanac, E.; Urlesberger, B.; Schwaberger, B.; Pichler, G. Accuracy of Pulse Oximetry in the Presence of Fetal Hemoglobin—A Systematic Review. *Children* **2021**, *8*, 361. [CrossRef] [PubMed]
13. Baik-Schneditz, N.; Schwaberger, B.; Mileder, L.; Höller, N.; Avian, A.; Urlesberger, B.; Pichler, G. Cardiac Output and Cerebral Oxygenation in Term Neonates during Neonatal Transition. *Children* **2021**, *8*, 439. [CrossRef] [PubMed]
14. Healy, D.B.; Dempsey, E.M.; O'Toole, J.M.; Schwarz, C.E. In-Silico Evaluation of Anthropomorphic Measurement Variations on Electrical Cardiometry in Neonates. *Children* **2021**, *8*, 936. [CrossRef] [PubMed]
15. Pawar, R.; Gavade, V.; Patil, N.; Mali, V.; Girwalkar, A.; Tarkasband, V.; Loya, S.; Chavan, A.; Nanivadekar, N.; Shinde, R.; et al. Neonatal Multisystem Inflammatory Syndrome (MIS-N) Associated with Prenatal Maternal SARS-CoV-2: A Case Series. *Children* **2021**, *8*, 572. [CrossRef] [PubMed]

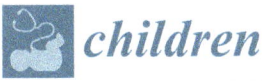

Review

The Role of Lung Ultrasound in the Management of the Critically Ill Neonate—A Narrative Review and Practical Guide

Lukas Aichhorn [1,*], Erik Küng [1], Lisa Habrina [1], Tobias Werther [1], Angelika Berger [1], Berndt Urlesberger [2] and Bernhard Schwaberger [2]

1. Comprehensive Center for Paediatrics, Department of Paediatrics and Adolescent Medicine, Division of Neonatology, Paediatric Intensive Care & Neuropaediatrics, Medical University of Vienna, Währinger Gürtel 18-20, 1090 Vienna, Austria; erik.kueng@meduniwien.ac.at (E.K.); lisa.habrina@meduniwien.ac.at (L.H.); tobias.werther@meduniwien.ac.at (T.W.); angelika.berger@meduniwien.ac.at (A.B.)
2. Department of Paediatrics and Adolescent Medicine, Division of Neonatology, Medical University of Graz, Auenbruggerplatz 34/2, 8036 Graz, Austria; berndt.urlesberger@medunigraz.at (B.U.); bernhard.schwaberger@medunigraz.at (B.S.)
* Correspondence: lukas.aichhorn@meduniwien.ac.at; Tel.: +43-1-40400-64020

Abstract: Lung ultrasound makes use of artifacts generated by the ratio of air and fluid in the lung. Recently, an enormous increase of research regarding lung ultrasound emerged, especially in intensive care units. The use of lung ultrasound on the neonatal intensive care unit enables the clinician to gain knowledge about the respiratory condition of the patients, make quick decisions, and reduces exposure to ionizing radiation. In this narrative review, the possibilities of lung ultrasound for the stabilization and resuscitation of the neonate using the ABCDE algorithm will be discussed.

Keywords: lung ultrasound; neonatal resuscitation; transition process; respiratory distress syndrome

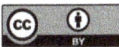

1. Introduction

On a daily basis, neonatologists are confronted with the challenging task of achieving the optimal care for term and preterm neonates. In particular, the stressful situation of resuscitation of infants often requires quick and decisive action with potentially crucial decisions regarding the current condition, but also the long-term outcome of the patient, based on limited information. The majority of these emergency situations in neonatology are respiratory conditions, often during the process of neonatal transition [1,2].

In the last decade, the use of lung ultrasound (LUS) has gained momentum in various specialties, not only to reduce exposure to radiation but because of the broad spectrum of diagnostic possibilities of this formerly underappreciated technique, especially in neonatal intensive care units (NICU) [3].

Many aspects of the management of critically ill neonates are controversial. As a consequence, a large number of protocols for the postnatal stabilization of infants have been proposed, to the extent that almost every institution has developed its own guideline and standard of practice for this purpose. In adult patients, ultrasound has become an integral part of emergency medicine [4] and pre-hospital care [5] over the past two decades with the corresponding standardization of protocols. However, only with recent publication of the International Evidence-Based Guidelines on Point of Care Ultrasound by the European Society of Paediatric and Neonatal Intensive Care, ultrasound found its way into paediatric and neonatal intensive care units in a standardized form [6]. The Paediatric Life Support (PLS) guidelines by the European resuscitation council mention ultrasound for situations like confirmation of proper tracheal tube position, management of circulatory failure or diagnosis of tension pneumothorax, pneumonia and pericardial tamponade. However, the European Resuscitation Council Guidelines 2021 for Newborn resuscitation and support of transition of infants at birth (NLS Guidelines) do not consider ultrasound, mainly due to a lack of evidence for term and preterm infants [7]. Several methods for opening and securing the airway mentioned in the NLS Guidelines can be assessed using ultrasound.

In our units, we started using a standardized LUS protocol, starting first in Vienna in 2016 [8], since LUS has been proven to be an effective, reliable, cheap—and frankly—a reasonably easy way to gain knowledge about the respiratory condition of a patient [3,9,10].

In this narrative review we want to share our insights, experiences and evidence-based information about the benefits of LUS in the management of the critically ill neonate. We will provide a guide through the stabilization process using the ABCDE algorithm. The PLS guidelines use A, B, C, D and E as mnemonic to assess the critically ill child and neonate, where A stands for airway, B for breathing, C for circulation, D for disability and E for other emergencies or environment [7].

Lung ultrasound makes use of *artifacts* generated by the ratio of air and fluid in the lung. For a long time, maybe even because of this particular feature, LUS has not been in the focus of research. One of the first reports of using LUS was published in 1951 by Stuhlfauth et al., who reported typical reflections in cases of pneumothorax. Since then, several studies were published with limited impact [11–13]. After gaining momentum in adult critical care medicine in the early 21st century, "International evidence-based recommendations for point of care lung ultrasound" were published in 2012 [6]. The paper provided the reader with evidence-based recommendations regarding the application of LUS in case of pneumothorax, interstitial syndrome, lung consolidation and pleural effusion. In the following years and especially recently, triggered by the SARS-CoV-2 pandemic, an enormous increase of research regarding LUS has emerged.

In this review, we focus on point of care LUS examinations performed by neonatologists in the intensive care setting, therefore we chose the term neonatologist-performed-LUS (NPLUS) in analogy to the common term of neonatologist-performed echocardiography (NPE).

The detailed description of the signs used in LUS for the neonate as well as certain applications of NPLUS have been sufficiently described elsewhere and are beyond the scope of this review [3,8,9,14,15]. However, for better understanding we briefly want to address the most important signs:

The first step in lung ultrasound is looking for lung sliding, which represents the movement of parietal and visceral pleura. In a healthy lung, a thin, regular pleural line is seen, with horizontal, hyperechogenic reverberation artefacts underneath, known as A-Lines. In case of a shift from a healthy lung to a less aerated lung, usually B-Lines emerge. Those can be identified as a well-defined comet-tail artefact, which erases A-Lines and moves with lung sliding. Newborns present initially with B-Lines, with a declining number of B-Lines in case of a normal transition during the first hours of life. In case of a very poorly or not aerated lung area, consolidations may be observed. In this case, hypoechoic areas, or even hepatization of the lung occurs. A lung ultrasound examination of a healthy neonate is seen in Supplementary file Video S1.

Furthermore, determination of a LUS-score has been proven to help the clinician make decisions based on the lung ultrasound findings. First described by Brat et al. in neonates, the score was later modified in several ways, but the principle remains the same: For each scanned area, artefacts or even patterns are classified or graded, usually from 0-3. The score of each area is added together, resulting in a score that basically inversely reflects lung aeration [3,16].

Our goal is to provide recommendations about the use of NPLUS especially for the critically ill neonate using the ABCDE algorithm.

2. A—Airway

Establishing and maintaining an open airway is essential to achieve postnatal transition and spontaneous breathing, or for further resuscitative actions to be effective [17]. Several methods, including head tilt, jaw thrust, suctioning of secretions, supraglottic devices and tracheal intubation are used to ensure open airways [18]. To assess the treatment response to each method, vital sign monitoring, clinical examination and point of care ultrasound can be used.

Intuitively, point of care ultrasound may be considered to be slower than clinical examination, but studies in adults have shown the contrary. In a prospective randomized study in 106 adult patients undergoing trauma resuscitation, ultrasound was faster in identifying esophageal intubation and confirmation of tracheal intubation compared to five-point auscultation and capnography [19].

In our experience, bilateral ventilation can be assessed within 15 s by verifying lung sliding. However, studies are lacking to provide evidence for a recommendation regarding the use of ultrasound to assess an open airway or tube placement during neonatal resuscitation.

2.1. Continuous Positive Airway Pressure

In spontaneously breathing preterm infants, it is recommended to consider continuous positive airway pressure (CPAP) as the initial method of ventilatory support after delivery—using either mask or nasal prongs [17]. NPLUS can be used for the diagnosis of conditions treated with CPAP, such as transient tachypnea of the newborn or respiratory distress syndrome [20].

2.2. Assisted Ventilation

In adult patients, several studies have shown that scanning for lung sliding using ultrasound is superior to clinical assessment in detecting effective ventilation [21,22]. For this purpose, the major sign in ultrasound is bilateral lung sliding [23]. Effective ventilation—regardless of the device—always results in visible lung sliding in the ventilated lungs. Furthermore, it allows the person performing manual ventilation to have visual feedback.

In experienced hands, confirmation of ventilation by ultrasound is faster compared to auscultation [19]. In neonates, lung sliding presents identical as in paediatric or adult patients, and due to the presence of B-Lines, recognition of lung sliding may be even easier in this patient cohort. However, evidence regarding the feasibility of assessment of effective ventilation using NPLUS is missing for neonates.

In adults, ultrasound assessment of the anterior neck soft tissues by measuring the minimum distance from the hyoid bone to skin surface showed promising results in predicting difficult mask ventilation and difficult laryngoscopy [24]. This correlation still needs to be examined in neonates, and findings may help identifying patients, in whom a difficult mask ventilation must be anticipated.

2.3. Assessment of Laryngeal Anatomy

Ultrasound allows for direct visualization of the laryngeal anatomy, vocal cords and arytenoid cartilages, and due to the dynamic character of an ultrasound exam, it can be used for assessment of glottic opening and vocal cord movement.

Ultrasound can play an important role in the diagnosis of vocal cord palsy and laryngomalacia without exposing the child to the risks of an invasive endoscopy [25,26].

In a recently published article, Oulego-Erroz et al. used ultrasound to diagnose laryngomalacia in an infant with stridor who required respiratory support. The authors successfully captured the collapse of arytenoids and narrowing of the glottic opening when the infant was agitated. The finding was confirmed by endoscopy [27].

2.4. Laryngeal Mask

A laryngeal mask can be used in infants above 34 weeks gestation when problems with establishing effective ventilation with a facemask occur, intubation is not possible, or as an alternative to tracheal intubation [17]. Correct positioning of a laryngeal mask is usually assessed by capnography, appropriate chest excursion, and the absence of an audible leak [28]. In 2015, Kim et al. demonstrated that it is possible to correctly identify rotated laryngeal masks in paediatric patients by assessing the symmetry of arytenoid elevations in transversal view using ultrasound. Using the same method, Song et al. were able to confirm laryngeal mask placement by ultrasound to be quick, non-invasive and reliable in adults [29]. Although no study assessed ultrasound for the detection of the correct position of laryngeal masks in neonates, the signs are the same as in paediatric patients. Evidence for a recommendation regarding the laryngeal mask placement during resuscitation in neonates is lacking.

2.5. Tracheal Intubation

In adult patients, ultrasound was shown to be useful in airway management including the identification of vocal cord palsy, predicting the optimal size of endotracheal, double lumen tubes including tracheostomy-tubes, evaluating the position of breathing tubes in trachea, main-stem bronchus, or esophagus, in pre-anesthetic airway evaluation and percutaneous cricothyroidotomy [30,31]. Some of these applications have already been studied in paediatric patients and neonates, but data is limited, especially in neonates.

Chest X-ray is considered gold standard for determination of endotracheal tube location and is recommended by the NLS Guidelines [17]. However, it contributes to cumulative radiation exposure, is often time-consuming and requires manipulation of the patient [32]. Verification of endotracheal tube position was shown to be possible using ultrasound in neonates back in 1986 by Slovis and Poland, who were able to directly visualize the tip of the tube in 16 infants. They reported that a distance of less than 1 cm between the tip of the tube and the aortic arch to be too low in the chest. This method was later shown to have 94% (95% CI: 85–98%) concordance with a tube positioned below the third thoracic vertebra in chest-X-ray in 56 cases in 29 neonates with birthweights between 370–3750 g [33]. The most common technique to assess correct endotracheal tube placement in neonates is measuring the distance between the tip of the tube and the superior aspect of the right pulmonary artery, because the carina cannot be reliably identified, and the superior aspect of the right pulmonary artery is approximately at the level of the bottom of the carina on midsagittal view (see Supplementary file Video S2) [32,34,35]. It is important to note that the tip-to-carina distance in chest-X-ray does not account for the angulation of the trachea to horizontal plane of 20° in supine position [34]. This assessment takes between 5 and 19 min and has significant agreement with chest-X-ray in neonates with bodyweights between 560–4935 g (95% CI: 0.92–0.98, $n = 40$), between 485–3345 g ($r^2 = 0.68$, $n = 30$), and with mean bodyweight of 2037 g ($r^2 = 0.61$, 95% CI: 0.26–0.79, $n = 40$) [32,34–36]. Overall, ultrasound interpretation of the endotracheal tube position in neonates correlates with the radiography position in 73–100% of cases with over 90% concordance with chest-X-ray in the four largest studies performed [37].

While direct visualization of the tip of the tube is accurate, in critical situations time is essential and assessment of bilateral lung sliding may be sufficient for assessment of the placement of the endotracheal tube, as shown by Fajardo-Escolar et al. in a preterm neonate with esophageal atresia. Even during resuscitation of a neonate, esophageal intubation can be detected using transversal view of the trachea and neck [37–39]. In our experience, assessment for bilateral lung sliding can be performed within one minute.

2.6. Ultrasound Guided Tracheal Intubation

In 2012 Fiadjoe et al. used real-time ultrasound of the vocal cords while performing a jaw thrust and inserting a hockey-stick-shaped styletted tube in the midline of the patients pharynx under direct vision until it was visible in ultrasound to successfully intubate a 14-month old child and called this technique ultrasound guided tracheal intubation [40]. This technique was later reported by Moustafa et al. to be 99%, 132/133 (72%, 96/133 on the first attempt) effective needing 57 s in adult patients [41]. This high efficacy was later confirmed by Ma et al., who found a 93.3% (28/30) success rate [42].

All studies used a hypoechoic shadowing and widening of the vocal cords in transversal view as proof of endotracheal intubation [41–43].

Although this technique was only studied in case reports in neonates, it is a promising alternative in patients with difficult airways, especially when resources are limited.

2.7. Airway Obstruction

Airway obstruction can be caused by inappropriate positioning with decreased airway tone and/or laryngeal adduction, or due to mucus, vernix, meconium, or blood clots [17]. By using NPLUS, not only effective ventilation by bilateral lung sliding can be recognized, but this method also provides the clinician with additional information regarding the cause for deterioration and produces an objective and reproducible image.

2.8. DOPES

The PLS Guidelines state that sudden rapid deterioration of a child with ventilatory support (via mask or tracheal tube) is a time-critical event that demands immediate action and recommends "DOPES" as a mnemonic for displacement of the device, obstruction of the airway, pneumothorax, equipment failure or stomach for abdominal compartment [7]. In assessing for "DOPES", ultrasound can be used for the first four letters simultaneously by searching for bilateral lung sliding. If present, the lung is bilaterally ventilated, excluding displacement of the device or obstruction of the airway and pneumothorax and most cases of equipment failure.

3. B—Breathing

The focus of LUS concerns the B-part in the ABCDE algorithm. Based on different clinical situations, we try to describe the possibilities of NPLUS in this category.

3.1. NPLUS in the Delivery Room

The choice of appropriate measures for the management of the initial stabilization process of preterm and term neonates is an important aspect in neonatology. Changes in aeration and subsequent hemodynamic changes happen quickly and must be evaluated consistently. Ventilation strategy, and evaluation of adequate lung aeration are key aspects in which ultrasound can be useful.

One of the most crucial steps in interpreting NPLUS is the appearance of the pleural line and lung sliding, as mentioned above. Recognition of lung sliding can be used to determine ventilation, rule out pneumothorax or identify the lung point as indicated in the Bedside Lung Ultrasound in Emergency (BLUE) Protocol or Sonographic Assessment of liFe-threatening Emergencies (SAFE) Algorithm [3,9].

Several studies analyzed the usefulness and reliability of NPLUS in the delivery room. Blank et al. used NPLUS to depict and analyze the initiation of breathing in term and late preterm infants. The authors captured one of the first four breaths in 35 infants and even the first breath in 28 infants. Using a modified, semiquantitative score with several different types of patterns, including "type 0" which occurs prior to establishment of the pleural line. The authors concluded that after the first four breaths, all infants had a visible pleural line, and that fluid clearance happens quickly with establishment of inspiratory efforts. NPLUS can be used to confirm initial penetration of air into the lungs and may support the decision to use different ventilation strategies. A white lung in the delivery room has been predictive for further need of respiratory support and surfactant therapy in this study [44]. In a more recent study, Blank et al. analyzed LUS videos of term and late preterm infants during the first day to describe the transition process, confirming that fluid clearance can be seen during the first few minutes of life with complete clearance after 4 h of life [45]. In another study, NPLUS was performed in the delivery room in 52 very—or extremely preterm infants. Findings included an excellent specificity for surfactant application, and even after 5–10 min, NPLUS outperformed the widely used FiO_2 threshold for prediction of surfactant therapy [46]. Raimondi et al. described fluid clearance in neonates >33 weeks using 3 types of patterns (white lung, prevalence of B-Lines, prevalence of A-Lines) and presented the shift from white lung to prevalence of A-Lines. White lung pattern performed as a predictor for NICU admission with a sensitivity of 77.1% and specificity of 100% [47].

In our experience, it is challenging to use NPLUS to visualize the first few breaths routinely due to practical reasons (positioning of the ultrasound machine, timing of examination, lack of new information due to clinical features). However, we use NPLUS for diagnostic purposes when signs of respiratory insufficiency, and/or tachypnoea occur, or in situations without sufficient ventilation.

3.2. Infants with Respiratory Distress: Respiratory Distress Syndrome vs. Transient Tachypnea of the Newborn

Respiratory distress is one of the most common reasons for admission to the NICU, therefore it is of great interest to differentiate between respiratory distress syndrome (RDS) with need for surfactant and transient tachypnea of the newborn (TTN) with delayed fluid clearance [48,49]. Several studies address the role of NPLUS in this situation. One of the first observations in this matter was described by Copetti and is called the "double lung point" which is seen in TTN [50]. This sign describes the boundary between coalescent B-Lines or white lung and aerated lung with A-Lines. However, more recent studies have shown that specificity and sensitivity of this sign was lower than described first. When respiratory distress occurs due to TTN, NPLUS would typically show a white lung with a great variability in different lung fields, disappearance of A-Lines, double lung point, irregular pleural line and pleural effusion in 20% of cases, while the occurrence of consolidations would point to RDS, MAS or pneumonia [51–53]. Ultrasound is as accurate as chest-X-ray in detecting TTN [54].

However, when RDS is present, sonographic findings differ from TTN: In RDS, typical findings are bilateral white lungs without spared areas or a boundary to a better aerated lung, consolidations, and a thickened, irregular pleural line [3]. One has to keep in mind that TTN and RDS are not always exclusively present and there might be mixed forms, which need a continuous clinical evaluation. See Supplementary file Video S3 for an infant with RDS, and Supplementary file Video S4 for an infant presenting with TTN.

3.3. Extremely Preterm Infant After Delivery—LUS and the Need for Surfactant and Ventilation

There is excellent evidence for the use of NPLUS to recognize the need for ventilation and surfactant replacement in preterm infants as described below.

In 2008, Copetti et al. studied NPLUS in infants and emphasized its value in detecting RDS, proposing that LUS may be helpful for guiding surfactant administration [10]. Two years later, the authors demonstrated that surfactant therapy in very preterm infants with a white lung in NPLUS did not improve interstitial fluid clearance [55]. Raimondi et al. studied 54 newborns (mean gestational age 32 weeks) who were admitted to the NICU with nasal CPAP and showed that a sonographic white lung predicted intubation within 24 h with a sensitivity of 88.9% and sensitivity of 100% [56].

De Martino et al. included 133 extremely preterm infants in a prospective trial and were able to show that NPLUS can be used to predict the need for surfactant. The authors demonstrated that it is possible to guide surfactant therapy using a LUS Score with a sensitivity of 82% and specificity of 92%, and they also provided data for the prediction of a second dose of surfactant [57]. In summary, the authors concluded that NPLUS guided surfactant administration is a reasonable alternative to FiO_2 criteria. This hypothesis was confirmed in the ULTRASURF study by Rodriguez-Fanjul et al., in which 56 infants were randomized in two groups, receiving ultrasound-guided or FiO_2-guided surfactant treatment, respectively. They concluded that the ultrasound-guided group received surfactant earlier and thus was exposed to less supplemental oxygen than the FiO_2-guided group [58].

The European consensus guidelines on the management of respiratory distress syndrome, updated in 2019, recommend surfactant therapy in infants requiring 6 cmH_2O nasal CPAP and an FiO_2 above 0.3 [59]. There is evidence that the use of the proposed LUS score has an excellent positive predictive value for the need of surfactant treatment and may lead to earlier administration of surfactant in children who need this treatment. Although

NPLUS is a comparatively easy ultrasound examination, it still is an observer-dependent method, opposed to the FiO_2 criteria, and one has to be aware of the possibility of differences in management due to inexperienced observers and/or incorrect exam results.

3.4. Meconium Aspiration

In infants who require intensive care due to meconium aspiration, NPLUS findings are characterized by atelectases, irregular pleural line, and spared areas, since meconium is distributed unevenly in the lungs and unaffected areas are ventilated properly or are even overdistended. The typical LUS pattern in MAS combines a broad range of signs as seen on Supplementary file Video S5 [3,15].

3.5. Pneumothorax

Detection and exclusion of pneumothorax are one of the most practical diagnostic features of NPLUS with extensive data regarding sensitivity and specificity [14,60,61]. NPLUS is as accurate as chest-X-ray in the detection of pneumothorax in neonates [62]. Exclusion of pneumothorax is achieved by observation of lung sliding and/or the occurrence of B-Lines. Detection of PTX is possible by absence of lung sliding, detection of the lung point, which can be seen as the boundary between the seashore-sign and stratosphere-sign (also called barcode-sign) in M-mode, as well as mirrored ribs, as seen in Supplementary file Video S6 and Image S1 [63]. In summary, detection of PTX using NPLUS showed excellent specificity and sensitivity.

A further value of NPLUS in pneumothorax commonly used within our units is the possibility of quick and repeated follow-up examinations. Once the lung point is found, the skin can be marked at that exact point and can be re-assessed later with information regarding changes of the size of the pneumothorax (the more lateral the point can be found in supine position, the greater is the dimension of the pneumothorax).

3.6. NPLUS in Infants with Bronchopulmonary Dysplasia

While respiratory distress is the most common reason for admission to the NICU, bronchopulmonary dysplasia (BPD) is the most common chronic disease following prematurity with increasing BPD rates in high-income countries [64].

Infants with BPD can deteriorate quickly due to structural abnormalities, reduced lung volume, high airway resistance and comorbidities of prematurity, resulting in emergency situations where respiratory status has to be evaluated quickly [65]. Increased ventilatory support may lead to pneumothorax, overdistension, bullae and other complications of invasive and non-invasive ventilation.

NPLUS can be helpful in the assessment of infants with BPD with acute respiratory deterioration. BPD is associated with a higher incidence of RSV infection rates, higher mortality and longer hospital stay [66]. In this context, NPLUS is a reliable tool for diagnosis and follow-up in acute bronchiolitis cases [67]. Findings are primarily consolidations in the posterior chest and pleural effusion, and there is a good correlation between oxygen support and NPLUS findings [68].

On the other hand, regarding the chronic aspect of the disease, there is solid data about the value of NPLUS for the prediction of BPD. Some recent prospective trials analyzed NPLUS scores of infants, who later developed BPD and found good predictive accuracy [69,70]. See Supplementary file Video S7 for an infant with BPD.

3.7. Pneumonia

NPLUS shows high diagnostic accuracy for the diagnosis of pneumonia in term and preterm neonates and in the paediatric population [71,72]. Typical signs are consolidations, which are usually larger than in bronchiolitis or RDS, air bronchograms, and pleural effusion [73,74].

3.8. Diaphragm Movement

Respiratory distress can be caused by abnormal diaphragmatic motion due to diaphragmatic paralysis. M-Mode can be used to assess diaphragmatic movement, achieved by scanning in the subxiphoid plane [75]. A prospective study of 400 healthy children described reference values for diaphragmatic excursion, with values of 6.4 and 6.6 mm excursion for the right and left hemidiaphragm, respectively [76]. Paradox or no movement can lead to the diagnosis of diaphragmatic paralysis in infants with signs of respiratory distress.

3.9. Congenital Malformations

Congenital pulmonary airway malformation and congenital diaphragmatic hernia (CDH) are rare malformations and frequently diagnosed antenatally. NPLUS can be used to confirm antenatally diagnosed, or to detect previously unknown cystic lung lesions. Presence of parenchymatous organs or bowel movement inside the thorax leads to the diagnosis of CDH (see Supplementary file Video S8) [77,78].

4. C—Circulation

Management of a critically ill infant with circulatory failure, in accordance with the ABCDE approach, should always include proper management of airway, oxygenation and ventilation. After steps A and B, pulse rate, pulse volume, peripheral and end-organ perfusion (capillary refill time, urinary output, level of consciousness), blood pressure and preload need to be evaluated, mainly by clinical examination and echocardiography [79]. In the management of circulatory deterioration, one has to consider etiology, pathophysiology and comorbidities. The transition from a compensated state to decompensation may occur rapidly and be unpredictable [7].

As mentioned above, the current paediatric CPR guidelines recommend performing point-of-care ultrasound by competent providers to identify reversible causes of cardiac arrest (tension pneumothorax, tamponade, hypovolemia). However, its application should not increase hands-off time or impact quality of CPR. Therefore, it is crucial for the team to plan and anticipate the best possible time for sonographic imaging [7,80].

Current evidence supports use of ultrasound for various diagnostic and procedural applications, including diagnosis and monitoring of common pulmonary diseases, hemodynamic instability, patent ductus arteriosus and persistent pulmonary hypertension of the newborn [81].

NPLUS in Neonates with Congenital Heart Disease and after Cardiac Surgery

Pulmonary overflow is one of the most common complications in patients with congenital heart disease with an incidence of approximately 48–60% [82]. NPLUS may be helpful in newborns with congenital heart disease to assess pulmonary overflow during the first days of life. Neonates with congenital heart disease who tend to develop pulmonary overflow had a higher LUS score at 72 h of life with a good correlation with echocardiography findings and with a better sensitivity and negative predictive value than chest X-ray [83].

Cardiorespiratory complications are common after cardiac surgery. Cardiopulmonary bypass during cardiac surgery generates a systemic capillary leak syndrome with pulmonary edema. NPLUS is a useful tool in monitoring these patients. The use of LUS reduces the exposure to ionizing radiation [8,84].

Diaphragmatic paralysis after cardiac surgery is a major differential diagnosis to consider in case of respiratory insufficiency in NICU patients. Assessment of the diaphragm with NPLUS is described above.

Furthermore, after cardiac surgery, a common reason for clinical deterioration may be pleural effusion or pneumothorax while a chest drainage is still in place. In this situation, NPLUS is helpful for diagnosis and treatment, and therapeutic interventions can be evaluated immediately.

5. Future Perspectives and Limitations

As mentioned earlier, the application of bedside LUS in the intensive care setting has gained enormous momentum during the last decade, additionally triggered by the SARS-CoV-2 pandemic. Despite the popularity of bedside ultrasound, more evidence, especially regarding the usefulness NPLUS and associated benefits for term and preterm infants is required, in order to generate recommendations and/or guidelines for the application of NPLUS in neonates. A glance into the literature about paediatric and adult intensive care medicine helps us understand possible applications and future directions when it comes to the further implementation of "visual medicine" in the emergency or intensive care setting. As discussed in the airway-section of this review, there is only limited data on sonography-based assessment of the airway, such as before and after intubation. Lung sliding is a basic, both visual and objective way of confirming effective ventilation, and more studies are needed to assess the benefits or disadvantages of this method in neonatal emergency situations.

Proper training in ultrasound is a key challenge when it comes to implementation of this method. In the hands of an experienced clinician, a NPLUS exam takes only about two minutes in order to gain important information like lung sliding or pleural effusion. The greatest limitation of ultrasound is the interobserver variability, as it is an observer dependent examination, and especially in the emergency setting, misinterpretation of NPLUS can lead to delayed or even wrong decisions (e.g., placement of a drainage, administration of surfactant, intubation). On the other hand, NPLUS is a comparatively simple diagnostic technique with a steep learning curve and consists mainly of pattern-recognition. Therefore, we consider a theoretical course of 30–60 min and 25 NPLUS examinations under supervision as sufficient for a clinician to count as experienced in NPLUS, based on suggestions by Rouby et al. and Benchouli et al. [85,86].

The development and availability of handheld and/or wireless ultrasound probes gives the neonatologist the opportunity to be more flexible and even quicker when a question about the respiratory status of an infant occurs and sonographic assessment is desired [87]. As mentioned above, the regular use of NPLUS has the potential to reduce the infant's exposure to radiation significantly [88].

Since we started performing NPLUS as a routine diagnostic tool in our units, we naturally used it increasingly also in emergency settings. It helped us recognize or rule out pneumothorax, visualize ventilation or atelectases, effusions, or consolidations in less than one minute. More experienced sonographers use NPLUS for assessment of tracheal tube placement, more sophisticated questions such as diagnosis of congenital malformations, diaphragmatic movement, and pneumomediastinum as well as assessment of laryngeal anatomy. Furthermore, due to its dynamic properties, NPLUS is an excellent tool for frequent follow-up exams, and visualization of respiratory conditions.

Supplementary Materials: The following are available online at https://www.mdpi.com/article/10.3390/children8080628/s1. Video S1: Lung ultrasound in anterior view of a healthy neonate. Video S2: Midsagittal view of a neonate at 26 4/7 weeks gestation with an endotracheal tube (ETT) in correct position as confirmed by chest-X-ray. Below the non-ossified sternum, the thymus and the aorta, the hyperechogenic rough line connecting the tip of the endotracheal tube (ETT) with the carina located below the right pulmonary artery (RPA) is the trachea. In practice, the endotracheal tube (ETT) can be identified by the black shadow below or by slightly moving the tube while performing the ultrasound scan. Video S3: Preterm infant with RDS: evenly distributed, confluent B-Lines and thickened pleural line Video S4: Preterm infant with TTN: Unevenly distributed B-Lines, especially in inferior regions, sudden appearance of A-Lines in superior regions, therefore presence of double lung point. Video S5: Video of an infant with MAS. Unevenly distributed areas with irregular pleural line, consolidations, B-Lines, and pleural effusion Video S6: Lung point in M-Mode of a neonate with pneumothorax. The lung point is a highly specific sign for pneumothorax and is found at the margin of pneumothorax and expanded lung. Video S7: Extremely preterm infant at 2 weeks after birth with early signs of bronchopulmonary dysplasia. Typical findings are a thickened pleural line, confluent B-Lines and consolidations in the lower, posterior regions Video S8: Preterm infant with prenatally diagnosed CDH. In a postnatally performed NPLUS exam, bowel movements can be seen to confirm the diagnosis Image S1: Neonate with pneumothorax in B-Mode. Stratosphere sign and mirrored ribs are typical signs of pneumothorax in neonates.

Author Contributions: Conceptualization, B.S., L.A., E.K. and L.H.; methodology, L.A., B.S.; writing—original draft preparation, L.A., E.K., L.H.; writing—review and editing, B.S., B.U., T.W., A.B.; visualization, L.A., L.H., E.K.; supervision, B.S.; All authors have read and agreed to the published version of the manuscript.

Funding: This research received no external funding.

Institutional Review Board Statement: Ethical review and approval were waived for this study, due to the study design of a narrative review.

Informed Consent Statement: Patient consent was waived due to the study design of a narrative review.

Conflicts of Interest: The authors declare no conflict of interest.

References

1. Morton, S.U.; Brodsky, D. Fetal Physiology and the Transition to Extrauterine Life. *Clin. Perinatol.* **2016**, *43*, 395–407. [CrossRef]
2. Sinha, S.K.; Donn, S.M. Fetal-to-neonatal maladaptation. *Semin. Fetal Neonatal Med.* **2006**, *11*, 166–173. [CrossRef] [PubMed]
3. Raimondi, F.; Yousef, N.; Migliaro, F.; Capasso, L.; De Luca, D. Point-of-care lung ultrasound in neonatology: Classification into descriptive and functional applications. *Pediatr. Res.* **2018**, *20*, 1–8. [CrossRef] [PubMed]
4. Whitson, M.R.; Mayo, P.H. Ultrasonography in the emergency department. *Crit. Care* **2016**, *20*. [CrossRef] [PubMed]
5. Bøtker, M.T.; Jacobsen, L.; Rudolph, S.S.; Knudsen, L. The role of point of care ultrasound in prehospital critical care: A systematic review. *Scand. J. Trauma Resusc. Emerg. Med.* **2018**, *26*, 51. [CrossRef]
6. Singh, Y.; Tissot, C.; Fraga, M.V.; Yousef, N.; Cortes, R.G.; Lopez, J.; Sanchez-de-Toledo, J.; Brierley, J.; Colunga, J.M.; Raffaj, D.; et al. International evidence-based guidelines on Point of Care Ultrasound (POCUS) for critically ill neonates and children issued by the POCUS Working Group of the European Society of Paediatric and Neonatal Intensive Care (ESPNIC). *Crit. Care* **2020**, *24*, 65. [CrossRef] [PubMed]
7. Van de Voorde, P.; Turner, N.M.; Djakow, J.; de Lucas, N.; Martinez-Mejias, A.; Biarent, D.; Bingham, R.; Brissaud, O.; Hoffmann, F.; Johannesdottir, G.B.; et al. European Resuscitation Council Guidelines 2021: Paediatric Life Support. *Resuscitation* **2021**, *161*, 327–387. [CrossRef] [PubMed]
8. Küng, E.; Ptacek, L.; Werther, T.; Reithmayr, S.; Aichhorn, L. *Neonatologie: Lungenultraschall Standard (Version 2.1)*; Zenodo: Geneva, Switzerland, 2020. [CrossRef]
9. Lichtenstein, D.A.; Mauriat, P. Lung Ultrasound in the Critically Ill Neonate. *Curr. Pediatr. Rev.* **2012**, *8*, 217–223. [CrossRef]
10. Copetti, R.; Cattarossi, L.; Macagno, F.; Violino, M.; Furlan, R. Lung Ultrasound in Respiratory Distress Syndrome: A Useful Tool for Early Diagnosis. *Neonatology* **2008**, *94*, 52–59. [CrossRef]
11. Stuhlfauth, K. Reflex effects of ultrasonics on the pneumothorax lung. *Dtsch. Med. Wochenschr.* **1951**, *76*, 537–539. [CrossRef]
12. Joyner, C.R.; Miller, L.D.; Dudrick, S.J.; Eskin, D.J.; Bloom, P. Reflected ultrasound in the study of diseases of the chest. *Trans. Am. Clin. Climatol. Assoc.* **1967**, *78*, 28–37.
13. Joyner, C.R.; Herman, R.J.; Reid, J.M. Reflected ultrasound in the detection and localization of pleural effusion. *JAMA* **1967**, *200*, 399–402. [CrossRef] [PubMed]
14. Lichtenstein, D.A.; Menu, Y. A Bedside Ultrasound Sign Ruling Out Pneumothorax in the Critically Ill. *Chest* **1995**, *108*, 1345–1348. [CrossRef] [PubMed]
15. Corsini, I.; Parri, N.; Gozzini, E.; Coviello, C.; Leonardi, V.; Poggi, C.; Giacalone, M.; Bianconi, T.; Tofani, L.; Raimondi, F.; et al. Lung Ultrasound for the Differential Diagnosis of Respiratory Distress in Neonates. *Neonatology* **2019**, *115*, 77–84. [CrossRef]
16. Brat, R.; Yousef, N.; Klifa, R.; Reynaud, S.; Aguilera, S.S.; De Luca, D. Lung Ultrasonography Score to Evaluate Oxygenation and Surfactant Need in Neonates Treated With Continuous Positive Airway Pressure. *JAMA Pediatr.* **2015**, *169*, e151797. [CrossRef] [PubMed]
17. Madar, J.; Roehr, C.C.; Ainsworth, S.; Ersdal, H.; Morley, C.; Rüdiger, M.; Skåre, C.; Szczapa, T.; te Pas, A.; Trevisanuto, D.; et al. European Resuscitation Council Guidelines 2021: Newborn resuscitation and support of transition of infants at birth. *Resuscitation* **2021**, *161*, 291–326. [CrossRef]
18. von Ungern-Sternberg, B.S.; Erb, T.O.; Frei, F.J. Management der oberen Atemwege beim spontan atmenden Kind: Eine Herausforderung für den Anästhesisten. *Anaesthesist* **2006**, *55*, 164–170. [CrossRef]
19. Mishra, P.; Bhoi, S.; Sinha, T. Integration of point-of-care ultrasound during rapid sequence intubation in trauma resuscitation. *J. Emergencies Trauma Shock* **2018**, *11*, 92–97. [CrossRef]
20. Raimondi, F.; Yousef, N.; Rodriguez Fanjul, J.; De Luca, D.; Corsini, I.; Shankar-Aguilera, S.; Dani, C.; Di Guardo, V.; Lama, S.; Mosca, F.; et al. A Multicenter Lung Ultrasound Study on Transient Tachypnea of the Neonate. *Neonatology* **2019**, *115*, 263–268. [CrossRef]

21. Álvarez-Díaz, N.; Amador-García, I.; Fuentes-Hernández, M.; Dorta-Guerra, R. Comparación entre la ecografía pulmonar transtorácica y el método clínico para confirmar la posición del tubo de doble luz izquierdo en anestesia torácica. Estudio piloto. *Rev. Española Anestesiol. Y Reanim.* **2015**, *62*, 305–312. [CrossRef]
22. Pfeiffer, P.; Rudolph, S.S.; Børglum, J.; Isbye, D.L. Temporal comparison of ultrasound vs. auscultation and capnography in verification of endotracheal tube placement: Lung ultrasound for ET tube verification. *Acta Anaesthesiol. Scand.* **2011**, *55*, 1190–1195. [CrossRef]
23. Marciniak, B.; Fayoux, P.; Hébrard, A.; Krivosic-Horber, R.; Engelhardt, T.; Bissonnette, B. Airway Management in Children: Ultrasonography Assessment of Tracheal Intubation in Real Time? *Anesth. Analg.* **2009**, *108*, 461–465. [CrossRef] [PubMed]
24. Alessandri, F.; Antenucci, G.; Piervincenzi, E.; Buonopane, C.; Bellucci, R.; Andreoli, C.; Alunni Fegatelli, D.; Ranieri, M.V.; Bilotta, F. Ultrasound as a new tool in the assessment of airway difficulties: An observational study. *Eur. J. Anaesthesiol.* **2019**, *36*, 509–515. [CrossRef]
25. Daniel, S.J.; Bertolizio, G.; McHugh, T. Airway ultrasound: Point of care in children—The time is now. *Pediatr. Anesth.* **2020**, *30*, 347–352. [CrossRef] [PubMed]
26. Friedman, E.M. Role of Ultrasound in the Assessment of Vocal Cord Function in Infants and Children. *Ann. Otol. Rhinol. Laryngol.* **1997**, *106*, 199–209. [CrossRef] [PubMed]
27. Oulego-Erroz, I.; Terroba-Seara, S.; Alonso-Quintela, P.; Benavent-Torres, R.; Castro-Vecino, P.D.; Martínez-Saez de Jubera, J. Bedside Airway Ultrasound in the Evaluation of Neonatal Stridor. *J. Pediatr.* **2020**, *227*, 321–323. [CrossRef]
28. Kim, J.; Kim, J.Y.; Kim, W.O.; Kil, H.K. An Ultrasound Evaluation of Laryngeal Mask Airway Position in Pediatric Patients: An Observational Study. *Anesth. Analg.* **2015**, *120*, 427–432. [CrossRef]
29. Song, K.; Yi, J.; Liu, W.; Huang, S.; Huang, Y. Confirmation of laryngeal mask airway placement by ultrasound examination: A pilot study. *J. Clin. Anesth.* **2016**, *34*, 638–646. [CrossRef]
30. You-Ten, K.E.; Siddiqui, N.; Teoh, W.H.; Kristensen, M.S. Point-of-care ultrasound (POCUS) of the upper airway. *Can. J. Anesth.* **2018**, *65*, 473–484. [CrossRef]
31. Osman, A.; Sum, K.M. Role of upper airway ultrasound in airway management. *J. Intensiv. Care* **2016**, *4*, 52. [CrossRef]
32. Zaytseva, A.; Kurepa, D.; Ahn, S.; Weinberger, B. Determination of optimal endotracheal tube tip depth from the gum in neonates by X-ray and ultrasound. *J. Matern. Fetal Neonatal Med.* **2020**, *33*, 2075–2080. [CrossRef] [PubMed]
33. Chowdhry, R.; Dangman, B.; Pinheiro, J.M.B. The concordance of ultrasound technique versus X-ray to confirm endotracheal tube position in neonates. *J. Perinatol.* **2015**, *35*, 481–484. [CrossRef]
34. Dennington, D.; Vali, P.; Finer, N.N.; Kim, J.H. Ultrasound Confirmation of Endotracheal Tube Position in Neonates. *Neonatology* **2012**, *102*, 185–189. [CrossRef] [PubMed]
35. Najib, K.; Pishva, N.; Amoozegar, H.; Pishdad, P.; Fallahzadeh, E. Ultrasonographic confirmation of endotracheal tube position in neonates. *Indian Pediatr.* **2016**, *53*, 886–888. [CrossRef] [PubMed]
36. Sethi, A.; Nimbalkar, A.; Patel, D.; Kungwani, A.; Nimbalkar, S. Point of care ultrasonography for position of tip of endotracheal tube in neonates. *Indian Pediatr.* **2014**, *51*, 119–121. [CrossRef] [PubMed]
37. Boretsky, K.R. Images in Anesthesiology: Point-of-care Ultrasound to Diagnose Esophageal Intubation. *Anesthesiology* **2018**, *129*, 190. [CrossRef]
38. Fajardo-Escolar, A.P.; Bonilla-Ramírez, A.J.; Winograd Gómez, V. Ultrasound-guided selective intubation in a preterm neonate undergoing type-C esophageal athresia correction. *Case report: Colomb. J. Anesthesiol.* **2018**, *46*, 75–78. [CrossRef]
39. Sim, S.-S.; Sun, J.-T.; Fan, C.-M.; Tsai, K.-C. The utility of ultrasonography to confirm proper endotracheal tube placement in neonates. *Resuscitation* **2016**, *106*, e19–e20. [CrossRef] [PubMed]
40. Fiadjoe, J.E.; Stricker, P.; Gurnaney, H.; Nishisaki, A.; Rabinowitz, A.; Gurwitz, A.; McCloskey, J.J.; Ganesh, A. Ultrasound-guided Tracheal Intubation. *Anesthesiology* **2012**, *117*, 1389–1391. [CrossRef]
41. Moustafa, M.A.; Arida, E.A.; Zanaty, O.M.; El-tamboly, S.F. Endotracheal intubation: Ultrasound-guided versus fiberscope in patients with cervical spine immobilization. *J. Anesth.* **2017**, *31*, 846–851. [CrossRef]
42. Ma, Y.; Wang, Y.; Shi, P.; Cao, X.; Ge, S. Ultrasound-guided versus Shikani optical stylet-aided tracheal intubation: A prospective randomized study. *BMC Anesthesiol.* **2020**, *20*, 221. [CrossRef] [PubMed]
43. Kundra, P.; Padala, S.R.A.N.; Jha, A.K. Ultrasound guided tracheal intubation with a styleted tracheal tube in anticipated difficult airway. *J. Clin. Monit. Comput.* **2021**, *35*, 285–287. [CrossRef] [PubMed]
44. Blank, D.A.; Rogerson, S.R.; Kamlin, C.O.F.; Fox, L.M.; Lorenz, L.; Kane, S.C.; Polglase, G.R.; Hooper, S.B.; Davis, P.G. Lung ultrasound during the initiation of breathing in healthy term and late preterm infants immediately after birth, a prospective, observational study. *Resuscitation* **2017**, *114*, 59–65. [CrossRef]
45. Blank, D.A.; Kamlin, C.O.F.; Rogerson, S.R.; Fox, L.M.; Lorenz, L.; Kane, S.C.; Polglase, G.R.; Hooper, S.B.; Davis, P.G. Lung ultrasound immediately after birth to describe normal neonatal transition: An observational study. *Arch. Dis. Child. Fetal Neonatal Ed.* **2018**, *103*, F157–F162. [CrossRef]
46. Badurdeen, S.; Kamlin, C.O.F.; Rogerson, S.R.; Kane, S.C.; Polglase, G.R.; Hooper, S.B.; Davis, P.G.; Blank, D.A. Lung ultrasound during newborn resuscitation predicts the need for surfactant therapy in very- and extremely preterm infants. *Resuscitation* **2021**, *162*, 227–235. [CrossRef]
47. Raimondi, F.; Migliaro, F.; Sodano, A.; Umbaldo, A.; Romano, A.; Vallone, G.; Capasso, L. Can neonatal lung ultrasound monitor fluid clearance and predict the need of respiratory support? *Crit. Care* **2012**, *16*, R220. [CrossRef] [PubMed]

48. Haidari, E.S.; Lee, H.C.; Illuzzi, J.L.; Phibbs, C.S.; Lin, H.; Xu, X. Hospital variation in admissions to neonatal intensive care units by diagnosis severity and category. *J. Perinatol.* **2021**, *41*, 468–477. [CrossRef]
49. Battersby, C.; Michaelides, S.; Upton, M.; Rennie, J.M. Term admissions to neonatal units in England: A role for transitional care? A retrospective cohort study. *BMJ Open* **2017**, *7*, e016050. [CrossRef]
50. Copetti, R.; Cattarossi, L. The 'Double Lung Point': An Ultrasound Sign Diagnostic of Transient Tachypnea of the Newborn. *Neonatology* **2007**, *91*, 203–209. [CrossRef] [PubMed]
51. Liu, J.; Wang, Y.; Fu, W.; Yang, C.-S.; Huang, J.-J. Diagnosis of Neonatal Transient Tachypnea and Its Differentiation From Respiratory Distress Syndrome Using Lung Ultrasound. *Medicine* **2014**, *93*, e197. [CrossRef]
52. Liu, J.; Chen, X.-X.; Li, X.-W.; Chen, S.-W.; Wang, Y.; Fu, W. Lung Ultrasonography to Diagnose Transient Tachypnea of the Newborn. *Chest* **2016**, *149*, 1269–1275. [CrossRef]
53. Vergine, M.; Copetti, R.; Brusa, G.; Cattarossi, L. Lung Ultrasound Accuracy in Respiratory Distress Syndrome and Transient Tachypnea of the Newborn. *Neonatology* **2014**, *106*, 87–93. [CrossRef]
54. International Liaison Committee on Lung Ultrasound (ILC-LUS) for the International Consensus Conference on Lung Ultrasound (ICC-LUS); Volpicelli, G.; Elbarbary, M.; Blaivas, M.; Lichtenstein, D.A.; Mathis, G.; Kirkpatrick, A.W.; Melniker, L.; Gargani, L.; Noble, V.E.; et al. International evidence-based recommendations for point-of-care lung ultrasound. *Intensive Care Med.* **2012**, *38*, 577–591. [CrossRef]
55. Cattarossi, L.; Copetti, R.; Poskurica, B.; Miserocchi, G. Surfactant administration for neonatal respiratory distress does not improve lung interstitial fluid clearance: Echographic and experimental evidence. *J. Perinat. Med.* **2010**, *38*, 557–563. [CrossRef]
56. Raimondi, F.; Migliaro, F.; Sodano, A.; Ferrara, T.; Lama, S.; Vallone, G.; Capasso, L. Use of Neonatal Chest Ultrasound to Predict Noninvasive Ventilation Failure. *Pediatrics* **2014**, *134*, e1089–e1094. [CrossRef]
57. De Martino, L.; Yousef, N.; Ben-Ammar, R.; Raimondi, F.; Shankar-Aguilera, S.; De Luca, D. Lung Ultrasound Score Predicts Surfactant Need in Extremely Preterm Neonates. *Pediatrics* **2018**, *142*, e20180463. [CrossRef] [PubMed]
58. Rodriguez-Fanjul, J.; Jordan, I.; Balaguer, M.; Batista-Muñoz, A.; Ramon, M.; Bobillo-Perez, S. Early surfactant replacement guided by lung ultrasound in preterm newborns with RDS: The ULTRASURF randomised controlled trial. *Eur. J. Pediatr.* **2020**, *179*, 1913–1920. [CrossRef]
59. Sweet, D.G.; Carnielli, V.; Greisen, G.; Hallman, M.; Ozek, E.; te Pas, A.; Plavka, R.; Roehr, C.C.; Saugstad, O.D.; Simeoni, U.; et al. European Consensus Guidelines on the Management of Respiratory Distress Syndrome—2019 Update. *Neonatology* **2019**, *115*, 432–450. [CrossRef] [PubMed]
60. Alrajab, S.; Youssef, A.M.; Akkus, N.I.; Caldito, G. Pleural ultrasonography versus chest radiography for the diagnosis of pneumothorax: Review of the literature and meta-analysis. *Crit. Care* **2013**, *17*, R208. [CrossRef] [PubMed]
61. Cattarossi, L.; Copetti, R.; Brusa, G.; Pintaldi, S. Lung Ultrasound Diagnostic Accuracy in Neonatal Pneumothorax. *Can. Respir. J.* **2016**, *2016*, 6515069. [CrossRef]
62. Fei, Q.; Lin, Y.; Yuan, T.-M. Lung Ultrasound, a Better Choice for Neonatal Pneumothorax: A Systematic Review and Meta-analysis. *Ultrasound Med. Biol.* **2021**, *47*, 359–369. [CrossRef]
63. Küng, E.; Aichhorn, L.; Berger, A.; Werther, T. Mirrored Ribs: A Sign for Pneumothorax in Neonates. *Pediatr. Crit. Care Med.* **2020**, *21*, e944–e947. [CrossRef] [PubMed]
64. Lui, K.; Lee, S.K.; Kusuda, S.; Adams, M.; Vento, M.; Reichman, B.; Darlow, B.A.; Lehtonen, L.; Modi, N.; Norman, M.; et al. Trends in Outcomes for Neonates Born Very Preterm and Very Low Birth Weight in 11 High-Income Countries. *J. Pediatr.* **2019**, *215*, 32–40.e14. [CrossRef] [PubMed]
65. van Mastrigt, E.; Kakar, E.; Ciet, P.; den Dekker, H.T.; Joosten, K.F.; Kalkman, P.; Swarte, R.; Kroon, A.A.; Tiddens, H.A.W.M.; de Jongste, J.C.; et al. Structural and functional ventilatory impairment in infants with severe bronchopulmonary dysplasia. *Pediatr. Pulmonol.* **2017**, *52*, 1029–1037. [CrossRef]
66. Groothuis, J.R.; Gutierrez, K.M.; Lauer, B.A. Respiratory syncytial virus infection in children with bronchopulmonary dysplasia. *Pediatrics* **1988**, *82*, 199–203.
67. Basile, V.; Di Mauro, A.; Scalini, E.; Comes, P.; Lofù, I.; Mostert, M.; Tafuri, S.; Manzionna, M.M. Lung ultrasound: A useful tool in diagnosis and management of bronchiolitis. *BMC Pediatr.* **2015**, *15*, 63. [CrossRef]
68. Di Mauro; Ammirabile; Quercia; Panza; Capozza; Manzionna; Laforgia Acute Bronchiolitis: Is There a Role for Lung Ultrasound? *Diagnostics* **2019**, *9*, 172. [CrossRef] [PubMed]
69. Alonso-Ojembarrena, A.; Serna-Guerediaga, I.; Aldecoa-Bilbao, V.; Gregorio-Hernández, R.; Alonso-Quintela, P.; Concheiro-Guisán, A.; Ramos-Rodríguez, A.; de las Heras-Martín, M.; Rodeño-Fernández, L.; Oulego-Erroz, I. The Predictive Value of Lung Ultrasound Scores in Developing Bronchopulmonary Dysplasia: A Prospective Multicenter Diagnostic Accuracy Study. *Chest* **2021**, in press. [CrossRef]
70. Hoshino, Y.; Arai, J.; Miura, R.; Takeuchi, S.; Yukitake, Y.; Kajikawa, D.; Kamakura, T.; Horigome, H. Lung Ultrasound for Predicting the Respiratory Outcome in Patients with Bronchopulmonary Dysplasia. *Am. J. Perinatol.* **2020**. [CrossRef]
71. Tusor, N.; De Cunto, A.; Basma, Y.; Klein, J.L.; Meau-Petit, V. Ventilator-associated pneumonia in neonates: The role of point of care lung ultrasound. *Eur. J. Pediatr.* **2021**, *180*, 137–146. [CrossRef]
72. Hegazy, L.M.; Rezk, A.R.; Sakr, H.M.; Ahmed, A.S. Comparison of Efficacy of LUS and CXR in the Diagnosis of Children Presenting with Respiratory Distress to Emergency Department. *Indian J. Crit. Care Med.* **2020**, *24*, 459–464. [CrossRef]

73. Liu, J.; Liu, F.; Liu, Y.; Wang, H.-W.; Feng, Z.-C. Lung Ultrasonography for the Diagnosis of Severe Neonatal Pneumonia. *Chest* **2014**, *146*, 383–388. [CrossRef]
74. Chen, S.-W.; Fu, W.; Liu, J.; Wang, Y. Routine application of lung ultrasonography in the neonatal intensive care unit. *Medicine* **2017**, *96*, e5826. [CrossRef]
75. Epelman, M.; Navarro, O.M.; Daneman, A.; Miller, S.F. M-mode sonography of diaphragmatic motion: Description of technique and experience in 278 pediatric patients. *Pediatr. Radiol.* **2005**, *35*, 661–667. [CrossRef]
76. El-Halaby, H.; Abdel-Hady, H.; Alsawah, G.; Abdelrahman, A.; El-Tahan, H. Sonographic Evaluation of Diaphragmatic Excursion and Thickness in Healthy Infants and Children. *J. Ultrasound Med.* **2016**, *35*, 167–175. [CrossRef]
77. Corsini, I.; Parri, N.; Coviello, C.; Leonardi, V.; Dani, C. Lung ultrasound findings in congenital diaphragmatic hernia. *Eur. J. Pediatr.* **2019**, *178*, 491–495. [CrossRef]
78. Yousef, N.; Mokhtari, M.; Durand, P.; Raimondi, F.; Migliaro, F.; Letourneau, A.; Tissières, P.; De Luca, D. Lung Ultrasound Findings in Congenital Pulmonary Airway Malformation. *Am. J. Perinatol.* **2018**, *35*, 1222–1227. [CrossRef] [PubMed]
79. Singh, Y. Echocardiographic Evaluation of Hemodynamics in Neonates and Children. *Front. Pediatr.* **2017**, *5*, 201. [CrossRef] [PubMed]
80. Blanco, P.; Martínez Buendía, C. Point-of-care ultrasound in cardiopulmonary resuscitation: A concise review. *J. Ultrasound* **2017**, *20*, 193–198. [CrossRef] [PubMed]
81. Miller, L.E.; Stoller, J.Z.; Fraga, M.V. Point-of-care ultrasound in the neonatal ICU. *Curr. Opin. Pediatr.* **2020**, *32*, 216–227. [CrossRef] [PubMed]
82. Rodríguez-Fanjul, J.; Llop, A.S.; Balaguer, M.; Bautista-Rodriguez, C.; Hernando, J.M.; Jordan, I. Usefulness of Lung Ultrasound in Neonatal Congenital Heart Disease (LUSNEHDI): Lung Ultrasound to Assess Pulmonary Overflow in Neonatal Congenital Heart Disease. *Pediatr. Cardiol.* **2016**, *37*, 1482–1487. [CrossRef] [PubMed]
83. Picano, E.; Scali, M.C.; Ciampi, Q.; Lichtenstein, D. Lung Ultrasound for the Cardiologist. *JACC Cardiovasc. Imaging* **2018**, *11*, 1692–1705. [CrossRef] [PubMed]
84. Liu, J.; Copetti, R.; Sorantin, E.; Lovrenski, J.; Rodriguez-Fanjul, J.; Kurepa, D.; Feng, X.; Cattaross, L.; Zhang, H.; Hwang, M.; et al. Protocol and Guidelines for Point-of-Care Lung Ultrasound in Diagnosing Neonatal Pulmonary Diseases Based on International Expert Consensus. *J. Vis. Exp.* **2019**, *145*. [CrossRef] [PubMed]
85. Rouby, J.-J.; Arbelot, C.; Gao, Y.; Zhang, M.; Lv, J.; An, Y.; Chunyao, W.; Bin, D.; Valente Barbas, C.S.; Dexheimer Neto, F.L.; et al. Training for Lung Ultrasound Score Measurement in Critically Ill Patients. *Am. J. Respir. Crit. Care Med.* **2018**, *198*, 398–401. [CrossRef]
86. Benchoufi, M.; Bokobza, J.; Chauvin, A.; Dion, E.; Baranne, M.-L.; Levan, F.; Gautier, M.; Cantin, D.; d'Humières, T.; Gil-Jardiné, C.; et al. Lung Injury in Patients with or Suspected COVID-19: A Comparison between Lung Ultrasound and Chest CT-Scanner Severity Assessments, an Observational Study. *medRxiv* **2020**. [CrossRef]
87. Schmid, M.; Dodt, C. Lungensonographie in der Notfall- und Intensivmedizin. *Med. Klin. Intensivmed. Und Notf.* **2018**, *113*, 616–624. [CrossRef]
88. Escourrou, G.; De Luca, D. Lung ultrasound decreased radiation exposure in preterm infants in a neonatal intensive care unit. *Acta Paediatr.* **2016**, *105*, e237–e239. [CrossRef]

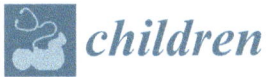

Brief Report

In Newborn Infants a New Intubation Method May Reduce the Number of Intubation Attempts: A Randomized Pilot Study

Marlies Bruckner [1,*], Nicholas M. Morris [1], Gerhard Pichler [1,2], Christina H. Wolfsberger [1], Stefan Heschl [3], Lukas P. Mileder [1], Bernhard Schwaberger [1], Georg M. Schmölzer [4,5] and Berndt Urlesberger [1,6]

1. Division of Neonatology, Department of Pediatrics and Adolescent Medicine, Medical University of Graz, Auenbruggerplatz 34/2, 8036 Graz, Austria; nicholas.morris@medunigraz.at (N.M.M.); gerhard.pichler@medunigraz.at (G.P.); christina.wolfsberger@medunigraz.at (C.H.W.); lukas.mileder@medunigraz.at (L.P.M.); bernhard.schwaberger@medunigraz.at (B.S.); berndt.urlesberger@medunigraz.at (B.U.)
2. Research Unit for Neonatal Macro- and Microcirculation, Medical University of Graz, Auenbruggerplatz 34/2, 8036 Graz, Austria
3. Department of Anesthesiology and Intensive Care Medicine, Pediatric Anesthesia, Medical University of Graz, Auenbruggerplatz 34/2, 8036 Graz, Austria; stefan.heschl@medunigraz.at
4. Centre for the Studies of Asphyxia and Resuscitation, Neonatal Research Unit, Royal Alexandra Hospital, 10240 Kingsway Avenue NW, Edmonton, AB T5H 3V9, Canada; georg.schmoelzer@me.com
5. Department of Pediatrics, Faculty of Medicine and Dentistry, University of Alberta, 11405-87 Avenue, Edmonton, AB T6G 1C9, Canada
6. Research Unit for Cerebral Development and Oximetry Research, Medical University of Graz, Auenbruggerplatz 34/2, 8036 Graz, Austria
* Correspondence: marlies.bruckner@medunigraz.at; Tel.: +43-316-3858-3724

Abstract: Severe desaturation or bradycardia often occur during neonatal endotracheal intubation. Using continuous gas flow through the endotracheal tube might reduce the incidence of these events. We hypothesized that continuous gas flow through the endotracheal tube during nasotracheal intubation compared to standard nasotracheal intubation will reduce the number of intubation attempts in newborn infants. In a randomized controlled pilot study, neonates were either intubated with continuous gas flow through the endotracheal tube during intubation (intervention group) or no gas flow during intubation (control group). Recruitment was stopped early due to financial and organizational issues. A total of 16 infants and 39 intubation attempts were analyzed. The median (interquartile range) number of intubation attempts and number of abandoned intubations due to desaturation and/or bradycardia were 1 (1–2) and 4 (2–5), ($p = 0.056$) and $n = 3$ versus $n = 20$, ($p = 0.060$) in the intervention group and control group, respectively. Continuous gas flow through the endotracheal tube during intubation seems to be favorable and there are no major unexpected adverse consequences of attempting this methodology.

Keywords: intubation; endotracheal tube; ventilation; acute respiratory failure; desaturation; neonatal intensive care unit; neonates

1. Introduction

The current intubation standard procedure includes sedation of the newborn infant, potentially leading to airway instability and diminishing breathing efforts. This causes a discontinuation of air/oxygen flow to the lungs before correct endotracheal tube (ETT) placement and might result in oxygen desaturation and/or bradycardia. During endotracheal intubation severe desaturation occurs in up to 51% of infants [1]. Furthermore, more than two intubation attempts are associated with an increased incidence of severe complications [2,3]. Providing continuous gas flow via the ETT itself during the intubation attempt might improve newborn infants' stability and thereby increase successful intubation rates.

We hypothesized that newborn infants requiring intubation who receive continuous gas flow during intubation (intervention group) will require less intubation attempts compared to the standard approach without gas flow (control group).

2. Materials and Methods

This randomized controlled pilot trial was carried out at the Division of Neonatology, Medical University of Graz, Austria, between October 2016 and October 2020 and registered at clinicaltrials.gov (identifier: NCT04089540). The Regional Committee on Biomedical Research Ethics of the Medical University of Graz approved the study protocol (EC number: 25–282ex12/13).

2.1. Study Poplulation

Term and preterm neonates admitted to neonatal intensive care units requiring intubation due to respiratory failure were eligible. Written parental informed consent was obtained prior to inclusion. Neonates with severe congenital malformations of the upper airway and hemodynamically significant congenital cardiovascular malformations were excluded.

2.2. Randomization and Blinding

Neonates were randomly assigned 1:1 to an intervention or control group by a computer-generated randomization software (www.randomizer.at), using a block randomization with a block size of 6. Blinding was not possible, considering the type of intervention.

2.3. Sample Size

A sample size of 40 infants was arbitrarily designated and authorized by the local ethics committee. Sample size calculations were not performed since no data from previous studies were available.

2.4. Interventions

The nasopharyngeal route for intubation was used according to the standard procedure. Infants routinely received 1 mg/kg Propofol (Fresenius Kabi, Bad Homburg vor der Höhe, Germany) intravenously for sedation shortly before intubation. Propofol application could be repeated if needed. In the intervention group, the Neopuff Infant T-Piece Resuscitator (Perivent, Fisher& Paykel Healthcare; New Zealand) was connected to the ETT with the default settings of positive-end expiratory pressure of 5 cmH$_2$O and gas flow of 6 L/min $\leq$ 1000 g, 7 L/min between 1000 and 2000 g, or 8 L/min > 2000 g birth weight. The fraction of inspired oxygen was adjusted for each patient during non-invasive mask ventilation prior to intubation, aiming for a target peripheral arterial oxygen saturation (SpO$_2$) of >89%. Continuous gas flow was provided through the ETT by an assisting staff member from insertion of the ETT into the nose until the ETT passed through the vocal cords. Once the ETT was placed in the trachea, continuous gas flow was discontinued and the ventilator was connected to start positive pressure ventilation (PPV). In the control group, no continuous gas flow was provided during intubation. Auscultation and/or exhaled carbon dioxide detection was used to assess correct ETT position. The duration of each intubation attempt was defined as the time from the removal of the face mask until the confirmation of correct ETT placement and was measured by a study team member using a stopwatch.

2.5. Intubation Attempt Abortion Criteria

Intubation attempts were stopped if SpO$_2$ was <80% and/or the heart rate was <100 beats/min for >5 s. In the intervention group, the ETT was kept inserted in the nostril while the other nostril and the mouth were held closed, and PPV was provided via the

ETT. In the control group the ETT was removed and non-invasive mask ventilation was performed until the neonate was stabilized.

2.6. Data Collection and Statistical Analysis

Demographics of study patients, intubation characteristics and the parameters of hospital stay were recorded. The primary outcome was the number of intubation attempts. The data are presented as mean (SD) for normally distributed continuous variables and median (IQR) when the distribution was skewed. We used intention-to-treat analysis and compared data using the Student's t-test for parametric and Mann-Whitney U test for non-parametric comparisons of continuous variables, and the Fisher's exact test for categorical variables. Statistical analyses were performed with IBM-SPSS-Statistics 24 Software (PSS Inc., Chicago, IL, USA.).

3. Results

Patient enrollment and allocation are demonstrated in the flow chart (Figure 1). Sixteen neonates were included; recruitment was stopped early due to financial and organizational issues (loss of equipoise within the recruiting team). Hence, we are reporting the data as a posteriori pilot study. Demographics, intubation parameters, and characteristics of hospital stay are presented in Table 1. Respiratory diagnoses of the included infants were respiratory distress syndrome ($n = 13$), meconium aspiration syndrome ($n = 1$) and pneumothorax ($n = 2$).

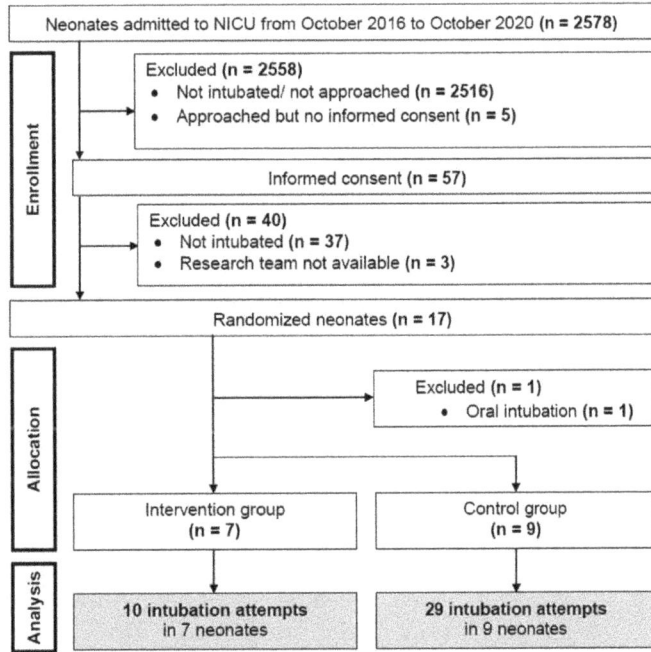

Figure 1. Flow Chart.

Table 1. Demographics and intubation characteristics. Data are expressed in n (%), median (IQR) or mean (SD) according to normal distribution. FiO_2 = Fraction of inspired oxygen.

	Study Group (n = 7)	Control Group (n = 9)	p-value
Demographics			
Gestational age (weeks)	30 (26–31)	32 (30–35)	0.222
Term infants (≥37 weeks gestation)	0 (0)	2 (22)	0.475
Female sex	2 (29)	5 (56)	0.608
Apgar 5 min	9 (8–9)	8 (8–9)	0.834
Postnatal age at intubation (hours)	15 (17)	36 (56)	0.873
Weight at intubation (grams)	1487 (819)	1857 (927)	0.461
Heart rate before intubation (beats/min)	151 (13)	145 (9)	0.292
Mean arterial blood pressure (mmHg) before intubation	44 (9)	42 (8)	0.694
Intubation			
Number of intubation attempts	1 (1–2)	4 (2–5)	0.056
Success on first intubation attempt	4 (57)	2 (22)	0.303
Duration until successful intubation (seconds)	204 (138–300)	858 (330–924)	0.114
Aborted intubations due to desaturation and/or bradycardia (n)	3	20	0.060
FiO2 during intubation	0.50 (0.40–0.75)	0.55 (0.40–0.70)	0.873
Gas flow (liters/minute)	6 (6–8)	8 (6–8)	0.289
Intravenous Propofol dosage (mg/kg)	1 (1–2)	2 (2–3)	0.072
Parameters of hospital stay			
Duration of invasive ventilation (days)	6 (2–7)	1 (0–3)	0.459
Duration of non-invasive ventilation (days)	14 (10–61)	6 (5–40)	0.153
Mortality (%)	0	0	1.000
Hospital stay (days)	46 (39–106)	30 (18–58)	0.187

3.1. Intubation Attempts

A total of 39 intubation attempts (intervention group n = 10, control group n = 29) were performed. The median (IQR) number of intubation attempts was 1 (1–2) and 4 (2–5) in the intervention and control group, respectively (p = 0.056) (Figure 2). The number of abandoned intubation attempts due to desaturation and/or bradycardia was n=3 in the intervention group vs. n =20 in the control group (p = 0.060).

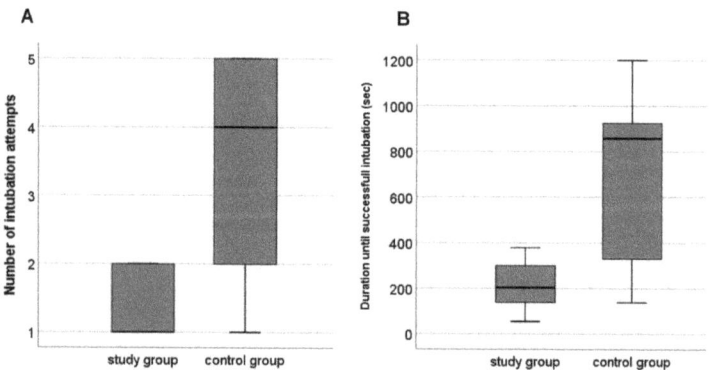

Figure 2. Boxplots of (A) number of intubation attempts and (B) duration until successful intubation in neonates intubated with the novel intubation method (study group) and the conventional intubation method (control group).

3.2. Secondary Outcomes

The first-pass success rate was 57% vs. 22% ($p = 0.303$) and the Propofol dose median (IQR) 1 (1–2) vs. 2 (2–3) mg/kg ($p = 0.072$) in the intervention compared to the control group, respectively. Duration until successful intubation was 204 (138–300) and 858 (330–924) sec in the intervention and control group, respectively ($p = 0.113$) (Table 1, Figure 2). There were no adverse effects in either groups.

4. Discussion

To the best of our knowledge, this is the first randomized controlled trial comparing continuous gas flow through the ETT during intubation with the standard procedure aiming to reduce intubation attempts in newborn infants. This study demonstrated that the concept of continuous gas flow through the ETT during intubation, and the initial results, seem to be favorable and that there are no major unexpected adverse consequences of attempting this methodology. Further on, continuous gas flow through the ETT might result in a reduction of the total number of intubation attempts, fewer abandoned intubation attempts, higher first-pass success rates and less Propofol administration. From a clinical perspective, the study team preferred the intervention intubation method and loss of equipoise was the consequence.

In pediatric patients, continuous oxygen flow through a nasal cannula results in longer periods of normoxemia compared to no oxygen flow during intubations in the operating room [4]. While we did not measure the time to desaturation, we suspect a shorter time until successful intubation and fewer abandoned intubation attempts due to desaturation and/or bradycardia in the intervention group, indicating improved cardiorespiratory stability during intubation. In our center infants routinely receive Propofol intravenously for sedation before intubation. Our standard operating procedure is based on a randomized controlled trial demonstrating no differences in heart rate when using the Propofol compared to the morphine, atropine, and suxam-ethonium regimen [5]. The SHINE trial is currently comparing the addition of a high-flow nasal cannula with standard care during neonatal intubation with a similar primary outcome (i.e., incidence of successful first attempt intubation without physiological instability) [6].

Successful neonatal intubation with the first attempt occurs in 64% of experienced professionals, but only in 20–26% of novice providers [2]. Thus, using continuous gas flow via the ETT might be an alternative technique especially for novice health care providers by which to reduce the risk for desaturation and/or bradycardia during intubation. As opportunities for endotracheal intubations of neonates are limited during pediatric training, the presented modified technique may lead to not only more stable infants, but also improved learning opportunities.

There are certain limitations to our study, which should be considered. The sample size was small and the study was stopped due to a change in the local intubation policy favoring less-invasive-surfactant-administration, which resulted in a lower intubation rate. We only report the p-values but do not mention significance, as this was a pilot trial with a small sample size and no power calculation. Hence, the results should be interpreted with caution. Furthermore, we only studied nasopharyngeal intubations, which represent the standard procedure at our unit. Using the same approach during oral intubation might yield different results. A strength of this study was the inclusion of small preterm infants, which are more prone to desaturation and/or bradycardia.

5. Conclusions

The concept of providing continuous gas flow through the ETT during nasopharyngeal intubation seems to be favorable without increased risk for major unexpected adverse events. This method might result in fewer intubation attempts and a higher rate of successful intubation on the first attempt and might reduce the number of abandoned intubations due to desaturation and/or bradycardia. Studies with greater sample sizes are urgently needed.

Author Contributions: Conceptualization, N.M.M., G.P., B.U.; methodology, M.B., N.M.M., G.P., B.U.; formal analysis, M.B., G.P., G.M.S.; investigation M.B., N.M.M., C.H.W., L.P.M., B.S.; resources, B.U.; data curation, M.B., G.P., G.M.S.; writing—original draft preparation, M.B., G.P., G.M.S.; writing—review and editing, M.B., N.M.M., G.P., C.H.W., L.P.M., B.S., G.M.S., B.U., S.H.; visualization, M.B., G.P., G.M.S.; supervision, G.P., B.U.; project administration, M.B., G.P. All authors have read and agreed to the published version of the manuscript.

Funding: We would like to thank the public for donating money to our funding agencies.

Institutional Review Board Statement: The study was conducted according to the guidelines of the Declaration of Helsinki, and approved by the Institutional Ethics Committee of Medical University of Graz (EC number: 25–282ex12/13).

Informed Consent Statement: Informed consent was obtained from all subjects involved in the study. Written informed consent has been obtained from the patients parents to publish this paper.

Data Availability Statement: The data presented in this study are available on request from the corresponding author.

Acknowledgments: We thank the parents for their trust, so we were allowed to investigate their infants. We also thank all the staff members, especially Evelyn Ziehenberger, for contributing to this study.

Conflicts of Interest: The authors declare no conflict of interest.

References

1. Foglia, E.E.; Ades, A.; Sawyer, T.; Glass, K.M.; Singh, N.; Jung, P.; Quek, B.H.; Johnston, L.C.; Barry, J.; Zenge, J.; et al. Neonatal Intubation Practice and Outcomes: An International Registry Study. *Pediatrics* **2019**, *143*, e20180902. [CrossRef] [PubMed]
2. Hatch, L.D.; Grubb, P.H.; Lea, A.S.; Walsh, W.F.; Markham, M.H.; Whitney, G.M.; Slaughter, J.C.; Stark, A.R.; Ely, E.W. Endotracheal Intubation in Neonates: A Prospective Study of Adverse Safety Events in 162 Infants. *J. Pediatr.* **2016**, *168*, 62–66. [CrossRef] [PubMed]
3. Fiadjoe, J.E.; Nishisaki, A.; Jagannathan, N.; Hunyady, A.I.; Greenberg, R.S.; Reynolds, P.I.; Matuszczak, M.E.; Rehman, M.A.; Polaner, D.M.; Szmuk, P.; et al. Airway management complications in children with difficult tracheal intubation from the Pediatric Difficult Intubation (PeDI) registry: A prospective cohort analysis. *Lancet Respir. Med.* **2016**, *4*, 37–48. [CrossRef]
4. Soneru, C.N.; Hurt, H.F.; Petersen, T.R.; Davis, D.D.; Braude, D.A.; Falcon, R.J. Apneic nasal oxygenation prolongs safe apnea time during pediatric intubations by learners. *Pediatr. Anesth.* **2019**, *29*, 628–634. [CrossRef] [PubMed]
5. Abdel-Latif, M.E.; Oei, J.; Lui, K. Propofol Compared with the Morphine, Atropine, and Suxamethonium Regimen as Induction Agents for Neonatal Endotracheal Intubation: A Randomized, Controlled Trial: In Reply. *Pediatrics* **2007**, *120*, 933. [CrossRef]
6. Hodgson, K.A.; Owen, L.S.; Kamlin, C.O.; Roberts, C.T.; Donath, S.M.; Davis, P.G.; Manley, B.J. A multicentre, randomised trial of stabilisation with nasal high flow during neonatal endotracheal intubation (the SHINE trial): A study protocol. *BMJ Open* **2020**, *10*, 1–6. [CrossRef] [PubMed]

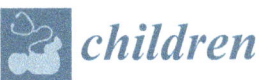

Article

Approach to the Connection between Meconium Consistency and Adverse Neonatal Outcomes: A Retrospective Clinical Review and Prospective In Vitro Study

Hueng-Chuen Fan [1,2,3,4], Fung-Wei Chang [5], Ying-Ru Pan [2], Szu-I Yu [2], Kuang-Hsi Chang [2], Chuan-Mu Chen [4,6,†] and Ching-Ann Liu [7,8,9,*]

1. Department of Pediatrics, Tungs' Taichung Metroharbor Hospital, Wuchi, Taichung 435, Taiwan; fanhuengchuen@yahoo.com.tw
2. Department of Medica research, Tungs' Taichung Metroharbor Hospital, Wuchi, Taichung 435, Taiwan; liz00049@yahoo.com.tw (Y.-R.P.); pride1223@gmail.com (S.-I.Y.); kuanghsichang@gmail.com (K.-H.C.)
3. Department of Rehabilitation, Jen-Teh Junior College of Medicine, Nursing and Management, Miaoli 356, Taiwan
4. Department of Life Sciences, Agricultural Biotechnology Center, National Chung Hsing University, Taichung 402, Taiwan; chchen1@dragon.nchu.edu.tw
5. Department of Obstetrics and Gynecology, Tri-Service General Hospital, National Defense Medical Center, Taipei 11490, Taiwan; doc30666@gmail.com
6. The iEGG and Animal Biotechnology Center, and Rong Hsing Research Center for Translational Medicine, National Chung Hsing University, Taichung 402, Taiwan
7. Bioinnovation Center, Buddhist Tzu Chi Medical Foundation, Hualien 970, Taiwan
8. Department of Medical Research, Hualien Tzu Chi Hospital, Hualien 970, Taiwan
9. Neuroscience Center, Hualien Tzu Chi Hospital, Hualien 970, Taiwan
* Correspondence: sagianne@gmail.com; Tel.: +886-3-8561825-15642
† The authors contributed equally to this study.

Abstract: Whether meconium-stained amniotic fluid (MSAF) serves as an indicator of fetal distress is under debate; however, the presence of MSAF concerns both obstetricians and pediatricians because meconium aspiration is a major contributor to neonatal morbidity and mortality, even with appropriate treatment. The present study suggested that thick meconium in infants might be associated with poor outcomes compared with thin meconium based on chart reviews. In addition, cell survival assays following the incubation of various meconium concentrations with monolayers of human epithelial and embryonic lung fibroblast cell lines were consistent with the results obtained from chart reviews. Exposure to meconium resulted in the significant release of nitrite from A549 and HEL299 cells. Medicinal agents, including dexamethasone, L-Nω-nitro-arginine methylester (L-NAME), and NS-398 significantly reduced the meconium-induced release of nitrite. These results support the hypothesis that thick meconium is a risk factor for neonates who require resuscitation, and inflammation appears to serve as the primary mechanism for meconium-associated lung injury. A better understanding of the relationship between nitrite and inflammation could result in the development of promising treatments for meconium aspiration syndrome (MAS).

Keywords: meconium-stained amniotic fluid (MSAF); meconium aspiration syndrome (MAS); cyclooxygenase-2 (COX-2); nitric oxide (NO); nitric oxide synthase (NOS)

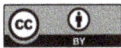

1. Introduction

Meconium is a black-green, odorless, rather sticky, and viscous material that can be found in the bowel of the developing fetus starting from 70–85 days of gestation [1–3]. Meconium contains bile acids and salts, mucus, pancreatic juices, cellular components exfoliated from the gastrointestinal tract, swallowed amniotic fluid, vernix caseosa, lanugo hairs, mucus glycoproteins, lipids, proteases, and blood that accumulates in the fetal colon throughout gestation [4,5]. When the meconium becomes excreted into the amniotic cavity, meconium-stained amniotic fluid (MSAF) can be detected [6–10]. MSAF can serve as an indicator of fetal bowel maturation [11] and can also represent a secondary fetal distress sign due to hypoxia [12–14]. Animal studies have revealed that hypoxia evokes a vagal response, stimulating colonic activity and relaxing the anal sphincter, promoting the release of meconium into the uterine cavity [15]. Animal studies also showed that fetal swallowing was suppressed by hypoxia, leading to a decrease in the normal ability to clear meconium from the amniotic fluid [16]. Therefore, hypoxia may result in excessive meconium excretion, disturb clearance, and prolong MSAF, which is associated with intrauterine fetal death, low APGAR scores [17], intrapartum fetal death [18], neurologic impairments [19,20], and meconium aspiration syndrome (MAS) [21].

Approximately 1% to 12% of neonates with MSAF will develop MAS [22–24], which is associated with various serious complications, such as persistent pulmonary hypertension (PPHN), long-term respiratory issues [7,25,26], neurodevelopmental problems [17,19,20,27–29], and mortality [6]. MAS is a multifaceted disease, characterized by airway obstruction, surfactant dysfunction, and pulmonary inflammation [30]. Aspirated meconium that obstructs the airway impacts the infant's oxygenation capacity [20,21], leading to the development of pneumothorax [22], pulmonary hypertension [23], and chemical pneumonitis [24], all of which can contribute to the occurrence of severe acute hypoxia, impaired neural development, and death [25,26]. However, routine intubation with suction is no longer recommended for the removal of meconium because these interventions have not been demonstrated to significantly reduce the incidence of MAS or MAS-related mortality [31,32], suggesting that other mechanisms may be responsible beyond airway obstruction.

Aspirated meconium can directly damage type II pneumocytes [24,33], and the enzymes found in meconium can cleave surfactants [33], leading to a significant decrease in surfactant levels. Moreover, aspirated meconium can alter surfactant fluidity [34] and ultrastructure [24], resulting in surfactant dysfunction. Although the administration of exogenous surfactant improved lung functions in an animal model of MAS [35], this approach is supported by limited data, and clinical trials of exogenous surfactant administration did not show significant reductions in MAS-associated mortality or other morbidities [36,37]. An important feature of newborn lungs exposed to meconium is the presence of an inflammatory response [38], in which inflammatory cells and cytokines, such as tumor necrosis factor (TNF)-α, interleukin (IL)-1β, IL-6, and IL-8, are activated by meconium to initiate pulmonary inflammation [30], and increased inflammatory indices are detected in cases of severe MAS [39]. Pathological examinations in MAS cases have revealed typical inflammatory pneumonitis, characterized by epithelial disruption, proteinaceous exudation with alveolar collapse, and cellular necrosis [40]. Together, these findings, combined with the clinical features of MAS [9,24,41–43], suggest that meconium causes profound functional alterations within the lungs, associated with an intense inflammatory reaction [33].

Nitric oxide (NO) is a ubiquitous gas that is involved in diverse physiological processes, including vasodilation, bronchodilation, neurotransmission, tumor surveillance, antimicrobial defense, and the regulation of inflammatory-immune processes [44–46]. Although inhaled NO can successfully treat MAS associated PPHN [47], NO inhalation was only associated with transient decreases in airway resistance and pulmonary pressure in animal models of MAS, suggesting that the underlying mechanisms associated with MAS extends beyond abnormal vascular constriction and may involve the lung parenchyma [48]. Moreover, NO can potentiate lung injury by promoting oxidative or nitrosative stress [49], inactivating surfactants, and stimulating inflammation [50]. NO is generated from L-arginine by three different NO synthases (NOS): neuronal NOS (nNOS; NOS-1), inducible NOS (iNOS; NOS-2), and endothelial NOS (eNOS; NOS-3) [51]. The role played by NO in meconium-induced lung injury remains unclear.

A pilot randomized control trial demonstrated a lack of significant differences in the outcomes of mild, moderate, and severe MAS when comparing cases treated with or without endotracheal suction [52], suggesting that meconium consistency has no effect on MAS prognosis; however, based on our own clinical experience, we suspected hypothesized that a potential connection exists between meconium consistency and MSAF prognosis. To investigate this hypothesis, we first examined the clinical data of neonates born with meconium from a local teaching hospital. Furthermore, we developed an in vitro model using human alveolar epithelial and bronchial cells to determine the effects of different meconium concentrations on lung cells.

2. Materials and Methods

2.1. Human Study
Data Sources

The medical records associated with live births delivered at Tungs' Taichung Metro-Harbor Hospital between 1 January 2013 and 31 December 2017 were reviewed, including the paper and electronic records of all infants admitted to the nursery, the sick neonate care unit, and the neonatal intensive care unit (NICU). Diagnoses were determined by qualified pediatricians according to the International Classification of Diseases, Clinical Modification, 9th Revision (ICD-9CM). Meconium consistency was categorized as either thick (dark green in color and with a pea soup consistency) or thin (lightly-stained yellow or greenish color) [53]. All enrolled subjects were de-identified and encrypted by the manager of the medical record at Tungs' Taichung MetroHarbor Hospital to protect patient privacy, and these data cannot be used either to trace individual patients or be linked to other census data, such as the cancer registry or the household registry. Due to the anonymized nature of the dataset, the need for informed consent was waived. This study was approved by the institutional review board at Tungs' Taichung MetroHarbor Hospital, Taiwan, ROC (IRB approval No.: 107048). All protocols used in the human study were performed in accordance with the ethical standards established by the 1964 Declaration of Helsinki and its later amendments or comparable ethical standards [54].

2.2. Cell Study

2.2.1. Preparation of Meconium

As the birth canal is not a sterile environment [55–59], we collected meconium from ten full-term, healthy neonates delivered via cesarean section to minimize potential contamination during delivery. Meconium was prepared according to a previously published method [60]. In brief, we obtained first-pass meconium samples within 30 min of passage, which were transferred from the diaper into a sterile container. These samples were pooled together and processed in a blender to achieve a uniform consistency. After being homogenized with 0.9% NaCl to a 20% (w/v) final concentration, the meconium was centrifuged at 5000 RPM for 20 min at 4 °C, the supernatant was filtered through an 8-μm filter (Millipore Co., Bedford, MA, USA), aliquoted into 2-mL sterile plastic bottles, and stored at –80 °C until use. For meconium collection, a parent's or guardian's permission and informed consent were required. This study was approved by the institutional review board at Tungs' Taichung MetroHarbor Hospital, Taiwan, ROC (IRB approval No.: 105047). All protocols used during the meconium collection process were performed in accordance with relevant guidelines and regulations [61].

2.2.2. Culture of Lung Cells

Alveolar epithelial cells from the human lung carcinoma cell line A 549 and lung cells from the human embryonic bronchial fibroblast cell line HEL 299 were purchased from the American Type Culture Collection (Manassas, VA, USA). All cells tested negative for *Mycoplasma* contamination before any experiments were conducted in this study. These cells were grown in monolayers at 37 °C in 5% CO_2 and 100% humidity using tissue culture dishes. A549 cells were maintained on RPMI1640 (Gibco BRL, Grand Island, NY, USA). HEL299 cells were maintained on Modified Eagle's Medium (MEM; Gibco BRL, Grand Island, NY, USA). Both media were supplemented with penicillin (1×10^5 U/L), streptomycin (100 mg/L), amphotericin B (0.25 mg/L), 2 mM L-glutamine (Invitrogen, Carlsbad, CA, USA), and 10% (v/v) fetal bovine serum (FBS, Hyclone Laboratories, Logan,

UT, USA). The same batch of FBS was used for all experiments. The culture medium was renewed every 2–3 days.

2.2.3. Meconium Stimulation

A549 and HEL 299 cells were plated into 96-well culture plates at a concentration of 1×10^5 cells/mL and incubated at 37 °C in 5% CO_2 for 24 h. After washing, A549 and HEL299 cells were incubated for an additional 24 h with serum-free RPMI1640 and MEM, respectively. A preliminary study showed that the percentages of cell death were similar when cells were exposed to meconium concentrations $\geq$20% at different time points (data not shown). Therefore, 20% meconium was used as a stock solution and was diluted with RPMI1640 or MEM to obtain various concentrations (0.1%, 1%, and 5%). Monolayers of cells were then incubated in a meconium-containing medium for various periods of time (1, 6, 12, 18, and 24 h). Control cells were incubated in a meconium-free medium in a similar manner. At each time point, the supernatant was collected and used to determine cell viability and nitrite production. The cells were washed twice with phosphate-buffered saline (PBS) and collected for RNA extraction.

2.2.4. Cell Viability

Cell viability was analyzed by measuring the activity of mitochondrial malate dehydrogenase (mMDH) using the WST-1 assay [62]. A549 and HEL299 cells were plated in 96-well plates, treated with or without meconium stimulation, and incubated with 10 µL of WST-1 reagent (BioVision, Milpitas, CA, USA) for 3 h at 37 °C. The amount of formazan generated, which was proportional to the number of viable cells, was calculated using a Multiskan™ FC Microplate Photometer (Molecular Devices) based on the absorbance signal at 440 nm. The absorbance was corrected using a background reading.

2.2.5. Nitrite Determination

Nitrite production was measured by a Griess assay, as previously described [63]. Briefly, the concentration of nitrite in A549 and HEL299 cells treated with or without meconium stimulation in the absence or presence of 2 mM L-NAME; 10^{-4}, 10^{-6}, 10^{-8}, or 10^{-10} M dexamethasone; or 25, 50, or 100 µM NS-398 in each well were measured by adding 100 µL Griess reagent (0.1% N-(1-Naphthyl) ethylenediamine in dH_2O and 1% sulfanilamide in 5% (v/v) phosphoric acid, mixed 1:1 immediately before use) to 100 µL of culture supernatant, followed by incubation at room temperature for 10 min. The absorbance at 540 nm was measured using a Multiskan™ FC Microplate Photometer (Molecular Devices). Nitrite concentrations in the culture supernatant were calculated based on a standard curve using known concentrations of sodium nitrite. The absorbance values were corrected using a background reading.

2.2.6. RNA Extraction and Real-Time Quantitative PCR

Total RNA was extracted from cultured A549 and HEL299 cells, isolated, and purified using TRIzol® RNA Isolation Reagents (Invitrogen, Liverpool, NY, USA). For the synthesis of the first-strand cDNA, 2 µg of total RNA was collected for a single-round reverse transcription reaction, performed using a High-Capacity cDNA Reverse Transcription Kit (Applied Biosystems, Foster City, CA, USA). cDNAs were exponentially doubled under conditions of 95 °C for 30 s, 40 cycles at 95 °C for 1 s, and 60 °C for 60 s, using the TaqMan probes PCR master mix (Applied Biosystems) and a Step-One™ Real-Time PCR System (Applied Biosystems). The simultaneous amplification of β_2-microglobulin (B2M) was used as an internal control against which to normalize the various mRNA levels in the samples and to quantify changes in gene expression levels using the $2^{-\Delta\Delta Ct}$ formula. The specific primers used in this study are shown in Table 1. All reactions were performed in at least triplicate and normalized to B2M gene expression levels. The data were analyzed using Bio-Rad CFX Manager 3.1 software (Bio-Rad) and are presented as fold changes in the normalized mRNA amounts of the meconium treatment group relative to those of the control group.

Table 1. Oligonucleotides primers for real-time RT-PCR analysis.

Gene Name	Sequence	Product (bp)	RefSeq No.
COX-2	Probe 56FAM 5′-ACATCCAGA-ZEN-TCACATTTGATTGACAGTCCA-3IABkFQ-3′ 5′- GCCATAGTCAGCATTGTAAGTTG -3′ 5′- GCACTACATACTTACCCACTTCA -3′	30	NM_000963
NOS-1	Probe 56FAM 5′-TCCTTAGCC-ZEN-GTCAAAACCTCCAGAG-3IABkFQ-32032 5′- AGACGCACGAAGATAGTTGAC-3′ 5′- CCGAAGCTCCAGAACTCAC-3′	25	NM_000963
NOS-2	Probe 56FAM 5′- TATTCAGCT -ZEN-GTGCCTTCAACCCCA -3IABkFQ-3′ 5′- GCAGCTCAGCCTGTACT-3′ 5′- CACCATCCTCTTTGCGACA-3′	24	NM_000625
NOS-3	Probe 56FAM 5′- TATTCAGCT -ZEN-GTGCCTTCAACCCCA -3IABk FQ-3′ 5′-ACGATGGTGACTTTGGCTA-3′ 5′-TGGAGGATGTGGCTGTCT-3′	23	NM_001160110
B2M	Probe 56FAM 5′- CCTGCCGTG -ZEN-TGAACCATGTGACT -3IABkFQ -3′ 5′- ACCTCCATGATGCTGCTTAC -3′ 5′- GGACTGGTCTTTCTATCTCTTGT -3′	23	99832111

COX-2: cyclooxygenase-2; NOS-1: nitric oxide synthase-1; NOS-2: nitric oxide synthase-2; NOS-3: nitric oxide synthase-3; B2M: β_2-microglobulin; RT-PCR: reverse transcriptase-polymerase chain reaction.

2.2.7. Library Preparation and Sequencing

The purified RNA was used to prepare a sequencing library using the TruSeq Stranded mRNA Library Prep Kit (Illumina, San Diego, CA, USA), following the manufacturer's recommendations. Briefly, mRNA was purified from total RNA (1 µg) by oligo (dT)-coupled magnetic beads and fragmented into small pieces under an elevated temperature. The first-strand cDNA was synthesized using reverse transcriptase and random primers. After the generation of double-strand cDNA and the adenylation of the 3′ ends of DNA fragments, the adaptors were ligated and purified using the AMPure XP system (Beckman Coulter, Beverly, Brea, CA, USA). The quality of the libraries was assessed using the Agilent Bioanalyzer 2100 system and a real-time PCR system. The qualified libraries were then sequenced on an Illumina NovaSeq 6000 platform with 150 bp paired-end reads, generated by Genomics, BioSci & Tech Co., New Taipei City, Taiwan.

2.2.8. Bioinformatics

Low-quality bases and sequences from adapters were removed from the raw data using the program Trimmomatic (version 0.39). The filtered reads were aligned to the reference genomes using Bowtie 2 (version 2.3.4.1). A user-friendly software, RSEM (version 1.2.28), was applied for the quantification of transcript abundance. Differentially expressed genes (DEGs) were identified by EBSeq (version 1.16.0) [64].

2.2.9. Statistical Analysis

Summary statistics are expressed as the frequency and percentage for categorical data and as the mean and standard deviation (SD) for continuous variables. Group differences in the distribution of delivery mode, preeclampsia, diabetes, antepartum hemorrhage, PROM, polyhydramnios, oligohydramnios, sex of the infant, hypoglycemia, NICU admission, CRAP use, intubation, ventilator use, and death were analyzed by the Fisher's exact test. Continuous variables, such as APGAR scores and maternal and gestational age, were compared between the thin and thick meconium groups using the Student's t-test. The survival percentages and the effects in cells exposed to various concentrations of meconium (0.5%, 1%, and 5%) and various treatment durations (1, 6, 12, 18, and 24 h) were evaluated using a one-way analysis of variance (ANOVA). The mRNA expression levels in cells with and without meconium treatment were analyzed by the paired Student's *t*-test. The nitrite levels in cells exposed to various meconium concentrations (0.5%, 1%, and 5%) for various treatment durations (1, 6, 12, 18, and 24 h), combined with various medicinal agents, were evaluated by one-way analysis of variance (ANOVA). A *p*-value < 0.05 was considered significant for all analyses (* $p < 0.05$ and ** $p < 0.005$). Statistical analyses were conducted using the statistical package SAS version 9.4 (SAS Institute Inc., Cary, NC, USA).

3. Results

3.1. Thick Meconium Is a Risk Factor for Neonates Receiving Resuscitation

A total of 8316 neonates were delivered at a local teaching hospital during this five-year study, including 3078 (37.01%) neonates delivered by cesarean section and 5238 (62.99%) neonates delivered vaginally. The charts for 1099 (13.22%) neonates recorded MSAF, or meconium-stained skin, nail, or umbilicus, including 454 (41.31%) neonates delivered by cesarean section and 645 (58.69%) neonates delivered vaginally. Among these, 95 (1.14%) neonates were deemed to have suffered from MAS and were admitted to the sick neonate care unit, and 12 neonates were admitted to the NICU. The male:female ratios were 598:501 in the MSAF group and approximately 1:1 (48: 49) in the MAS group.

To investigate the effects of exposure to different meconium consistencies among infants diagnosed with MAS, we divided the infants diagnosed with MAS into thin and thick meconium groups, based on the data obtained from the chart review, resulting in 72 cases classified into the thin meconium group and 23 cases classified into the thick meconium group. No significant differences were identified among maternal factors such as maternal age; delivery mode; or medical conditions, such as preeclampsia, diabetes, antepartum hemorrhage, PROM, polyhydramnios, and oligohydramnios. Several neonatal factors, including gestational age, birth, weight, sex of the infant, and the prevalence of hypoglycemia did not differ significantly between the two groups. However, the APGAR scores at 1 min and 5 min, the numbers of neonates who required NICU admission, CPAP use, intubation, or ventilator use, and the number of neonates who died showed significant differences between the two groups, suggesting that the presence of thick meconium may be significantly associated with receiving advanced life support (Table 2).

Table 2. Comparisons of variables between neonates delivered in the presence of thin or thick meconium.

	Thin Meconium N = 72	Thick Meconium N = 23	*p*-Value
Maternal factors			
Maternal age, years	30.38 ± 4.39	31.13 ± 5.41	0.46
Delivery mode, (CS/NSD)	17/55	8/15	0.29
Preeclampsia, N (%)	5 (6.94%)	2 (8.70%)	0.68
Diabetes, N (%)	6 (8.33%)	2 (8.70%)	1.00
Antepartum hemorrhage, N (%)	2 (2.78%)	1 (4.35%)	0.57
PROM, N (%)	8 (11.11%)	3 (13.04%)	0.72
Polyhydramnios, N (%)	4 (5.56%)	2 (8.70%)	0.35
Oligohydramnios, N (%)	3 (4.17%)	1 (4.35%)	1.00
Neonatal factors			
Gestational age, weeks	39.39 ± 3.01	39.13 ± 2.82	0.51
Birth weight, g	3039.24 ± 497.19	2836.35 ± 490.40	0.09
Sex (female/male)	36/36	12/11	1.00
APGAR1 min	7.80 ± 1.31	6.19 ± 2.64	0.01 *
APGAR5 min	9.01 ± 0.83	7.86 ± 2.22	0.02 *
Hypoglycemia, N (%)	3 (4.17%)	2 (8.70%)	1.00
NICU admission, N (%)	0	12 (52.17%)	<0.001 **
CPAP, N (%)	0	6 (26.09%)	<0.001 **
Intubation, N (%)	0	7 (30.43%)	<0.001 **
Ventilator, N (%)	0	6 (26.09%)	<0.001 **
Death, N (%)	0	2 (8.70%)	0.06

CS: *cesarean* section; NSD: normal spontaneous delivery; PROM: premature rupture of membranes; NICU: neonatal intensive care unit; CPAP: continuous positive airway pressure. *: $p < 0.05$; **: $p < 0.005$.

3.2. Thick Meconium with Longer Exposure Times Induces Lung Cell Death

The results of the cell viability assay demonstrated that A549 (Figure 1A) and HEL299 cells (Figure 1B) showed different responses following exposure to variable meconium concentrations and meconium exposure durations. Furthermore, we found that higher meconium concentrations or longer exposure times resulted in increased cell death, suggesting that the concentration and exposure time had a significant effect on lung cell viability.

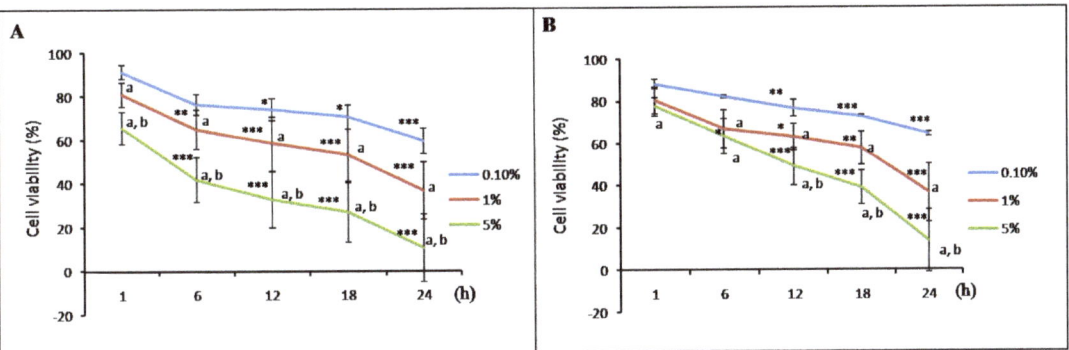

Figure 1. Cell viability of human lung cells, including (**A**) A549: alveolar epithelial cells and (**B**) HEL299: human embryonic lung tissue cells, exposed to 0.1%, 1%, and 5% human meconium concentrations for 1, 6, 12, 18, and 24 h (n_{Exp} = 5). The data represent the mean ± standard deviation. a: $p < 0.05$, versus the 0.1% group; b: $p < 0.05$ versus the 1% group; *: $p < 0.05$ versus at 1 h; **: $p < 0.005$ versus 1 h; ***: $p < 0.0005$ versus 1 h.

3.3. Meconium Induces NOS and COX Gene Expression

A significant amount of cell death was observed when A549 (Figure 1A) or HEL299 cells (Figure 1B) were exposed to meconium at concentrations higher than 0.1% with an exposure time equal to or longer than 6 h. To investigate the effects of meconium exposure on lung cell gene expression, a pilot RNA-seq study was performed using RNA samples from A549 and HEL299 cells following a 6 h exposure to 1% meconium. Meconium may activate inflammatory cells and induce cytokines to initiate pulmonary inflammation [24], and NOS and COX, which are the primary inflammatory mediators and are expressed in the airway epithelium, releasing NO and COX products during acute inflammatory responses [65]. The results of the RNA-seq showed greater fold changes in nitrite production-related genes, including *NOS-1*, and *NOS-2*, especially *NOS-2*, in the HEL299 cells than in A549 cells. The *COX-2* expression levels in both A549 and HEL299 cells were very high (Table 3). These genes were selected for further study, and their expression was validated by real-time RT-PCR. *NOS-1*, *NOS-2*, *NOS-3*, and *COX-2* expression was detectable in both A549 and HEL299 cells. Significant differences in *NOS-1* mRNA expression levels were observed between the HEL299 cells with meconium stimulation versus those without (Figure 2A). However, no significant differences in *NOS-1* mRNA expression levels were observed in A549 cells with or without meconium stimulation (Figure 2A). *NOS-2* (Figure 2B) and *COX-2* (Figure 2D) mRNA levels increased significantly following meconium stimulation in both in A549 cells and HEL299 cells. No significant differences were observed for *NOS-3* mRNA levels in A549 and HEL299 cells with and without meconium stimulation (Figure 2C).

Table 3. Human lung cell lines were treated with vehicle (1% NaCl) or 1% human meconium for 6 h, and gene expression levels were measured using RNA-seq analysis. Gene expression was analyzed using bioinformatics software to compare expression between meconium-treated and vehicle-treated A549 and HEL299 cells.

Cell Lines		A549	HEL299	
Name/Gene ID/MIM	Gene Description	Fold Increase		Map
NOS1/4842/163731	nitric oxide synthase 1(NOS-1)	0.9845475	1.6171549	12q24.22
NOS2/4843/163730	nitric oxide synthase 2 (NOS-2)	0.4949685	3.2921734	17q11.2
NOS3/4846/163729	nitric oxide synthase 3 (NOS-3)	1.1372183	1.1059593	7q36.1
PTGS2/5743/600262	cyclooxygenase-2 (COX-2)	22.952443	19.439566	1q31.1

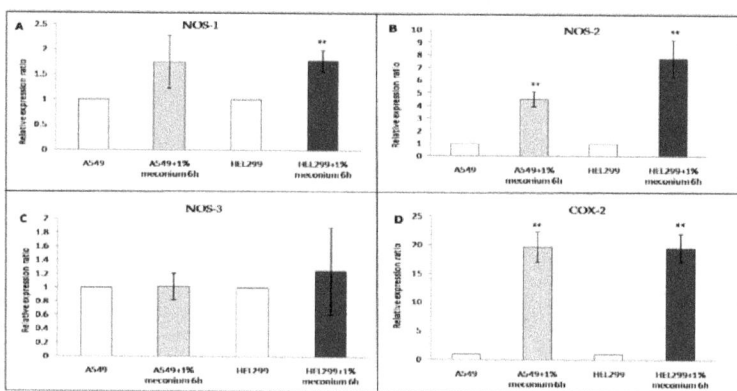

Figure 2. Meconium induces *NOS* and *COX* gene expression. A549 and HEL299 cells were incubated with or without 1% meconium for 6 h. The mRNA expression levels of *B2M* were used as an internal control. Mean relative expression levels for the genes (**A**) *NOS-1*, (**B**) *NOS-2*, (**C**) *NOS-3*, and (**D**) *COX-2*, before and after 1% meconium stimulation for 6 h in A549 and HEL299 cells (n_{Exp} = 4). The data represent the mean ± standard deviations. NOS: Nitric oxide synthases. COX: Cyclooxygenase. **: $p < 0.005$ versus cells without meconium stimulation.

3.4. Meconium Enhances Nitrite Production

Nitrite levels from A549 (Figure 3A) and HEL299 cells (Figure 3B) exposed to meconium at concentrations higher than 0.1% increased significantly compared with those in the control cells. Using 1% meconium, nitrite production significantly increased in the supernatant collected from A549 and HEL299 cells after 1, 6, 12, 18, and 24 h exposure compared with nitrite levels in the control cells. The results also showed that the nitrite production by HEL299 cells was significantly greater than that observed for A549 cells after 6 h of exposure to 1% meconium (nitrite levels in HEL299 after 6 h vs. nitrite levels in A549 after 6 h: 411.18 ± 36.41 vs. 238.13 ± 22.29, $p = 0.017$).

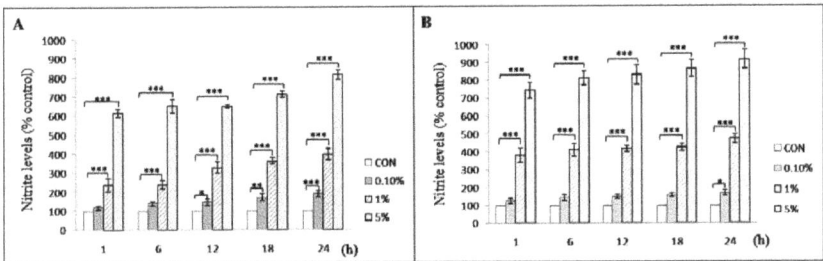

Figure 3. Effects of meconium concentrations on nitrite production in (**A**) A549 and (**B**) HEL299 cells. A549 and HEL299 cells were exposed for 1, 6, 12, 18, or 24 h to 0.1%, 1%, or 5% human meconium. (n_{Exp} = 4). The data represent the mean ± standard deviation. Nitrite levels were significantly higher in the supernatants of cells exposed to meconium compared with the values in control cells. *: $p < 0.05$; **: $p < 0.005$; ***: $p < 0.0005$.

3.5. Dexamethasone and COX-2 Inhibitor Treatment Significantly Reduced the Nitrite Production Induced by Meconium Stimulation

The effects of various medicinal agents on nitrite production were examined. The addition of 2 mM arginine increased nitrite production in HEL299 cells to a greater degree than in A549 cells following meconium exposure. The nitrite levels observed in HEL299 and A549 cells treated with 2 mML-NAME; 10^{-10}, 10^{-8}, 10^{-6}, or 10^{-4}M dexamethasone; or 25, 50, or 100 µM NS-398. L-NAME, dexamethasone, and NS-398 treatment were all able to significantly reduce nitrite production in A549 (Figure 4A) and HEL299 cells treated with 1% meconium for 6 h (Figure 4B).

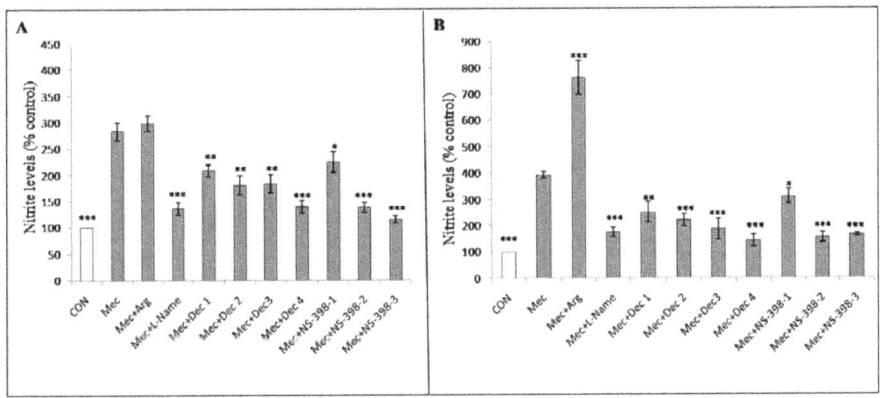

Figure 4. L-NAME, dexamethasone and NS-398 significantly reduced nitrite production following 1% meconium exposure for 6 h in (**A**) A549 and (**B**) HEL299 cells (n_{Exp} = 4). Nitrite levels were significantly higher in the supernatant of untreated cells exposed to meconium compared with those in control cells. The data represent the mean ± standard deviation. Mec: 1% meconium exposure for 6 h. Arg: 2mM L-arginine; L-NAME: 2mM L-Nω-nitro-arginine methylester; Dec 1: 10^{-10} M dexamethasone; Dec 2: 10^{-8} M dexamethasone; Dec 3: 10^{-6} M dexamethasone; Dec 4: 10^{-4} M dexamethasone; NS-398-1: 25 µM NS-398; NS-398-2: 50 µM NS-398; NS-398-3: 100 µM NS-398. *: $p < 0.05$; **:$p < 0.005$; ***: $p < 0.0005$.

4. Discussion

The presence of MSAF raises serious concerns, and meconium aspiration remains a major contributor to neonatal morbidity and mortality, despite appropriate treatment strategies [7,66]. In this study, the incidence of MSAF was 13.22%, which is within the reported range from 5–20% [6–10]. MAS is diagnosed in neonates born through MSAF who present with symptoms that cannot be otherwise explained [67]. In this study, the incidence rate of MAS was 1.14% among all neonates, which was within the reported range from

0.2–1.3% in China [68,69]. In the USA, the incidence rates for MAS range from 0.1 to 0.4% of births [29,70]. In France, the incidence of MAS was reported to be 0.2% [22]. In this study, 8.64% of neonates with MSAF exhibited airway symptoms, and 6.31% of MAS diagnosed neonates required ventilator support, in addition to an MAS diagnosed mortality rate of 2.1%. The literature has reported that between 4.2 and 62% of infants born through MSAF subsequently suffer from respiratory distress [22,71], and between 33 and 49.7% of MAS diagnosed neonates require ventilator support, with a 5–12% mortality rate [52,72,73]. The discrepancy between our results and those reported by others may be due to differences in ethnicity, socio-demographic variables, health institutions, or the provided level of medical care reported across different countries, case numbers, and study time points.

Although numerous studies have reported no significant differences in adverse neonatal outcomes associated with meconium consistency [52,74–76], our clinical experience [77], and the results of this retrospective analysis suggest that thick meconium may serve as a clinical risk for adverse neonatal outcomes, including low APGAR scores at 1 min and 5 min, neonatal death, or the need for NICU admission, resuscitation, CPAP use, or ventilator use. Our findings agree with the results of several papers [4,21,22,78–80]. Maternal factors, including maternal age, delivery mode, and the presence of medical conditions such as preeclampsia, diabetes, antepartum hemorrhage, PROM, polyhydramnios and oligohydramnios, and neonatal factors including gestational age, birth weight, sex of the infant, and the prevalence of hypoglycemia have all been reported to be associated with the presence of MSAF [14,21,22,25,78,81–85]. Because thin meconium is reported to be associated with chronic hypoxic stress, whereas thick meconium is reported to be associated with acute hypoxic stress or inflammation [13,79], we hypothesize that fetal asphyxia that occurs before or during delivery in both groups may represent a confounding factor that might neutralize the power of statistical analyses in both groups, leading to the lack of significant differences in maternal factors between the two groups.

Clinically, our results and those reported by others [14,21,22,25,78,81–85], showed that the presence of thick meconium was associated with higher rates of respiratory compromise, intubation at birth, and receiving ventilator support compared with thin MSAF. As a result, infants with thick MSAF have higher exposures to acute hypoxic events, leading to a higher risk of developing respiratory insufficiency. However, an interesting study proposed that the extent of lung destruction observed in MAS was not related to the aspiration of meconium but rather to the length and degree of asphyxia [86]. Infants who experience long and severe asphyxia usually demonstrate airway symptoms soon after delivery; however, some cases of MAS in this study and another study [87] developed in apparently healthy, meconium-stained neonates. Although we are not able to determine the occurrence of potential fetal asphyxia before or during labor among infants with MSAF, we hypothesize that inflammation in the airway may occur when an MSAF infant develops MAS, especially in the thick meconium group. The processes underlying inflammation in the airway at the cellular level are less well understood.

Our study showed that the cellular viabilities of both alveolar epithelial and bronchial cells were significantly reduced by stimulation with human meconium, and the severity of the response correlated with both exposure time and the meconium concentration, suggesting that meconium exerts a direct toxicity effect in alveolar and bronchial cells. Although bile salts and proteolytic enzymes, which are considered toxic components found in meconium, are capable of injuring the alveolar and bronchial structures [4,5], the consequent inflammation triggered by the meconium in the lungs may explain "postsurfactant slump" [88].

In this study, the results of the Figures 1, 3 and 4 demonstrated that A549 cells and HEL299 cells presented with different responses to the same meconium stimuli, suggesting that alveolar and bronchial cells might respond differently to meconium exposure, which was also compatible with the results of our RNA-seq and RT-PCR results. Although several papers have used A549 cells treated with meconium to simulate MAS in vitro [6,42,60,89], and A549 cells retain some characteristics of normal alveolar type II cells, A549 cells are in fact an adult human lung carcinoma cell line [90]. Additionally, bronchial tissue has been reported to be involved in the pathogenesis of MAS [50,91]; therefore, in this study, HEL299 cells, which are derived from fetal bronchial tissue, were used in combination with A549 cells to explore the effects of exposure to various concentrations of meconium.

RT-PCR showed that the mRNA expression of *NOS-1* was slightly elevated in A549 cells following 1% meconium exposure for 6 h, but this effect was not significant. Although NOS-3 is viewed as an important regulator of nitrite production in the perinatal lung vasculature [92], A549 and HEL299 cells do not contain any vascular components, so the changes in the mRNA expression levels of *NOS-3* were not significant following meconium stimulation. The levels of *NOS-2* mRNA significantly increased following meconium stimulation in both A549 cells and HEL299 cells. We hypothesize that *NOS-2* serves as the primary nitrite production mechanism in A549 cells in response to meconium stimulation, which is supported by the literature [93,94]. Moreover, in this study, the mRNA levels of *NOS-1* and *NOS-2* were significantly higher in HEL299 cells than in A549 cells in response to meconium stimulation, suggesting that fetal HEL299 cells could generate more nitrite than A549 cells even under identical meconium exposure conditions.

Nitrite production significantly increased in the supernatant derived from both A549 and HEL299 cells after 1, 6, 12, 18, and 24 h of 1% meconium exposure compared with nitrite production by control cells. Consistently, the amount of nitrite produced by HEL299 cells treated with 1% meconium for 6 h was significantly greater than that observed for A549 cells (Figure 3). Therefore, the association between elevated nitrite levels and reduced lung cell viability following meconium stimulation suggests that NO may play an important role in the pathogenesis of meconium-associated lung injury. The involvement of NO in meconium-associated lung injury has previously been studied [41,95–99]. Although the idea that elevated levels of NO might contribute to tissue damage is not new, our results showed HEL299 cells generated higher nitrite levels than A549 cells (Figure 3); therefore, previous experiments using A549 cells may not accurately represent the extent of lung injuries caused by meconium exposure.

Various studies of animals and cell lines examining the effects of meconium exposure have indicated the involvement of inflammatory mediators, such as NO and COX [41,95–98]. NO is required for vasodilation in PPHN and may cause other pathological changes in the body associated with the activation of inflammatory cells and cytokines, especially during lung injury [100,101]. In addition to NO, COX, also known as prostaglandin synthase, is a potent inflammatory mediator. Two mammalian COX enzyme isoforms have been identified, COX1 and COX2, which are considered constitutive and inducible, respectively [102]. The anti-inflammatory effects of non-steroidal anti-inflammatory drugs primarily act through their abilities to inhibit prostaglandin production, particularly through the inhibition of COX-2 activity [103]. COX is similar to NOS, including the expression of both constitutive forms, which are mostly involved in housekeeping tasks [104], and inducible forms, which shape the cellular response to stress and various bioactive agents [105]. For example, both NOS and COX in the airway epithelium become activated during acute inflammatory responses [65]. A number of studies have also suggested a role for COX in the cytotoxic effects of MAS [97,106]. Our RNA-seq and RT-PCR data showed that COX-2 mRNA levels in both A549 and HEL299 cells were highly expressed in response to meconium stimulation, and NS-398, a COX-2 specific inhibitor, has been shown to inhibit inflammation-related COX-2 activity [107]. Our results showed that the anti-inflammatory effect of NS-398 mitigated meconium-induced COX-2 over-expression, which, in turn, reduced the meconium-induced nitrite production in both A549 and HEL299 cells, suggesting that NS-398 may have an inhibitory effect against the cytotoxic effects of MAS. Furthermore, these data suggest that inflammation may represent a primary mechanism underlying lung injury induced by meconium aspiration.

L-NAME is a competitive inhibitor of NOS [108] and was able to prevent the release of NO from A549 and HEL299 cells in response to meconium stimulation. Although L-NAME has been shown to significantly decrease the levels of both nitrite and nitrate in cellular supernatants [96,109], L-NAME is also associated with teratogenic fetal limb defects and cannot be used for the treatment of MAS. As lung cells may produce NO from L-arginine due to NOS activity, L-arginine in this study was used as a positive control. Although corticosteroids are among the most effective anti-inflammatory agents used to treat many inflammatory diseases [110], the use of steroids is not recommended by the Cochrane database for the treatment of MAS [111], and a meta-analysis showed that steroid use did not decrease mortality or associated morbidities [112]. However, our experience and those reported by others have indicated that the outcomes of infants with MAS can be significantly improved by the administration of both systemic and inhaled steroids [113–115]. Intratracheally instilled steroid, either alone or with a surfactant, has resulted in a good response in an animal MAS model [116,117], and the use of steroids significantly attenuated pulmonary hemodynamic deterioration and structural lung damage caused by meconium aspiration in a piglet MAS model [50]. Moreover, NO and COX-2 production were inhibited by steroid treatment [118,119]. In this study, the nitrite levels induced by meconium exposure in both cell types could be significantly reduced by dexamethasone treatment, at a concentration as low as 10^{-10} M, suggesting that the use of dexamethasone may potentially protect against MAS-induced inflammation.

Because inhaled NO(INO) has a potent vasodilating effect, INO was approved by the FDA in 2000 as an effective regimen for the treatment of infants with MAS-associated PPHN [47,92]. Additionally, INO displays anti-inflammatory effects, including reducing cytokine synthesis, inactivating nuclear factor -κB (NF-κB), decreasing the expression of adhesion molecules, and preventing neutrophil adhesion and migration to the alveolar space [120]. In this study, NO, nitrite, nitrate, and NO-derived metabolites were generated when lung cells were stimulated with meconium. Although the generation of NO may be beneficial to lung cells, in plasma or other physiological fluids or buffers, NO becomes almost completely oxidized into nitrite, which remains stable for several hours [121]. Therefore, in many cases, the NO status in the blood does not accurately reflect the corresponding NO status of tissues of interest due to the use of different analysis tools and different samples [122]. Our results suggested that the mechanism underlying the meconium stimulation of lung cells involves inflammation, and meconium stimulation causes a significant decrease in lung cell proliferation (Figure 1). We suspect that the NO generated in this study may only represent a small portion of the generated nitrite found in lung cells stimulated by meconium. Therefore, the effects of INO on lung cells likely differ from the effects reflected by the nitrite data in this study.

The current study had a number of limitations. First, this study was performed as a retrospective study, and errors may be reflected in the medical records. Second, the sample size was small, and the duration of follow-up was only five years. Significant reductions in morbidity and mortality may have increased with a longer period of follow-up. Third, this was performed as a single-center study. Multi-center, international studies may provide a more convincing result. Fourth, infants who underwent rescue procedures may have had significantly lower APGAR scores than infants who did not. Therefore, we suggest that the relationship between the thick MSAF group and significantly low APGAR scores may require further investigation using a prospective study that includes more infants with thick MSAF to clarify this issue. Fifth, fetal alveolar cells may represent a better study material for MAS than fetal bronchial cells and adult alveolar lung cells. Sixth, inconsistencies in the mRNA expression levels for *NOS2* in A549 cells between the RNA-seq results (Table 3) and the real-time RT-PCR results (Figure 2B) may be due to an up-regulation in the cellular *NOS2* mRNA levels in response to stimulation, associated with an increase in the number of passages after thawing [123]. Seventh, the lack of an animal study was a limitation of our study, which may have provided a more comprehensive understanding of the effects of meconium on lung injury. Finally, this study was not randomized. These limitations may have introduced some bias during the analysis of the effects of meconium on neonatal lungs.

5. Conclusions

The clinical features of MAS are characterized by profound functional alterations within the lung, associated with an intense inflammatory reaction, and thick meconium causes a more severe fetal inflammatory response than thin meconium. Our clinical data showed that undesired morbidities, such as intensive birth resuscitation, ICU admission, intubation, ventilation, and death, which were observed for the thick meconium group, did not appear in the thin meconium group. Our in vitro studies showed that the thick meconium with longer exposure times markedly induced lung cell death and exposure to meconium resulted in the significant release of nitrite from lung cells. Taken together, these study results further confirm the inflammatory effects of meconium on lung cells while also suggesting future avenues of research regarding potential agents for counteracting these effects in infants.

Author Contributions: Conceptualization, H.-C.F., C.-M.C. and C.-A.L.; methodology, H.-C.F., F.-W.C., Y.-R.P., S.-I.Y. and K.-H.C.; investigation, F.-W.C. and Y.-R.P.; data curation, H.-C.F., Y.-R.P., S.-I.Y. and K.-H.C.; writing—original draft preparation, H.-C.F. and F.-W.C.; writing—review and editing, C.-M.C. and C.-A.L. supervision, C.-M.C. and C.-A.L. All authors have read and agreed to the published version of the manuscript.

Funding: This research received no external funding.

Institutional Review Board Statement: The study was conducted according to the guidelines of the Declaration of Helsinki and approved by the Institutional Review Board (clinical data analysis, approval number: 107048 and date of approval: 6th December 2018; meconium collection and preparation, approval number: 105047 and date of approval: 10 November 2016).

Informed Consent Statement: Subjects were de-identified and encrypted by the manager of the medical record, Tungs' Taichung MetroHarbor Hospital, to protect patient privacy, and these data cannot be used either to trace individual patients or be linked to other census data, such as the cancer registry or the household registry. Due to the anonymized nature of the dataset, the need for informed consent was waived. Regarding the meconium collection and preparation in this study, the family had to sign an informed consent before meconium collection. Written informed consent has been obtained from the patients to publish this paper.

Data Availability Statement: The data are not publicly available due to privacy.

Acknowledgments: This work was supported by grants from the Tungs' MetroHarbor Hospital (TTMHH-106R0003 and TTMHH-108c0006).

Conflicts of Interest: The authors declare no conflict of interest. The funders had no role in the design of the study; in the collection, analyses, or interpretation of data; in the writing of the manuscript, or in the decision to publish the results.

References

1. Antonowicz, I.; Shwachman, H. Meconium in health and in disease. *Adv. Pediatr.* **1979**, *26*, 275–310. [PubMed]
2. Holtzman, R.B.; Banzhaf, W.C.; Silver, R.K.; Hageman, J.R. Perinatal management of meconium staining of the amniotic fluid. *Clin. Perinatol.* **1989**, *16*, 825–838. [CrossRef]
3. Romero, R.; Yoon, B.H.; Chaemsaithong, P.; Cortez, J.; Park, C.W.; Gonzalez, R.; Behnke, E.; Hassan, S.S.; Chaiworapongsa, T.; Yeo, L. Bacteria and endotoxin in meconium-stained amniotic fluid at term: Could intra-amniotic infection cause meconium passage? *J. Matern. Fetal Neonatal Med.* **2014**, *27*, 775–788. [CrossRef] [PubMed]
4. Rahman, S.; Unsworth, J.; Vause, S. Meconium in labour. *Obstet. Gynaecol. Reprod. Med.* **2013**, *23*, 247–252. [CrossRef]
5. Romero, R.; Yoon, B.H.; Chaemsaithong, P.; Cortez, J.; Park, C.W.; Gonzalez, R.; Behnke, E.; Hassan, S.S.; Gotsch, F.; Yeo, L.; et al. Secreted phospholipase a2 is increased in meconium-stained amniotic fluid of term gestations: Potential implications for the genesis of meconium aspiration syndrome. *J. Matern. Fetal Neonatal Med.* **2014**, *27*, 975–983. [CrossRef]
6. Ahanya, S.N.; Lakshmanan, J.; Morgan, B.L.; Ross, M.G. Meconium passage in utero: Mechanisms, consequences, and management. *Obstet. Gynecol. Surv.* **2005**, *60*, 45–56. [CrossRef]
7. Dargaville, P.A.; Copnell, B.; Australian and New Zealand Neonatal Network. The epidemiology of meconium aspiration syndrome: Incidence, risk factors, therapies, and outcome. *Pediatrics* **2006**, *117*, 1712–1721. [CrossRef]
8. van Ierland, Y.; de Beaufort, A.J. Why does meconium cause meconium aspiration syndrome? Current concepts of mas pathophysiology. *Early Hum. Dev.* **2009**, *85*, 617–620. [CrossRef]

9. Zagariya, A.; Bhat, R.; Navale, S.; Vidyasagar, D. Cytokine expression in meconium-induced lungs. *Indian J. Pediatr.* **2004**, *71*, 195–201. [CrossRef] [PubMed]
10. Ziadeh, S.M.; Sunna, E. Obstetric and perinatal outcome of pregnancies with term labour and meconium-stained amniotic fluid. *Arch. Gynecol. Obstet.* **2000**, *264*, 84–87. [CrossRef]
11. Poggi, S.H.; Ghidini, A. Pathophysiology of meconium passage into the amniotic fluid. *Early Hum. Dev.* **2009**, *85*, 607–610. [CrossRef] [PubMed]
12. Ciftci, A.O.; Tanyel, F.C.; Karnak, I.; Buyukpamukcu, N.; Hicsonmez, A. In-utero defecation: Fact or fiction? *Eur. J. Pediatr. Surg.* **1999**, *9*, 376–380. [CrossRef] [PubMed]
13. Monen, L.; Hasaart, T.H.; Kuppens, S.M. The aetiology of meconium-stained amniotic fluid: Pathologic hypoxia or physiologic foetal ripening? *Early Hum. Dev.* **2014**, *90*, 325–328. [CrossRef] [PubMed]
14. Walsh, M.C.; Fanaroff, J.M. Meconium stained fluid: Approach to the mother and the baby. *Clin. Perinatol.* **2007**, *34*, 653–665. [CrossRef]
15. Westgate, J.A.; Bennet, L.; Gunn, A.J. Meconium and fetal hypoxia: Some experimental observations and clinical relevance. *BJOG* **2002**, *109*, 1171–1174. [CrossRef] [PubMed]
16. Sherman, D.J.; Ross, M.G.; Day, L.; Humme, J.; Ervin, M.G. Fetal swallowing: Response to graded maternal hypoxemia. *J. Appl. Physiol.* **1991**, *71*, 1856–1861. [CrossRef]
17. Ohana, O.; Holcberg, G.; Sergienko, R.; Sheiner, E. Risk factors for intrauterine fetal death (1988–2009). *J. Matern. Fetal Neonatal Med.* **2011**, *24*, 1079–1083. [CrossRef] [PubMed]
18. Brailovschi, Y.; Sheiner, E.; Wiznitzer, A.; Shahaf, P.; Levy, A. Risk factors for intrapartum fetal death and trends over the years. *Arch. Gynecol. Obstet.* **2012**, *285*, 323–329. [CrossRef]
19. Kalis, V.; Turek, J.; Hudec, A.; Rokyta, P.; Rokyta, Z.; Mejchar, B. Meconium and postnatal neurologic handicaps. *Ceska Gynekol.* **2001**, *66*, 369–377.
20. Redline, R.W. Severe fetal placental vascular lesions in term infants with neurologic impairment. *Am. J. Obstet. Gynecol.* **2005**, *192*, 452–457. [CrossRef]
21. Sheiner, E.; Hadar, A.; Shoham-Vardi, I.; Hallak, M.; Katz, M.; Mazor, M. The effect of meconium on perinatal outcome: A prospective analysis. *J. Matern. Fetal Neonatal Med.* **2002**, *11*, 54–59. [CrossRef]
22. Fischer, C.; Rybakowski, C.; Ferdynus, C.; Sagot, P.; Gouyon, J.B. A population-based study of meconium aspiration syndrome in neonates born between 37 and 43 weeks of gestation. *Int. J. Pediatr.* **2012**, *2012*, 321545. [CrossRef]
23. Gupta, V.; Bhatia, B.D.; Mishra, O.P. Meconium stained amniotic fluid: Antenatal, intrapartum and neonatal attributes. *Indian Pediatr.* **1996**, *33*, 293–297.
24. Monfredini, C.; Cavallin, F.; Villani, P.E.; Paterlini, G.; Allais, B.; Trevisanuto, D. Meconium aspiration syndrome: A narrative review. *Children* **2021**, *8*, 230. [CrossRef]
25. Bhutani, V.K. Developing a systems approach to prevent meconium aspiration syndrome: Lessons learned from multinational studies. *J. Perinatol.* **2008**, *28* (Suppl. S3), S30–S35. [CrossRef]
26. Olicker, A.L.; Raffay, T.M.; Ryan, R.M. Neonatal respiratory distress secondary to meconium aspiration syndrome. *Children* **2021**, *8*, 246. [CrossRef]
27. Beligere, N.; Rao, R. Neurodevelopmental outcome of infants with meconium aspiration syndrome: Report of a study and literature review. *J. Perinatol.* **2008**, *28* (Suppl. S3), S93–S101. [CrossRef]
28. Naeye, R.L. Can meconium in the amniotic fluid injure the fetal brain? *Obstet. Gynecol.* **1995**, *86*, 720–724. [CrossRef]
29. Thornton, P.D.; Campbell, R.T.; Mogos, M.F.; Klima, C.S.; Parsson, J.; Strid, M. Meconium aspiration syndrome: Incidence and outcomes using discharge data. *Early Hum. Dev.* **2019**, *136*, 21–26. [CrossRef]
30. Rawat, M.; Nangia, S.; Chandrasekharan, P.; Lakshminrusimha, S. Approach to infants born through meconium stained amniotic fluid: Evolution based on evidence? *Am. J. Perinatol.* **2018**, *35*, 815–822. [CrossRef]
31. Perlman, J.M.; Wyllie, J.; Kattwinkel, J.; Atkins, D.L.; Chameides, L.; Goldsmith, J.P.; Guinsburg, R.; Hazinski, M.F.; Morley, C.; Richmond, S.; et al. Part 11: Neonatal resuscitation: 2010 international consensus on cardiopulmonary resuscitation and emergency cardiovascular care science with treatment recommendations. *Circulation* **2010**, *122*, S516–S538. [CrossRef] [PubMed]
32. Wyllie, J.; Perlman, J.M.; Kattwinkel, J.; Atkins, D.L.; Chameides, L.; Goldsmith, J.P.; Guinsburg, R.; Hazinski, M.F.; Morley, C.; Richmond, S.; et al. Part 11: Neonatal resuscitation: 2010 international consensus on cardiopulmonary resuscitation and emergency cardiovascular care science with treatment recommendations. *Resuscitation* **2010**, *81* (Suppl. S1), e260–e287. [CrossRef] [PubMed]
33. Kopincova, J.; Calkovska, A. Meconium-induced inflammation and surfactant inactivation: Specifics of molecular mechanisms. *Pediatr. Res.* **2016**, *79*, 514–521. [CrossRef]
34. Lopez-Rodriguez, E.; Perez-Gil, J. Structure-function relationships in pulmonary surfactant membranes: From biophysics to therapy. *Biochim. Biophys. Acta* **2014**, *1838*, 1568–1585. [CrossRef] [PubMed]
35. Mikolka, P.; Kopincova, J.; Tomcikova Mikusiakova, L.; Kosutova, P.; Antosova, M.; Calkovska, A.; Mokra, D. Effects of surfactant/budesonide therapy on oxidative modifications in the lung in experimental meconium-induced lung injury. *J. Physiol. Pharmacol.* **2016**, *67*, 57–65. [PubMed]
36. El Shahed, A.I.; Dargaville, P.A.; Ohlsson, A.; Soll, R. Surfactant for meconium aspiration syndrome in term and late preterm infants. *Cochrane Database Syst. Rev.* **2014**, *2014*, CD002054. [CrossRef]

37. Polin, R.A.; Carlo, W.A.; Committee on Fetus and Newborn. Surfactant replacement therapy for preterm and term neonates with respiratory distress. *Am. Acad. Pediatr.* **2014**, *133*, 156–163.
38. Vidyasagar, D.; Lukkarinen, H.; Kaapa, P.; Zagariya, A. Inflammatory response and apoptosis in newborn lungs after meconium aspiration. *Biotechnol. Prog.* **2005**, *21*, 192–197. [CrossRef]
39. Hofer, N.; Jank, K.; Strenger, V.; Pansy, J.; Resch, B. Inflammatory indices in meconium aspiration syndrome. *Pediatr. Pulmonol.* **2016**, *51*, 601–606. [CrossRef]
40. Dargaville, P.A.; South, M.; McDougall, P.N. Surfactant and surfactant inhibitors in meconium aspiration syndrome. *J. Pediatr.* **2001**, *138*, 113–115. [CrossRef]
41. Davey, A.M.; Becker, J.D.; Davis, J.M. Meconium aspiration syndrome: Physiological and inflammatory changes in a newborn piglet model. *Pediatr. Pulmonol.* **1993**, *16*, 101–108. [CrossRef] [PubMed]
42. de Beaufort, A.J.; Bakker, A.C.; van Tol, M.J.; Poorthuis, B.J.; Schrama, A.J.; Berger, H.M. Meconium is a source of pro-inflammatory substances and can induce cytokine production in cultured a549 epithelial cells. *Pediatr. Res.* **2003**, *54*, 491–495. [CrossRef] [PubMed]
43. Zagariya, A.; Bhat, R.; Uhal, B.; Navale, S.; Freidine, M.; Vidyasagar, D. Cell death and lung cell histology in meconium aspirated newborn rabbit lung. *Eur. J. Pediatr.* **2000**, *159*, 819–826. [CrossRef] [PubMed]
44. Esposito, E.; Cuzzocrea, S. The role of nitric oxide synthases in lung inflammation. *Curr. Opin. Investig. Drugs* **2007**, *8*, 899–909. [PubMed]
45. Garthwaite, J.; Boulton, C.L. Nitric oxide signaling in the central nervous system. *Annu. Rev. Physiol.* **1995**, *57*, 683–706. [CrossRef] [PubMed]
46. Workman, A.D.; Carey, R.M.; Kohanski, M.A.; Kennedy, D.W.; Palmer, J.N.; Adappa, N.D.; Cohen, N.A. Relative susceptibility of airway organisms to antimicrobial effects of nitric oxide. *Int. Forum Allergy Rhinol.* **2017**, *7*, 770–776. [CrossRef]
47. Lai, M.Y.; Chu, S.M.; Lakshminrusimha, S.; Lin, H.C. Beyond the inhaled nitric oxide in persistent pulmonary hypertension of the newborn. *Pediatr. Neonatol.* **2018**, *59*, 15–23. [CrossRef] [PubMed]
48. Cuesta, E.G.; Diaz, F.J.; Renedo, A.A.; Ruanova, B.F.; de Heredia y Goya, J.L.; Sanchez, L.F.; Valls i Soler, A. Transient response to inhaled nitric oxide in meconium aspiration in newborn lambs. *Pediatr. Res.* **1998**, *43*, 198–202. [CrossRef]
49. Soukka, H.; Viinikka, L.; Kaapa, P. Involvement of thromboxane a2 and prostacyclin in the early pulmonary hypertension after porcine meconium aspiration. *Pediatr. Res.* **1998**, *44*, 838–842. [CrossRef]
50. Holopainen, R.; Aho, H.; Laine, J.; Peuravuori, H.; Soukka, H.; Kaapa, P. Human meconium has high phospholipase a2 activity and induces cellular injury and apoptosis in piglet lungs. *Pediatr. Res.* **1999**, *46*, 626–632. [CrossRef]
51. Mattila, J.T.; Thomas, A.C. Nitric oxide synthase: Non-canonical expression patterns. *Front. Immunol.* **2014**, *5*, 478. [CrossRef] [PubMed]
52. Nangia, S.; Sunder, S.; Biswas, R.; Saili, A. Endotracheal suction in term non vigorous meconium stained neonates—A pilot study. *Resuscitation* **2016**, *105*, 79–84. [CrossRef] [PubMed]
53. Bhat, R.Y.; Rao, A. Meconium-stained amniotic fluid and meconium aspiration syndrome: A prospective study. *Ann. Trop. Paediatr.* **2008**, *28*, 199–203. [CrossRef] [PubMed]
54. Helsinki Declaration of the World Medical Association (WMA). Ethical principles of medical research involving human subjects. *Pol. Merkur Lekarski* **2014**, *36*, 298–301.
55. Backhed, F.; Roswall, J.; Peng, Y.; Feng, Q.; Jia, H.; Kovatcheva-Datchary, P.; Li, Y.; Xia, Y.; Xie, H.; Zhong, H.; et al. Dynamics and stabilization of the human gut microbiome during the first year of life. *Cell Host Microbe* **2015**, *17*, 852. [CrossRef]
56. Dominguez-Bello, M.G.; Costello, E.K.; Contreras, M.; Magris, M.; Hidalgo, G.; Fierer, N.; Knight, R. Delivery mode shapes the acquisition and structure of the initial microbiota across multiple body habitats in newborns. *Proc. Natl. Acad. Sci. USA* **2010**, *107*, 11971–11975. [CrossRef]
57. Jimenez, E.; Marin, M.L.; Martin, R.; Odriozola, J.M.; Olivares, M.; Xaus, J.; Fernandez, L.; Rodriguez, J.M. Is meconium from healthy newborns actually sterile? *Res. Microbiol.* **2008**, *159*, 187–193. [CrossRef]
58. Nagpal, R.; Tsuji, H.; Takahashi, T.; Kawashima, K.; Nagata, S.; Nomoto, K.; Yamashiro, Y. Sensitive quantitative analysis of the meconium bacterial microbiota in healthy term infants born vaginally or by cesarean section. *Front. Microbiol.* **2016**, *7*, 1997. [CrossRef]
59. Stinson, L.F.; Keelan, J.A.; Payne, M.S. Characterization of the bacterial microbiome in first-pass meconium using propidium monoazide (pma) to exclude nonviable bacterial DNA. *Lett. Appl. Microbiol.* **2019**, *68*, 378–385. [CrossRef]
60. Zagariya, A.; Bhat, R.; Chari, G.; Uhal, B.; Navale, S.; Vidyasagar, D. Apoptosis of airway epithelial cells in response to meconium. *Life Sci.* **2005**, *76*, 1849–1858. [CrossRef]
61. WMA Declaration of Taipei on Ethical Considerations Regarding Health Databases and Biobanks. 2016. Available online: https://www.Wma.Net/policies-post/wma-declaration-of-taipei-on-ethical-considerations-regarding-health-databases-and-biobanks/ (accessed on 7 September 2021).
62. Galas, R.J., Jr.; Liu, J.C. Surface density of vascular endothelial growth factor modulates endothelial proliferation and differentiation. *J. Cell Biochem.* **2014**, *115*, 111–120. [CrossRef]
63. Patil, R.H.; Naveen Kumar, M.; Kiran Kumar, K.M.; Nagesh, R.; Kavya, K.; Babu, R.L.; Ramesh, G.T.; Chidananda Sharma, S. Dexamethasone inhibits inflammatory response via down regulation of ap-1 transcription factor in human lung epithelial cells. *Gene* **2018**, *645*, 85–94. [CrossRef] [PubMed]

64. Garber, M.; Grabherr, M.G.; Guttman, M.; Trapnell, C. Computational methods for transcriptome annotation and quantification using rna-seq. *Nat. Methods* **2011**, *8*, 469–477. [CrossRef] [PubMed]
65. Watkins, D.N.; Garlepp, M.J.; Thompson, P.J. Regulation of the inducible cyclo-oxygenase pathway in human cultured airway epithelial (a549) cells by nitric oxide. *Br. J. Pharmacol.* **1997**, *121*, 1482–1488. [CrossRef]
66. Edwards, E.M.; Lakshminrusimha, S.; Ehret, D.E.Y.; Horbar, J.D. Nicu admissions for meconium aspiration syndrome before and after a national resuscitation program suctioning guideline change. *Children* **2019**, *6*, 68. [CrossRef] [PubMed]
67. Fanaroff, A.A. Meconium aspiration syndrome: Historical aspects. *J. Perinatol.* **2008**, *28* (Suppl. S3), S3–S7. [CrossRef]
68. Hui, R.; Jing-Jing, P.; Yun-Su, Z.; Xiao-Yu, Z.; Xiao-Qing, C.; Yang, Y. Surfactant lavage for neonatal meconium aspiration syndrome—An updated meta-analysis. *J. Chin. Med. Assoc.* **2020**, *83*, 761–773. [CrossRef]
69. Sun, J.; Qu, S.; Zhang, C.; Xiang, Z.; Fu, Z.; Yao, L. Neonatal mortality rate and risk factors in northeast china: Analysis of 5277 neonates in 2005. *Clin. Exp. Obstet. Gynecol.* **2014**, *41*, 512–516.
70. Whitfield, J.M.; Charsha, D.S.; Chiruvolu, A. Prevention of meconium aspiration syndrome: An update and the baylor experience. *Bayl. Univ. Med. Cent. Proc.* **2009**, *22*, 128–131. [CrossRef]
71. Burke-Strickland, M.; Edwards, N.B. Meconium aspiration in the newborn. *Minn. Med.* **1973**, *56*, 1031–1035.
72. Liu, W.F.; Harrington, T. Delivery room risk factors for meconium aspiration syndrome. *Am. J. Perinatol.* **2002**, *19*, 367–378. [CrossRef] [PubMed]
73. Swarnam, K.; Soraisham, A.S.; Sivanandan, S. Advances in the management of meconium aspiration syndrome. *Int. J. Pediatr.* **2012**, *2012*, 359571. [CrossRef]
74. Gauchan, E.; Basnet, S.; Malla, T. Meconium aspiration syndrome and neonatal outcome: A prospective study. *Am. J. Public Health Res.* **2015**, *3*, 48–52.
75. Louis, D.; Sundaram, V.; Mukhopadhyay, K.; Dutta, S.; Kumar, P. Predictors of mortality in neonates with meconium aspiration syndrome. *Indian Pediatr.* **2014**, *51*, 637–640. [CrossRef] [PubMed]
76. Matalon, R.; Wainstock, T.; Walfisch, A.; Sheiner, E. Exposure to meconium-stained amniotic fluid and long-term neurological-related hospitalizations throughout childhood. *Am. J. Perinatol.* **2020**. online ahead of print. [CrossRef]
77. Lu, Y.C.; Wang, C.C.; Lee, C.M.; Hwang, K.S.; Hua, Y.M.; Yuh, Y.S.; Chiu, Y.L.; Hsu, W.F.; Chou, Y.L.; Huang, S.W.; et al. Reevaluating reference ranges of oxygen saturation for healthy full-term neonates using pulse oximetry. *Pediatr. Neonatol.* **2014**, *55*, 459–465. [CrossRef]
78. Khazardoost, S.; Hantoushzadeh, S.; Khooshideh, M.; Borna, S. Risk factors for meconium aspiration in meconium stained amniotic fluid. *J. Obstet. Gynaecol.* **2007**, *27*, 577–579. [CrossRef] [PubMed]
79. Kitsommart, R.; Thammawong, N.; Sommai, K.; Yangnoy, J.; Bowornkitiwong, W.; Paes, B. Impact of meconium consistency on infant resuscitation and respiratory outcomes: A retrospective-cohort study and systematic review. *J. Matern. Fetal Neonatal Med.* **2020**, *34*, 4141–4147. [CrossRef]
80. Lama, S.; Mahato, S.K.; Chaudhary, N.; Agrawal, N.; Pathak, S.; Kurmi, O.P.; Bhatia, B.; Agarwal, K.N. Clinico-radiological observations in meconium aspiration syndrome. *JNMA J. Nepal Med. Assoc.* **2018**, *56*, 510–515. [CrossRef] [PubMed]
81. Hernandez, C.; Little, B.B.; Dax, J.S.; Gilstrap, L.C., 3rd; Rosenfeld, C.R. Prediction of the severity of meconium aspiration syndrome. *Am. J. Obstet. Gynecol.* **1993**, *169*, 61–70. [CrossRef]
82. Hovi, M.; Raatikainen, K.; Heiskanen, N.; Heinonen, S. Obstetric outcome in post-term pregnancies: Time for reappraisal in clinical management. *Acta Obstet. Gynecol. Scand.* **2006**, *85*, 805–809. [CrossRef]
83. Maayan-Metzger, A.; Leibovitch, L.; Schushan-Eisen, I.; Strauss, T.; Kuint, J. Meconium-stained amniotic fluid and hypoglycemia among term newborn infants. *Fetal Pediatr. Pathol.* **2012**, *31*, 283–287. [CrossRef]
84. Pariente, G.; Peles, C.; Perri, Z.H.; Baumfeld, Y.; Mastrolia, S.A.; Koifman, A.; Weintraub, A.Y.; Hershkovitz, R. Meconium-stained amniotic fluid—Risk factors and immediate perinatal outcomes among sga infants. *J. Matern. Fetal Neonatal Med.* **2015**, *28*, 1064–1067. [CrossRef]
85. Xu, H.; Mas-Calvet, M.; Wei, S.Q.; Luo, Z.C.; Fraser, W.D. Abnormal fetal heart rate tracing patterns in patients with thick meconium staining of the amniotic fluid: Association with perinatal outcomes. *Am. J. Obstet. Gynecol.* **2009**, *200*, 283.e1–283.e7. [CrossRef]
86. Mazor, M.; Hershkovitz, R.; Bashiri, A.; Maymon, E.; Schreiber, R.; Dukler, D.; Katz, M.; Shoham-Vardi, I. Meconium stained amniotic fluid in preterm delivery is an independent risk factor for perinatal complications. *Eur. J. Obstet. Gynecol. Reprod. Biol.* **1998**, *81*, 9–13. [CrossRef]
87. Wiswell, T.E.; Bent, R.C. Meconium staining and the meconium aspiration syndrome. Unresolved issues. *Pediatr. Clin. N. Am.* **1993**, *40*, 955–981. [CrossRef]
88. Katz, L.A.; Klein, J.M. Repeat surfactant therapy for postsurfactant slump. *J. Perinatol.* **2006**, *26*, 414–422. [CrossRef] [PubMed]
89. Jeng, M.J.; Soong, W.J.; Lee, Y.S.; Tsao, P.C.; Yang, C.F.; Chiu, S.Y.; Tang, R.B. Meconium exposure dependent cell death and apoptosis in human alveolar epithelial cells. *Pediatr. Pulmonol.* **2010**, *45*, 816–823. [CrossRef]
90. Foster, K.A.; Oster, C.G.; Mayer, M.M.; Avery, M.L.; Audus, K.L. Characterization of the a549 cell line as a type ii pulmonary epithelial cell model for drug metabolism. *Exp. Cell Res.* **1998**, *243*, 359–366. [CrossRef]
91. Korhonen, K.; Soukka, H.; Halkola, L.; Peuravuori, H.; Aho, H.; Pulkki, K.; Kero, P.; Kaapa, P.O. Meconium induces only localized inflammatory lung injury in piglets. *Pediatr. Res.* **2003**, *54*, 192–197. [CrossRef]

92. Porta, N.F.; Steinhorn, R.H. Pulmonary vasodilator therapy in the nicu: Inhaled nitric oxide, sildenafil, and other pulmonary vasodilating agents. *Clin. Perinatol.* **2012**, *39*, 149–164. [CrossRef]
93. Nathan, C.; Xie, Q.W. Nitric oxide synthases: Roles, tolls, and controls. *Cell* **1994**, *78*, 915–918. [CrossRef]
94. Pfeilschifter, J.; Eberhardt, W.; Beck, K.F. Regulation of gene expression by nitric oxide. *Pflug. Arch.* **2001**, *442*, 479–486. [CrossRef] [PubMed]
95. Fontanilla, R.; Zagariya, A.; Vidyasagar, D. Meconium-induced release of nitric oxide in rabbit alveolar cells. *J. Perinatol.* **2008**, *28* (Suppl. S3), S123–S126. [CrossRef] [PubMed]
96. Khan, A.M.; Lally, K.P.; Elidemir, O.; Colasurdo, G.N. Meconium enhances the release of nitric oxide in human airway epithelial cells. *Biol. Neonate* **2002**, *81*, 99–104. [CrossRef] [PubMed]
97. Kytola, J.; Uotila, P.; Kaapa, P. Meconium stimulates cyclooxygenase-2 expression in rat lungs. *Prostaglandins Leukot. Essent. Fat. Acids* **1999**, *60*, 107–110. [CrossRef] [PubMed]
98. Li, Y.H.; Yan, Z.Q.; Brauner, A.; Tullus, K. Meconium induces expression of inducible no synthase and activation of nf-kappab in rat alveolar macrophages. *Pediatr. Res.* **2001**, *49*, 820–825. [CrossRef]
99. Sharma, J.N.; Al-Omran, A.; Parvathy, S.S. Role of nitric oxide in inflammatory diseases. *Inflammopharmacology* **2007**, *15*, 252–259. [CrossRef] [PubMed]
100. Adhikari, N.K.; Burns, K.E.; Friedrich, J.O.; Granton, J.T.; Cook, D.J.; Meade, M.O. Effect of nitric oxide on oxygenation and mortality in acute lung injury: Systematic review and meta-analysis. *BMJ* **2007**, *334*, 779. [CrossRef]
101. Crosswhite, P.; Sun, Z. Nitric oxide, oxidative stress and inflammation in pulmonary arterial hypertension. *J. Hypertens.* **2010**, *28*, 201–212. [CrossRef]
102. Funk, C.D. Prostaglandins and leukotrienes: Advances in eicosanoid biology. *Science* **2001**, *294*, 1871–1875. [CrossRef] [PubMed]
103. Bacchi, S.; Palumbo, P.; Sponta, A.; Coppolino, M.F. Clinical pharmacology of non-steroidal anti-inflammatory drugs: A review. *Antiinflamm. Antiallergy Agents Med. Chem.* **2012**, *11*, 52–64. [CrossRef] [PubMed]
104. Sorokin, A. Nitric oxide synthase and cyclooxygenase pathways: A complex interplay in cellular signaling. *Curr. Med. Chem.* **2016**, *23*, 2559–2578. [CrossRef]
105. Cuzzocrea, S.; Salvemini, D. Molecular mechanisms involved in the reciprocal regulation of cyclooxygenase and nitric oxide synthase enzymes. *Kidney Int.* **2007**, *71*, 290–297. [CrossRef] [PubMed]
106. Uotila, P.J.; Kaapa, P.O. Cyclooxygenase-2 expression in human monocytes stimulated by meconium. *Lancet* **1998**, *351*, 878. [CrossRef]
107. Fan, H.C.; Wang, S.Y.; Peng, Y.J.; Lee, H.S. Valproic acid impacts the growth of growth plate chondrocytes. *Int. J. Environ. Res. Public Health* **2020**, *17*, 3675. [CrossRef]
108. Robbins, R.A.; Springall, D.R.; Warren, J.B.; Kwon, O.J.; Buttery, L.D.; Wilson, A.J.; Adcock, I.M.; Riveros-Moreno, V.; Moncada, S.; Polak, J.; et al. Inducible nitric oxide synthase is increased in murine lung epithelial cells by cytokine stimulation. *Biochem. Biophys. Res. Commun.* **1994**, *198*, 835–843. [CrossRef] [PubMed]
109. Belvisi, M.; Barnes, P.J.; Larkin, S.; Yacoub, M.; Tadjkarimi, S.; Williams, T.J.; Mitchell, J.A. Nitric oxide synthase activity is elevated in inflammatory lung disease in humans. *Eur. J. Pharmacol.* **1995**, *283*, 255–258. [CrossRef]
110. Barnes, P.J. How corticosteroids control inflammation: Quintiles prize lecture 2005. *Br. J. Pharmacol.* **2006**, *148*, 245–254. [CrossRef]
111. Ward, M.; Sinn, J. Steroid therapy for meconium aspiration syndrome in newborn infants. *Cochrane Database Syst. Rev.* **2003**, *2003*, CD003485. [CrossRef]
112. Yeung, T.; Jasani, B.; Shah, P.S. Steroids for the management of neonates with meconium aspiration syndrome: A systematic review and meta-analysis. *Indian Pediatr.* **2021**, *58*, 370–376. [CrossRef] [PubMed]
113. Basu, S.; Kumar, A.; Bhatia, B.D.; Satya, K.; Singh, T.B. Role of steroids on the clinical course and outcome of meconium aspiration syndrome—A randomized controlled trial. *J. Trop. Pediatr.* **2007**, *53*, 331–337. [CrossRef]
114. Tripathi, S.; Saili, A. The effect of steroids on the clinical course and outcome of neonates with meconium aspiration syndrome. *J. Trop. Pediatr.* **2007**, *53*, 8–12. [CrossRef]
115. Tripathi, S.; Saili, A.; Dutta, R. Inflammatory markers in meconium induced lung injury in neonates and effect of steroids on their levels: A randomized controlled trial. *Indian J. Med. Microbiol.* **2007**, *25*, 103–107. [CrossRef]
116. Mikolka, P.; Mokra, D.; Kopincova, J.; Tomcikova-Mikusiakova, L.; Calkovska, A. Budesonide added to modified porcine surfactant curosurf may additionally improve the lung functions in meconium aspiration syndrome. *Physiol. Res.* **2013**, *62*, S191–S200. [CrossRef] [PubMed]
117. Mokra, D.; Mokry, J.; Drgova, A.; Petraskova, M.; Bulikova, J.; Calkovska, A. Intratracheally administered corticosteroids improve lung function in meconium-instilled rabbits. *J. Physiol. Pharmacol.* **2007**, *58* (Suppl. S5), 389–398.
118. Hong, H.; Jang, B.C. Prednisone inhibits the il-1beta-induced expression of cox-2 in hei-oc1 murine auditory cells through the inhibition of erk-1/2, jnk-1 and ap-1 activity. *Int. J. Mol. Med.* **2014**, *34*, 1640–1646. [CrossRef]
119. Linehan, J.D.; Kolios, G.; Valatas, V.; Robertson, D.A.; Westwick, J. Effect of corticosteroids on nitric oxide production in inflammatory bowel disease: Are leukocytes the site of action? *Am. J. Physiol. Gastrointest. Liver Physiol.* **2005**, *288*, G261–G267. [CrossRef]
120. Levine, A.B.; Punihaole, D.; Levine, T.B. Characterization of the role of nitric oxide and its clinical applications. *Cardiology* **2012**, *122*, 55–68. [CrossRef]

121. Bryan, N.S.; Grisham, M.B. Methods to detect nitric oxide and its metabolites in biological samples. *Free Radic. Biol. Med.* **2007**, *43*, 645–657. [CrossRef]
122. Bryan, N.S. Nitrite in nitric oxide biology: Cause or consequence? A systems-based review. *Free Radic. Biol. Med.* **2006**, *41*, 691–701. [CrossRef] [PubMed]
123. Pechkovsky, D.V.; Zissel, G.; Goldmann, T.; Einhaus, M.; Taube, C.; Magnussen, H.; Schlaak, M.; Muller-Quernheim, J. Pattern of nos2 and nos3 mrna expression in human a549 cells and primary cultured aec ii. *Am. J. Physiol. Lung Cell. Mol. Physiol.* **2002**, *282*, L684–L692. [CrossRef] [PubMed]

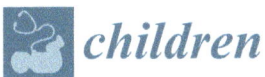

Article

Randomized Trial of Oxygen Saturation Targets during and after Resuscitation and Reversal of Ductal Flow in an Ovine Model of Meconium Aspiration and Pulmonary Hypertension

Amy L. Lesneski [1], Payam Vali [2], Morgan E. Hardie [2], Satyan Lakshminrusimha [2,*], and Deepika Sankaran [2]

1 Department of Stem Cell Research, University of California, Davis, Sacramento, CA 95817, USA; allesneski@ucdavis.edu
2 Department of Pediatrics, University of California, Davis, Sacramento, CA 95817, USA; pvali@ucdavis.edu (P.V.); mehardie@ucdavis.edu (M.E.H.); dsankaran@ucdavis.edu (D.S.)
* Correspondence: slakshmi@ucdavis.edu

Citation: Lesneski, A.L.; Vali, P.; Hardie, M.E.; Lakshminrusimha, S.; Sankaran, D. Randomized Trial of Oxygen Saturation Targets during and after Resuscitation and Reversal of Ductal Flow in an Ovine Model of Meconium Aspiration and Pulmonary Hypertension. *Children* **2021**, *8*, 594. https://doi.org/10.3390/children8070594

Academic Editor: Bernhard Schwaberger

Received: 9 June 2021
Accepted: 12 July 2021
Published: 14 July 2021

Publisher's Note: MDPI stays neutral with regard to jurisdictional claims in published maps and institutional affiliations.

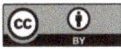

Copyright: © 2021 by the authors. Licensee MDPI, Basel, Switzerland. This article is an open access article distributed under the terms and conditions of the Creative Commons Attribution (CC BY) license (https://creativecommons.org/licenses/by/4.0/).

Abstract: Neonatal resuscitation (NRP) guidelines suggest targeting 85–95% preductal SpO_2 by 10 min after birth. Optimal oxygen saturation (SpO_2) targets during resuscitation and in the post-resuscitation management of neonatal meconium aspiration syndrome (MAS) with persistent pulmonary hypertension (PPHN) remains uncertain. Our objective was to compare the time to reversal of ductal flow from fetal pattern (right-to-left), to left-to-right, and to evaluate pulmonary (Q_{PA}), carotid (Q_{CA}) and ductal (Q_{DA}) blood flows between standard (85–94%) and high (95–99%) SpO_2 targets during and after resuscitation. Twelve lambs asphyxiated by endotracheal meconium instillation and cord occlusion to induce MAS and PPHN were resuscitated per NRP guidelines and were randomized to either standard (85–94%) or high (95–99%) SpO_2 targets. Out of twelve lambs with MAS and PPHN, six each were randomized to standard and high SpO_2 targets. Median [interquartile range] time to change in direction of blood flow across the ductus arteriosus from right-to-left, to left-to-right was significantly shorter with high SpO_2 target (7.4 (4.4–10.8) min) compared to standard SpO_2 target (31.5 (21–66.2) min, $p = 0.03$). Q_{PA} was significantly higher during the first 10 min after birth with higher SpO_2 target. At 60 min after birth, the Q_{PA}, Q_{CA} and Q_{DA} were not different between the groups. To conclude, targeting SpO_2 of 95–99% during and after resuscitation may hasten reversal of ductal flow in lambs with MAS and PPHN and transiently increase Q_{PA} but no differences were observed at 60 min. Clinical studies comparing low and high SpO_2 targets assessing hemodynamics and neurodevelopmental outcomes are warranted.

Keywords: meconium aspiration; oxygen saturation targets; neonatal resuscitation; persistent pulmonary hypertension of the newborn; asphyxia; ductus arteriosus; pulmonary blood flow; post-resuscitation

1. Introduction

Successful transition of the fetus to extrauterine life involves a rapid increase in pulmonary blood flow (Q_{PA}) during the first few breaths after birth, allowing the lungs to establish as the site of gas exchange. A failure of this transition can lead to persistent pulmonary hypertension of the newborn (PPHN), characterized by sustained elevation of pulmonary vascular resistance (PVR), right-to-left shunting of blood across the foramen ovale and ductus arteriosus, and reduced Q_{PA} [1]. These newborns experience severe respiratory distress and labile hypoxemia soon after birth.

Oxygen (O_2) mediates decrease in PVR after birth and has been used to correct the hypoxemia in PPHN, along with strategies to improve lung inflation with respiratory support [2,3]. Current neonatal resuscitation guidelines recommend initiating ventilation with 21% O_2 with subsequent O_2 titration to target goal preductal pulse oximetry O_2 saturation (SpO_2) ranges corresponding to the minute of life, to achieve 85–95% SpO_2 by

10 min after birth. This strategy has been associated with optimal hemodynamics and gas exchange during resuscitation [4]. Rawat et al. reported that targeting 95–99% SpO_2 in the post-resuscitation period lowered PVR and improved cerebral O_2 delivery, while targeting 85–89% SpO_2 increased PVR, and decreased Q_{PA} and cerebral O_2 delivery in a term ovine model of meconium aspiration syndrome (MAS) with PPHN [5]. However, flow across the ductus arteriosus (Q_{DA}) was not evaluated in this study and ductal flow is a major contributor to Q_{PA} [6]. The optimal preductal SpO_2 target range during resuscitation and post-resuscitation period that hastens reversal of shunting across the patent ductus arteriosus (PDA) from the fetal pattern to the postnatal pattern of left-to-right remains unknown.

We hypothesized that the time to reversal of shunting across the PDA is shorter with high SpO_2 target of 95–99% compared to standard SpO_2 target of 85–94%. Our objective was to compare the time to reversal of shunt across the PDA from the fetal (right-to-left) to the postnatal (left-to-right) pattern between standard (85–94%) and high (95–99%) SpO_2 target ranges during resuscitation and the post-resuscitation period in a term ovine asphyxiated model of MAS and PPHN. We also evaluated the changes in Q_{PA}, Q_{DA} and carotid blood flow (Q_{CA}), and gas exchange at 10 min and 60 min after birth between low and high SpO_2 targets as secondary outcomes.

2. Materials and Methods

The protocol was approved by the Institutional Animal Care and Use Committee (IACUC, protocol #20267) at the University of California Davis, CA, USA. This protocol involves a perinatal model of MAS and PPHN in term newborn lambs that has been extensively described previously [5,7]. All experiments were performed in accordance with animal ethical guidelines (ARRIVE) [8]. Time-dated near-term (139–141 days) gestation pregnant ewes from Van Laningham Farm (Arbuckle, CA, USA) underwent cesarean section following overnight fasting, after endotracheal intubation under general anesthesia with IV diazepam and ketamine, and inhaled 2% isoflurane, as previously described [9].

2.1. Fetal Instrumentation

The fetal lamb was partially exteriorized and intubated with a 4.5-mm cuffed endotracheal tube (ETT), the lung fluid was passively drained by gravity, and the ETT was occluded to prevent entry of air. The lamb was instrumented under maternal anesthesia after subcutaneous bupivacaine infiltration. Catheters were inserted into the right carotid artery and right jugular vein for preductal arterial blood draws, invasive blood pressure and heart rate monitoring, and IV access respectively. A flow probe (Transonics, Ithaca, NY, USA) was placed around the left carotid artery to measure blood flow. A left thoracotomy was performed, and flow probes were placed around the left pulmonary artery and ductus arteriosus to measure blood flows. Subsequently, the thoracotomy and neck incisions were closed in layers. The baseline hemodynamics were recorded and arterial blood gases were obtained.

2.2. Meconium Instillation, Asphyxia and Resuscitation

Fetal lambs were asphyxiated following instrumentation by umbilical cord occlusion (by manual compression) for 5 min or until heart rate decreased below 40 beats per minute. Meconium (5 mL/kg of 20% meconium suspended in ewe amniotic fluid) was simultaneously instilled into their endotracheal tube as previously described [7,10]. During asphyxiation, the lambs gasped and spontaneously aspirated the meconium into their lungs. The cord compression was released for 2 min to allow hemodynamic recovery, followed by another 5-min cord occlusion.

Lambs were randomized to standard SpO_2 target (85–94%) or high SpO_2 target (95–99%) using opaque envelopes prior to the beginning of the study (incision for cesarean section). The lambs were then delivered and ventilated with peak inflation pressures (PIP) of 30–35 cm H_2O, PEEP of 5 cm H_2O, rate of 40 breaths per minute and inspired O_2 of 21%

that was then titrated based on preductal SpO$_2$ per Neonatal Resuscitation Program (NRP) guidelines during resuscitation to achieve a goal of 85–94% (standard target arm) [11] or titrated to achieve a goal of 95–99% SpO$_2$ after delivery (high target arm). The titration of oxygen was proportional to the difference between observed SpO$_2$ and target SpO$_2$ and was performed every minute. The endotracheal tube was connected to a ventilator and PaCO$_2$ was targeted in the 40–60 mm Hg range to allow permissive hypercapnia. The resuscitators were not blinded to the intervention. Hemodynamics were continuously monitored, and arterial blood gases were obtained at baseline, 10-min and subsequently at 15-min intervals. Lambs were monitored for up to 60 min and were finally euthanized using IV pentobarbital (Fatal-Plus, Vortech Pharmaceuticals, Dearborn, MI, USA).

2.3. Primary and Secondary Outcomes

Primary outcome measures were time to reversal of ductal shunt (from right-to-left to left-to-right) from the time of delivery.

Secondary outcome measures were changes in Q_{PA}, Q_{DA} and Q_{CA}, and gas exchange at 10 min and 60 min after birth between standard and high SpO$_2$ targets. Cerebral oxygen delivery (mL/kg/min) was calculated by multiplying carotid artery oxygen content (CaO$_2$ = (1.34 × Hemoglobin in g/dL × SaO$_2$%/100%) + (partial pressure of O$_2$ in mm Hg × 0.0031)) and left carotid artery blood flow (mL/kg/min).

2.4. Data Collection and Analysis

Hemodynamic variables were continuously monitored and recorded using BIOPAC systems data acquisition software (Goleta, CA, USA). Blood gases were analyzed using a blood gas analyzer (Radiometer ABL90 FLEX, Denmark). By convention, the right-to-left direction of Q_{DA} was labeled as negative and left-to-right direction of Q_{DA} was labeled as positive. Categorical data were analyzed using chi-squared test with Fisher's exact test as appropriate, parametric continuous data were analyzed using unpaired *t*-test, and changes in Q_{DA} and Q_{PA} over time were compared using repeated measures ANOVA. The median time to reversal of shunting (non-parametric) was compared between standard and high SpO$_2$ targets using Wilcoxon rank sum test. Statistical significance was defined as $p < 0.05$.

3. Results

Out of twelve near-term lambs that were asphyxiated, six were randomized to standard SpO$_2$ target and the remaining six were randomized to high SpO$_2$ target. Hemodynamic and arterial blood gas characteristics at fetal baseline prior to asphyxia were similar between the study groups (Table 1).

3.1. Time to Reversal of Shunt across the PDA

Median (interquartile range) time to transition from right-to-left to exclusive left-to-right shunting across the ductus arteriosus was significantly shorter with high SpO$_2$ target (7.4 (4.4–10.8) min) compared to standard SpO$_2$ target (31.5 (12–66.2) min, $p = 0.03$, Figure 1). The mean Q_{DA} (left-to-right) flow was increased with the high SpO$_2$ targets from 0.5 to 10 min by ANOVA repeated measures. The Q_{DA} significantly increased from fetal baseline to 5-min after birth in both standard and high SpO$_2$ targets ($p < 0.05$) and decreased significantly by 60 min in high SpO$_2$ target ($p < 0.05$).

Table 1. Comparison of fetal baseline hemodynamic and arterial blood gas parameters and end-asphyxia hemodynamic parameters in a near-term ovine model of meconium aspiration syndrome (MAS) and persistent pulmonary hypertension (PPHN) randomized to standard (85–94%) and high (95–99%) preductal SpO_2 target groups.

Parameter	Standard SpO_2 Target (85–94%, n = 6)	High SpO_2 Target (95–99%, n = 6)
Weight (kg)	3.4 ± 0.8	3.3 ± 0.4
Gestational Age (days)	139.7 ± 0.7	139.3 ± 0.8
Parameters at Fetal Baseline		
Hemoglobin, g/dL	13.88 ± 2.47	11.93 ± 1.52
pH	7.18 ± 0.08	7.19 ± 0.06
$PaCO_2$ (mm Hg)	74.73 ± 12.58	64.95 ± 5.17
PaO_2 (mm Hg)	22.08 ± 6.22	28.38 ± 4.51
Cerebral Oxygen Delivery (mL/kg/min)	4.26 ± 2.17	2.40 ± 0.64
Lactate (mmol/L)	2.20 ± 0.53	2.37 ± 0.96
Heart Rate (bpm)	155.17 ± 21.95	164.23 ± 21.50
Mean Arterial Blood Pressure (mm Hg)	55.52 ± 4.42	61.11 ± 3.8
Mean Ductal Blood Flow (mL/kg/min)	−125.89 ± 64.77	−84.33 ± 36.09
Mean Pulmonary Artery Blood Flow (mL/kg/min)	25.21 ± 8.25	49.39 ± 23.59
Duration of Asphyxia (min)	13.43 ± 0.63	15.32 ± 1.82
Parameters at End of Asphyxia		
Mean Carotid Artery Blood Flow (mL/kg/min)	24.0 (5.5)	21.2 (4.4)
Mean Ductal Blood Flow (mL/kg/min)	−18.3 (6.9)	−15 (7.7)
Mean Pulmonary Artery Blood Flow (mL/kg/min)	18.3 (2.7)	29.4 (13.2)

Data presented as mean ± standard deviation. Data were not different by unpaired t test. $PaCO_2$ = arterial carbon dioxide pressure; PaO_2 = arterial oxygen pressure; SpO_2 = oxygen saturation.

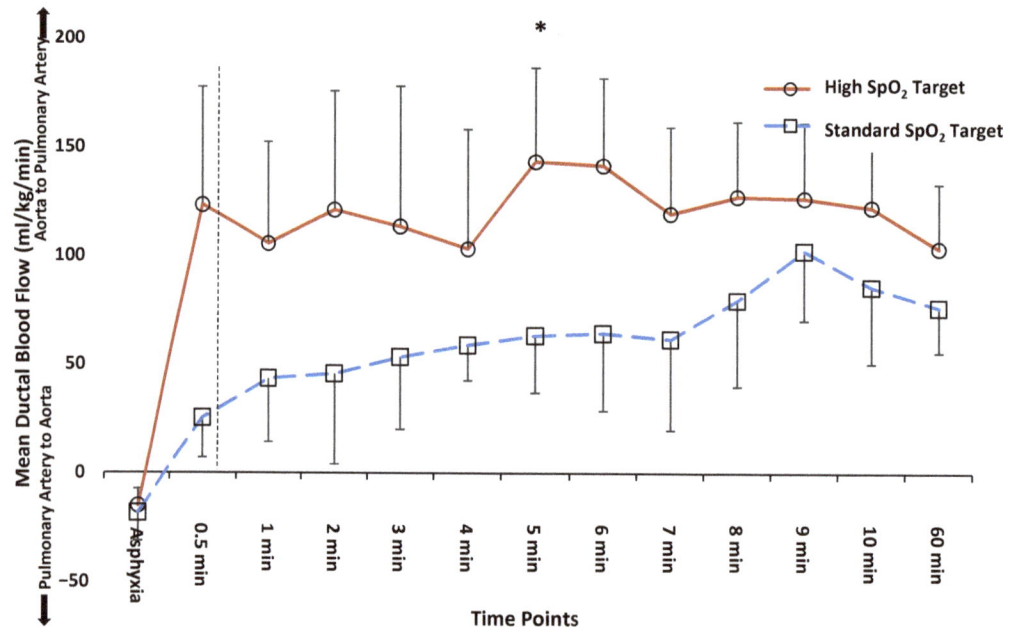

Figure 1. Mean ductus arteriosus blood flow (Q_{DA}) and direction of flow over timepoints from asphyxia, 0.5 min and up to 60 min after delivery between the two oxygen target groups. Delivery of lamb is indicated by the dashed, vertical line. Positive flow indicates left-to-right shunting from aorta to the pulmonary artery. Negative flow indicates right-to-left shunting

from pulmonary artery to the aorta. Median (interquartile range) time for exclusive left-to-right ductal shunting post-delivery was significantly shorter in the high SpO$_2$ target group (median 7.4 vs. 31.5 min, by Wilcoxon rank sum test). * $p < 0.05$, left-to-right ductal flow was significantly higher with high SpO$_2$ target compared to standard SpO$_2$ target ($p = 0.002$, ANOVA repeated measures). However, by 60 min after delivery, the Q$_{DA}$ was not different between the two SpO$_2$ targets. The QDA significantly increased in both high and standard SpO$_2$ targets from fetal baseline to 5-min after birth, and significantly decreased by 60 min after birth in the high SpO$_2$ target.

3.2. Comparison of Hemodynamics and Arterial Blood Gas Parameters at 5 and 10 min after Birth

During the first 10 min after delivery, the Q$_{DA}$ (left-to-right, Figure 1, $p = 0.002$) and Q$_{PA}$ (Figure 2, $p = 0.048$) were significantly higher with high SpO$_2$ target compared to standard SpO$_2$ target by ANOVA repeated measures. The Q$_{PA}$ significantly decreased from 5-min to 60-min after birth with high SpO$_2$ target. The hemodynamic parameters at 5 min and at 10 min time points after delivery are depicted in Tables 2 and 3 respectively and were not different. The arterial blood gas parameters were not different at 10-min after delivery (Table 3). Although the PaO$_2$ and SpO$_2$ were higher in the high SpO$_2$ target group, these differences did not reach statistical significance.

Table 2. Comparison of hemodynamics at 5 min after birth in a perinatal lamb model of MAS and PPHN.

Parameter	Standard SpO$_2$ Target (85–94%, n = 6)	High SpO$_2$ Target (95–99%, n = 6)
Heart Rate (bpm)	182.12 ± 12.14	170.78 ± 13.08
Mean Arterial Blood Pressure (mm Hg)	52.91 ± 18.79	65.38 ± 8.81
Mean Carotid Flow (Q$_{CA}$, mL/kg/min)	34.10 ± 14.84	20.22 ± 8.47

Data presented as mean and standard deviation. Positive flow indicates left-to-right ductus arteriosus blood flow. There was no significant difference between the two SpO$_2$ targets at 5-min timepoint by unpaired t-test.

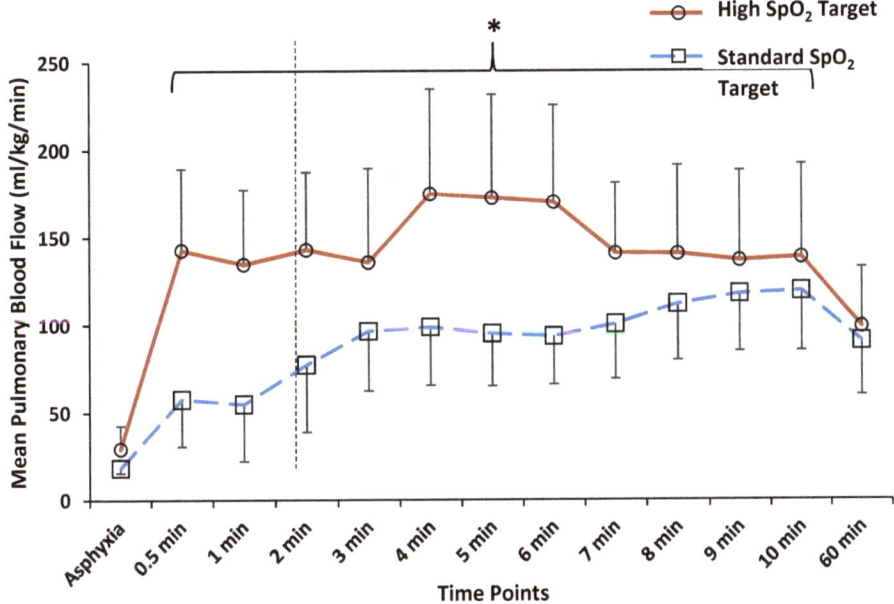

Figure 2. Mean pulmonary blood flow (Q$_{PA}$) during the immediate post-natal period in a lamb model of meconium aspiration syndrome (MAS) and persistent pulmonary hypertension (PPHN). Delivery of lamb is indicated by the dashed, vertical line. The Q$_{PA}$ was significantly higher from 0.5 min to 10 min after delivery with high SpO$_2$ target compared to standard SpO$_2$ target ($p = 0.048$). However, by 60 min after delivery, the Q$_{PA}$ was not different between the two SpO$_2$ targets. * $p < 0.05$.

Table 3. Comparison of hemodynamics and oxygenation at 10 min after birth in a perinatal lamb model of MAS and PPHN.

Parameter	Standard SpO$_2$ Target (85–94%, n = 6)	High SpO$_2$ Target (95–99%, n = 6)
Hemoglobin, g/dL	13.18 ± 1.95	11.9 ± 1.40
pH	7.05 ± 0.24	7.11 ± 0.19
PaCO$_2$ (mm Hg)	79.48 ± 48.89	64.5 ± 42.89
PaO$_2$ (mm Hg)	53.42 ± 22.97	60.13 ± 2.55
SaO$_2$ (%)	89.7 ± 4.32	93.9 ± 3.96
SpO$_2$ (%)	77.75 ± 30.61	91.33 ± 6.51
CaO$_2$ (mL O$_2$/dL)	15.98 ± 2.14	15.14 ± 1.62
Cerebral Oxygen Delivery (mL/kg/min)	4.78 ± 2.23	3.69 ± 0.47
Lactate (mmol/L)	6.02 ± 1.97	5.90 ± 1.75
Heart Rate (bpm)	176.0 ± 13.22	162.55 ± 31.18
Mean Arterial Blood Pressure (mmHg)	59.34 ± 9.497	65.67 ± 8.98
Mean Carotid Flow (Q$_{CA}$, mL/kg/min)	29.17 ± 12.31	20.44 ± 7.32
Inspired O$_2$ (%) at 10 min	40.75 ± 39.5	30.67 ± 16.74

Data presented as mean and standard deviation. No significant differences in parameters between the standard and high SpO$_2$ target groups at 10-min time point by unpaired t-test.

3.3. Comparison of Hemodynamics and Arterial Blood Gas Parameters at 60 min after Birth

There was no significant difference in mean Q$_{CA}$, Q$_{DA}$, or Q$_{PA}$ blood flows at 60 min after birth (Table 4). One lamb randomized in the standard SpO$_2$ group maintained a bidirectional Q$_{DA}$ shunt throughout the study period. There were no significant differences in inspired O$_2$ concentration, arterial O$_2$ content, cerebral O$_2$ delivery or PaO$_2$ between the standard and high SpO$_2$ target groups at 60 min after birth. However, the pH was higher ($p = 0.046$) and PaCO$_2$ was lower ($p = 0.042$) with high SpO$_2$ target at the 60 min timepoint. An illustration summarizing the hemodynamics and gas exchange at 60 min after birth is presented as Figure 3A,B.

Table 4. Comparison of hemodynamics and oxygenation comparisons at 60 min after birth in a perinatal lamb model of MAS and PPHN.

Parameter	Standard SpO$_2$ Target (85–94%, n = 6)	High SpO$_2$ Target (95–99%, n = 6)
Hemoglobin, g/dL	12.32 ± 3.17	11.85 ± 1.08
pH	7.12 ± 0.11	7.25 ± 0.09 †
PaCO$_2$ (mmHg)	61.23 ± 15.42	44.08 ± 7.07 †
PaO$_2$ (mmHg)	48.14 ± 21.76	65.08 ± 18.77
SaO$_2$ (%)	86.66 ± 12.29	94.68 ± 3.55
SpO$_2$ (%)	88.4 ± 7.3	95.33 ± 2.50
CaO$_2$ (mlO$_2$/dL)	14.96 ± 4.22	15.23 ± 1.44
Cerebral Oxygen Delivery (ml/kg/min)	2.54 ± 0.68	2.12 ± 0.9
Lactate (mmol/L)	4.25 ± 1.94	4.07 ± 1.75
Heart Rate (bpm)	167.76 ± 32.46	154.56 ± 9.94
Mean Arterial Blood Pressure (mmHg)	53.41 ± 14.30	71.51 ± 8.14 †
Mean Carotid Flow (Q$_{CA}$-mL/kg/min)	16.01 ± 4.96	14.28 ± 7.21
Inspired O$_2$ (%) at 60 min	41.5 ± 13.25	64.66 ± 31.51

PaCO$_2$ = arterial carbon dioxide pressure; PaO$_2$ = arterial oxygen pressure; SaO$_2$ = arterial oxygen saturation from blood gas; SpO$_2$ = preductal pulse oximeter oxygen saturation; CaO$_2$ = arterial oxygen content. † Significantly different from the 85–94% target group; $p < 0.05$, unpaired student t-test, unequal variances.

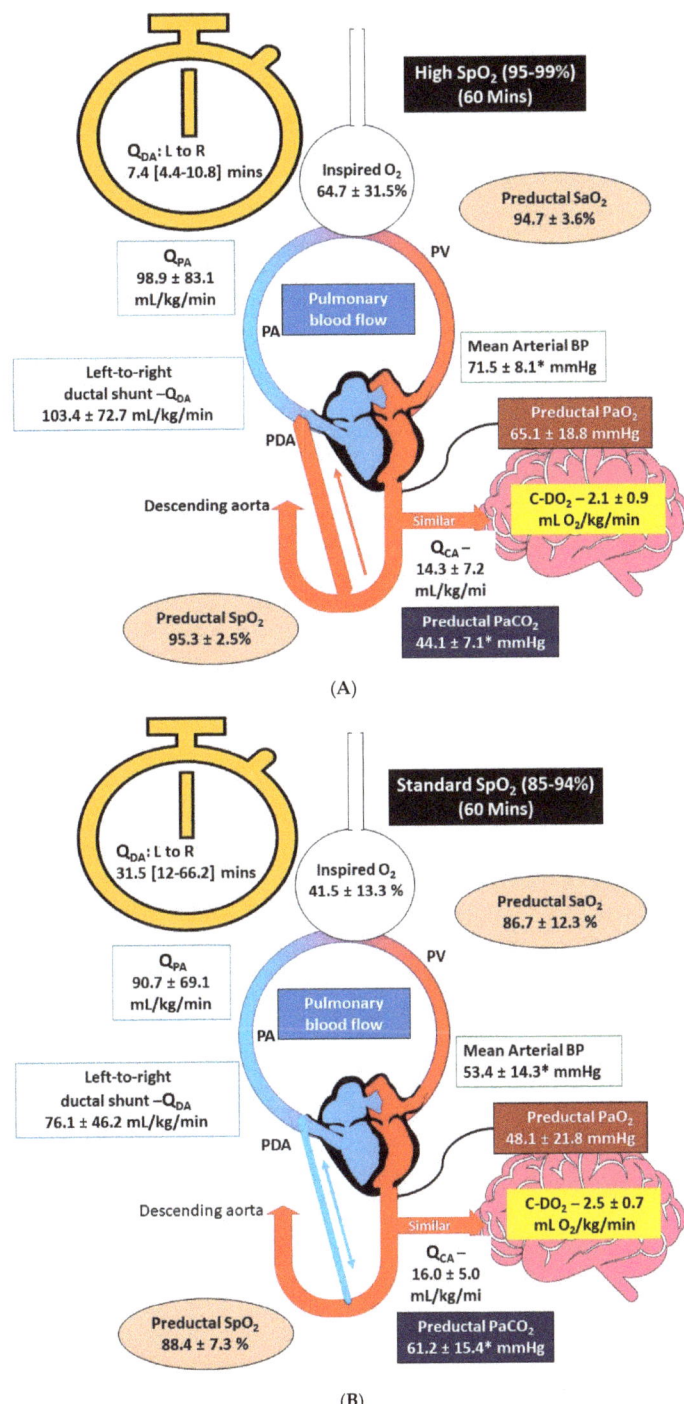

Figure 3. (**A**) Graphical summary of the results demonstrating the hemodynamics and gas exchange at 60 min after birth with high (95–99%) oxygen saturation (SpO$_2$) targets in an ovine model of meconium

aspiration and pulmonary hypertension. Median time to reversal of shunting was 7.4 (4.4–10.8) min after birth. The inspired oxygen concentration, preductal SpO$_2$ and arterial oxygen saturation (SaO$_2$), left-to-right ductal shunting (Q$_{DA}$), left pulmonary artery blood flow (Q$_{PA}$), left carotid artery blood flow (Q$_{CA}$), cerebral O$_2$ delivery (C-DO$_2$) and arterial partial pressure of carbon dioxide (PaCO$_2$) are shown. Shorter time to reversal of Q$_{DA}$ shunt to left-to-right, transiently increased Q$_{DA}$ and Q$_{PA}$ from 0.5–10 min after birth, and lower PaCO$_2$ at 60 min were observed with high SpO$_2$ target. * $p < 0.05$ compared to standard SpO$_2$ target group in (**B**). (**B**) Graphical summary of the results demonstrating the hemodynamics and gas exchange at 60 min after birth with standard (85–94%) oxygen saturation (SpO$_2$) targets in an ovine model of meconium aspiration and pulmonary hypertension. Median time to reversal of shunting was 31.5 (12–66.2) min after birth. The inspired oxygen concentration, preductal SpO$_2$ and arterial oxygen saturation (SaO$_2$), left-to-right ductal shunting (Q$_{DA}$), left pulmonary artery blood flow (Q$_{PA}$), left carotid artery blood flow (Q$_{CA}$), cerebral O2 delivery (C-DO$_2$) and arterial partial pressure of carbon dioxide (PaCO$_2$) are shown. Longer time to reversal of Q$_{DA}$ shunt to left-to-right and higher PaCO$_2$ at 60 min were observed with standard SpO$_2$ target. * $p < 0.05$ compared to high SpO$_2$ target group shown in (**A**).

4. Discussion

Neonatal PPHN is commonly associated with parenchymal lung disease such as MAS [1]. Mortality rates of 4–33% have been reported for neonatal PPHN [12]. Right-to-left shunting via the PDA and PFO resulting in labile hypoxemia is characteristic of PPHN. Supplemental O$_2$ can decrease PVR thus improving Q$_{PA}$, hastening reversal of extrapulmonary shunting to left-to-right. We demonstrate quicker reversal of ductal shunting to left-to-right with higher (95–99%) compared to the lower (85–94%) SpO$_2$ target during resuscitation and in the post-resuscitation period.

The American Academy of Pediatrics (AAP) NRP Textbook of Neonatal Resuscitation recommends initiating resuscitation with 21% O$_2$, titrating inspired O$_2$ to achieve the target SpO$_2$ range for every minute, and finally 85–95% by 10 min after birth. Maintaining SpO$_2$ within the range recommended by NRP by actively titrating the inspired O$_2$ led to effective oxygenation and Q$_{PA}$ in an ovine model of MAS [4]. However, there is wide variation among neonatologists in their preference of SpO$_2$ targets immediately after the initial resuscitation period [13,14]. In a recent animal study by Rawat et al., higher SpO$_2$ target of 95–99% resulted in lower PVR, higher Q$_{PA}$, higher cerebral O$_2$ delivery with lower lactate levels, but was associated with higher inspired O$_2$ and higher lung 3-nitrotyrosine, a marker of oxidative stress compared to lower ranges of target SpO$_2$ [5]. However, the authors did not evaluate direction of ductal flow and Q$_{DA}$ in that study.

During neonatal resuscitation, O$_2$ needs to be titrated judiciously to avoid hypo or hyperoxia. Kapadia et al. reported that post-resuscitation hyperoxia with perinatal acidemia is associated with higher incidence of moderate to severe hypoxic ischemic encephalopathy [15]. Thus, it is prudent to decrease supplemental O$_2$ in a timely manner to avoid hyperoxemia. We show that the benefits of targeting higher SpO$_2$ are transient and Q$_{PA}$ is identical between the two study groups by 60 min after birth. We also observed lower PaCO$_2$ in the high SpO$_2$ target group at 60 min after birth. We speculate that the higher SpO$_2$ target may have caused a transient surge in Q$_{PA}$ (Figure 2) that might have contributed to better gas exchange and lower PaCO$_2$ (Figure 3A,B). Additionally, the initial increase in left-to-right Q$_{DA}$ and increase in Q$_{PA}$ were not persistent at 60 min after birth (Figures 1 and 2). We speculate that reduction in Q$_{PA}$ could be secondary to transient effect of increased inspired O$_2$ on PVR or ductal constriction limiting Q$_{DA}$ leading to lower Q$_{PA}$. As the ductal flow remained steady between 5 min and 60 min after birth (Figure 1), we suspect that the PDA remained patent at 60 min in these lambs. We speculate that higher SpO$_2$ target is associated with earlier ductal narrowing and less cardiac dysfunction with quicker cardiovascular recovery from the asphyxial insult resulting in better mean arterial pressures (MAPs). Whereas in the standard SpO$_2$ target group, there may be slower ductal constriction and cardiovascular recovery from the asphyxial insult resulting in lower MAPs. Higher volume of shunt from the aorta-to-pulmonary artery is likely to expose ductal tissue to higher PaO_2 and hasten narrowing of the ductus. Furthermore, the diastolic BP were higher with high SpO_2 target at 60 min after delivery when compared to standard SpO_2 target (65 ± 13 vs. 45 ± 6, $p = 0.02$), possibly due to ductal constriction, thus contributing to higher MAPs.

Our study has several limitations. The severity of asphyxia was mild to moderate. Despite this, we did demonstrate significant degree of hypoxemia, low Q_{PA} and right-to-left shunting across the PDA following delivery in all the lambs (Tables 1 and 2 and Figure 1). We did not measure the pulmonary artery and left atrial pressures, and hence could not evaluate the PVR. In addition, we did not evaluate the shunting across the PFO. We had a small sample size and larger number of lambs might have led to different results. The markers of oxidative stress have not been evaluated. We did not recover the lambs and assess for long term outcomes. Although we targeted to achieve preductal SpO_2 within a narrow set range, the achieved SpO_2 was 88 ± 7% and 95 ± 3% in the standard and high SpO_2 target groups, respectively. This difficulty in achieving a set SpO_2 target range has previously been demonstrated in randomized trials in preterm infants [16,17].

To our knowledge, this is the first comparison of time to reversal of ductal shunting in PPHN between standard and high SpO_2 targets during resuscitation and in the post-resuscitation period. The novel aspect of this study is the measurement of Q_{DA} along with the direction of flow in a large mammalian model of MAS and PPHN closely mimicking human cardiopulmonary physiology. The lambs underwent meconium aspiration by spontaneous aspiration with negative pressure in the perinatal period during transition rather forceful instillation of meconium in the postnatal (1–3 days, often the case in piglet models) period [18]. Although an ovine model of PPHN can be induced by prenatal ductal ligation, we are unable to assess Q_{DA} in that model. Finally, the randomized study design is a major strength of this study.

5. Conclusions

In this term lamb model of MAS and PPHN, targeting SpO_2 at a higher range (95–99%) during resuscitation and in the immediate post-resuscitation period, led to a quicker transition to left-to-right shunting across the PDA but did not result in sustained increase in pulmonary blood flow. These findings support the current NRP recommendations to target preductal SpO_2 between 85–95% by 10 min. Clinical trials evaluating hemodynamics and long-term neurocognitive outcomes in term neonates comparing current recommended range to higher SpO_2 targets are warranted in patients at risk of PPHN such as MAS with asphyxia and congenital diaphragmatic hernia.

Author Contributions: A.L.L.: data extraction and analysis, conducting experiments, and writing the manuscript. P.V.: conducting experiments, critiquing, and revising the manuscript. M.E.H.: conducting experiments, data extraction, critiquing and revising the manuscript. S.L.: concept, procuring funds, conducting experiments, writing, critiquing, and revising the manuscript. D.S.: conducting studies, analysis of data, writing, critiquing and revising the manuscript. All authors have read and agreed to the published version of the manuscript.

Funding: This research was funded by NICHD 5R01 HD072929 (S.L.), Children's Miracle Network at University of California, Davis, First Tech Federal Credit Union and UC Davis Pediatrics, and Canadian Pediatric Society NRP research grant (D.S.).

Institutional Review Board Statement: The study was conducted according to the guidelines of the Declaration of Helsinki and approved by the Institutional Animal Care and Use Committee (IACUC) at the University of California Davis, Davis, CA, USA (protocol #20267).

Informed Consent Statement: Not applicable.

Data Availability Statement: The data presented in this study are available in this article.

Conflicts of Interest: The authors declare no conflict of interest. S.L. is a member of the AAP NRP steering committee. The views expressed in this article are his own and does not represent the official position of AAP or NRP. The funders had no role in the design of the study; in the collection, analyses, or interpretation of data; in the writing of the manuscript, or in the decision to publish the results.

References

1. Lakshminrusimha, S.; Keszler, M. Persistent Pulmonary Hypertension of the Newborn. *Neoreviews* **2015**, *16*, e680–e692. [CrossRef] [PubMed]
2. Morin, F.C., 3rd; Egan, E.A.; Ferguson, W.; Lundgren, C.E. Development of pulmonary vascular response to oxygen. *Am. J. Physiol. Heart Circ. Physiol.* **1988**, *254*, H542–H546. [CrossRef] [PubMed]
3. Teitel, D.F.; Iwamoto, H.S.; Rudolph, A.M. Changes in the Pulmonary Circulation during Birth-Related Events. *Pediatr. Res.* **1990**, *27*, 372–378. [CrossRef] [PubMed]
4. Rawat, M.; Chandrasekharan, P.K.; Swartz, D.D.; Mathew, B.; Nair, J.; Gugino, S.F.; Koenigsknecht, C.; Vali, P.; Lakshminrusimha, S. Neonatal resuscitation adhering to oxygen saturation guidelines in asphyxiated lambs with meconium aspiration. *Pediatr. Res.* **2016**, *79*, 583–588. [CrossRef] [PubMed]
5. Rawat, M.; Chandrasekharan, P.; Gugino, S.F.; Koenigsknecht, C.; Nielsen, L.; Wedgwood, S.; Mathew, B.; Nair, J.; Steinhorn, R.; Lakshminrusimha, S. Optimal Oxygen Targets in Term Lambs with Meconium Aspiration Syndrome and Pulmonary Hypertension. *Am. J. Respir. Cell Mol. Biol.* **2020**, *63*, 510–518. [CrossRef] [PubMed]
6. Smolich, J.J.; Kenna, K.R.; Mynard, J.P. Antenatal betamethasone augments early rise in pulmonary perfusion at birth in preterm lambs: Role of ductal shunting and right ventricular outflow distribution. *Am. J. Physiol. Regul. Integr. Comp. Physiol.* **2019**, *316*, R716–R724. [CrossRef] [PubMed]
7. Lakshminrusimha, S.; Mathew, B.; Nair, J.; Gugino, S.F.; Koenigsknecht, C.; Rawat, M.; Nielsen, L.; Swartz, D.D. Tracheal suctioning improves gas exchange but not hemodynamics in asphyxiated lambs with meconium aspiration. *Pediatr. Res.* **2015**, *77*, 347–355. [CrossRef] [PubMed]
8. Kilkenny, C.; Browne, W.J.; Cuthill, I.C.; Emerson, M.; Altman, D.G. Improving bioscience research reporting: The ARRIVE guidelines for reporting animal research. *PLoS Biol.* **2010**, *8*, e1000412. [CrossRef] [PubMed]
9. Sankaran, D.; Chandrasekharan, P.K.; Gugino, S.F.; Koenigsknecht, C.; Helman, J.; Nair, J.; Mathew, B.; Rawat, M.; Vali, P.; Nielsen, L.; et al. Randomised trial of epinephrine dose and flush volume in term newborn lambs. *Arch. Dis. Child. Fetal Neonatal Ed.* **2021**. [CrossRef] [PubMed]
10. Sankaran, D.; Vali, P.; Chen, P.; Lesneski, A.L.; Hardie, M.E.; Alhassen, Z.; Wedgwood, S.; Wyckoff, M.H.; Lakshminrusimha, S. Randomized trial of oxygen weaning strategies following chest compressions during neonatal resuscitation. *Pediatr. Res.* **2021**, 1–9. [CrossRef]
11. American Academy of Pediatrics; Weiner, G.M.; American Heart Association; Zaichkin, J. *Textbook of Neonatal Resuscitation*, 7th ed.; American Academy of Pediatrics: Itasca, IL, USA, 2016.
12. Walsh-Sukys, M.C.; Tyson, J.E.; Wright, L.L.; Bauer, C.R.; Korones, S.B.; Stevenson, D.K.; Verter, J.; Stoll, B.J.; Lemons, J.A.; Papile, L.A.; et al. Persistent pulmonary hypertension of the newborn in the era before nitric oxide: Practice variation and outcomes. *Pediatrics* **2000**, *105*, 14–20. [CrossRef] [PubMed]
13. Nakwan, N.; Chaiwiriyawong, P. An international survey on persistent pulmonary hypertension of the newborn: A need for an evidence-based management. *J. Neonatal-Perinat. Med.* **2016**, *9*, 243–250. [CrossRef] [PubMed]
14. Alapati, D.; Jassar, R.; Shaffer, T.H. Management of Supplemental Oxygen for Infants with Persistent Pulmonary Hypertension of Newborn: A Survey. *Am. J. Perinatol.* **2017**, *34*, 276–282. [CrossRef] [PubMed]
15. Kapadia, V.S.; Chalak, L.F.; DuPont, T.L.; Rollins, N.K.; Brion, L.P.; Wyckoff, M.H. Perinatal asphyxia with hyperoxemia within the first hour of life is associated with moderate to severe hypoxic-ischemic encephalopathy. *J. Pediatr.* **2013**, *163*, 949–954. [CrossRef] [PubMed]
16. Askie, L.M.; Darlow, B.A.; Finer, N.; Schmidt, B.; Stenson, B.; Tarnow-Mordi, W.; Davis, P.G.; Carlo, W.A.; Brocklehurst, P.; Davies, L.C.; et al. Association Between Oxygen Saturation Targeting and Death or Disability in Extremely Preterm Infants in the Neonatal Oxygenation Prospective Meta-analysis Collaboration. *JAMA* **2018**, *319*, 2190–2201. [CrossRef] [PubMed]
17. Lakshminrusimha, S.; Manja, V.; Mathew, B.; Suresh, G.K. Oxygen targeting in preterm infants: A physiological interpretation. *J. Perinatol.* **2015**, *35*, 8–15. [CrossRef] [PubMed]
18. Wiswell, T.E.; Peabody, S.S.; Davis, J.M.; Slayter, M.V.; Bent, R.C.; Merritt, T.A. Surfactant therapy and high-frequency jet ventilation in the management of a piglet model of the meconium aspiration syndrome. *Pediatr. Res.* **1994**, *36*, 494–500. [CrossRef] [PubMed]

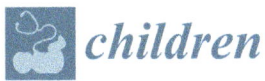

Article

Inhaled Nitric Oxide at Birth Reduces Pulmonary Vascular Resistance and Improves Oxygenation in Preterm Lambs

Satyan Lakshminrusimha [1,*], Sylvia F. Gugino [2,3], Krishnamurthy Sekar [4], Stephen Wedgwood [1], Carmon Koenigsknecht [2], Jayasree Nair [2] and Bobby Mathew [2]

[1] Departments of Pediatrics, University of California at Davis, UC Davis Children's Hospital, 2516 Stockton Blvd, Sacramento, CA 95817, USA; swedgwood@ucdavis.edu
[2] Department of Pediatrics, State University of New York at Buffalo, Buffalo, NY 14222, USA; sfgugino@buffalo.edu (S.F.G.); carmonko@buffalo.edu (C.K.); jnair@upa.chob.edu (J.N.); bmathew@upa.chob.edu (B.M.)
[3] Physiology and Biophysics, State University of New York at Buffalo, Buffalo, NY 14222, USA
[4] Department of Pediatrics, University of Oklahoma, Oklahoma City, OK 73013, USA; Krishnamurthy-Sekar@ouhsc.edu
* Correspondence: slakshmi@ucdavis.edu; Tel.: +1-(916)-734-5178

Abstract: Resuscitation with 21% O_2 may not achieve target oxygenation in preterm infants and in neonates with persistent pulmonary hypertension of the newborn (PPHN). Inhaled nitric oxide (iNO) at birth can reduce pulmonary vascular resistance (PVR) and improve PaO_2. We studied the effect of iNO on oxygenation and changes in PVR in preterm lambs with and without PPHN during resuscitation and stabilization at birth. Preterm lambs with and without PPHN (induced by antenatal ductal ligation) were delivered at 134 d gestation (term is 147–150 d). Lambs without PPHN were ventilated with 21% O_2, titrated O_2 to maintain target oxygenation or 21% O_2 + iNO (20 ppm) at birth for 30 min. Preterm lambs with PPHN were ventilated with 50% O_2, titrated O_2 or 50% O_2 + iNO. Resuscitation with 21% O_2 in preterm lambs and 50%O_2 in PPHN lambs did not achieve target oxygenation. Inhaled NO significantly decreased PVR in all lambs and increased PaO_2 in preterm lambs ventilated with 21% O_2 similar to that achieved by titrated O_2 (41 ± 9% at 30 min). Inhaled NO increased PaO_2 to 45 ± 13, 45 ± 20 and 76 ± 11 mmHg with 50% O_2, titrated O_2 up to 100% and 50% O_2 + iNO, respectively, in PPHN lambs. We concluded that iNO at birth reduces PVR and FiO_2 required to achieve target PaO_2.

Keywords: inhaled nitric oxide; resuscitation; prematurity; persistent pulmonary hypertension of newborn; pulmonary vascular resistance; hypoxic pulmonary vasoconstriction

1. Introduction

During fetal life, pulmonary vascular resistance (PVR) is high and PaO_2 levels are low compared to the postnatal period [1]. Oxygen is a potent and specific pulmonary vasodilator and plays an important role in decreasing PVR at birth [1]. After birth, PVR gradually decreases and oxygenation slowly improves over the first minutes of life. Current neonatal resuscitation guidelines recommend the use of 21% oxygen in the delivery room resuscitation of term infants [2]. However, controversy exists as to the optimal resuscitation gas in preterm infants [3]. Recent studies suggest that extremely preterm infants who were first resuscitated with 21% oxygen and titrated up to achieve target SpO_2 had higher mortality from respiratory failure compared to infants whose resuscitation was initiated with 100% oxygen and titrated down [4]. However, high initial inspired oxygen concentration (>65%) is not recommended during resuscitation of preterm infants due to the risk of oxidative stress [5,6]. Promoting pulmonary vasodilation without excessive supplemental oxygen can potentially facilitate the establishment of gas exchange in the lung without exposing the infant to oxygen toxicity.

Persistent pulmonary hypertension of the newborn (PPHN) [7] is a disorder characterized by elevated pulmonary vascular resistance (PVR), extra-pulmonary right-to-left shunting and hypoxemia. Inhaled nitric oxide (iNO) is a selective pulmonary vasodilator approved by the Food and Drug Administration in term infants with PPHN and acts by increasing cGMP in pulmonary arterial smooth muscle cells (PASMC). We hypothesized that ventilation with iNO at birth would reduce PVR and increase arterial partial pressure of oxygen both in preterm newborn lambs and in PPHN lambs, similar to that achieved by high FiO_2 (Figure 1). Our overall aim was to evaluate if iNO supplementation resulted in a reduced need for inspired oxygen as being secondary to a decrease in PVR in animal models with and without PPHN.

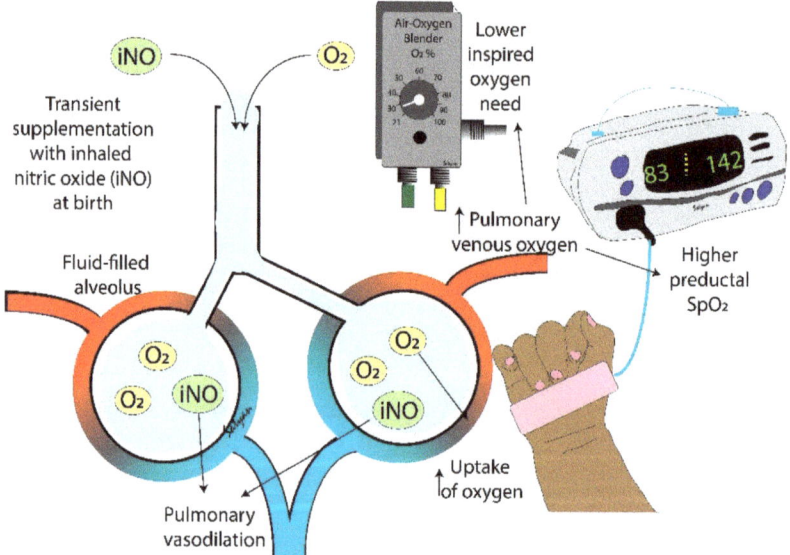

Figure 1. Hypothesis. Newly born, preterm infants have immature lungs filled with liquid. Administration of low concentrations of inspired oxygen alone may not be adequate to achieve target oxygen saturation (SpO_2). Transient supplementation with inhaled nitric oxide (iNO) during delivery room resuscitation and stabilization can promote pulmonary vasodilation and enhance gas exchange leading to a lower need for inspired oxygen and higher preductal SpO_2. Copyright Satyan Lakshminrusimha.

2. Materials and Methods

This study was approved by the University at Buffalo Institutional Animal Care and Use Committee. Time-dated pregnant ewes were procured from New Pasteur farms, Attica, NY. Lambs were delivered by caesarean section at 134 d gestation (term gestation in lambs is 147–150 days). We used the ovine in utero ductal ligation model to induce PPHN. Time-dated pregnant ewes were anesthetized as previously described [8] and fetal ductus arteriosus was ligated at 128 d gestational age [9]. The fetus was then placed back in the uterus for 8 days. On the day of delivery, preterm lambs (with and without PPHN) were partially exteriorized by cesarean section and catheters were placed in the jugular vein and carotid artery to obtain PaO_2 measurements at different levels of oxygen exposure with and without iNO. The dose of iNO was 20 ppm. We conducted the study in 2 phases:

I. Oxygenation studies: Preterm lambs with and without PPHN were intubated at birth and randomized to be ventilated with 21, 50 or 100% oxygen with or without iNO for 30 min. Preductal arterial gases were drawn every 5 min and recorded.

II. Pulmonary hemodynamic studies: In a subsequent set of experiments, we studied the effect of iNO on oxygenation and pulmonary vascular resistance. These lambs were exteriorized as described previously [8,9]. In addition to the placement of right carotid and jugular lines, we performed a thoracotomy and placed pulmonary arterial and left atrial catheters to measure pressures and a pulmonary arterial flow probe to measure blood flow. The flow probe was placed around the left pulmonary artery in lambs without PPHN to avoid the influence of blood flow through the patent ductus arteriosus (PDA). In lambs with PPHN, the flow probe was placed around the main pulmonary artery as the ductus arteriosus was ligated in utero to induce PPHN.

   a. Based on results from phase I oxygenation studies, preterm lambs without PPHN were exposed to 21% oxygen, titrated oxygen to maintain PaO_2 between 45 and 80 mmHg and titrated oxygen with iNO at 20 ppm.
   b. In lambs with PPHN, 21% oxygen was avoided as PaO_2 levels were low with this FiO_2 in phase I oxygenation studies. PPHN lambs were exposed to 50% oxygen, titrated oxygen to maintain PaO_2 between 45 and 80 mmHg and titrated oxygen with iNO at 20 ppm for 30 min.
   c. Lambs were effectively anesthetized during the period of instrumentation through the isoflurane inhalant administered to the ewe. The lambs were then delivered and ventilated at the following initial settings: 30 cm H_2O peak inspiratory pressure, 5 cm H_2O positive end expiratory pressure, and 40 respirations per minute. Sedation was maintained by administration of an initial propofol bolus (2 mg/kg) followed by a constant rate infusion given to effect. Additional doses of fentanyl at 1–5 mcg/kg were administered as needed for signs of discomfort. Maintenance IV fluid with dextrose and electrolytes was also provided. Arterial blood pressure, heart rate, and pulse oximetry were monitored and recorded. Ventilator settings were adjusted to maintain a $PaCO_2$ between 35 and 50 mmHg.
   d. Pulmonary vascular resistance was calculated as follows:

$$PVR = (\text{mean PA pressure} - \text{LA pressure})/\text{pulmonary blood flow in (mL·min}^{-1}\text{·kg}^{-1})$$

In lambs without PPHN, the left pulmonary arterial flow was used to calculate the "left" PVR. In lambs with PPHN, the main pulmonary arterial flow was used for this calculation.

3. Results

I. **Oxygenation studies**: Thirty-six preterm lambs without PPHN and 30 lambs with PPHN were included in this phase of the study (6 lambs in each group). There was a significant difference in birth weight between preterm lambs without PPHN (3059 ± 105 g) and lambs with PPHN (2576 ± 210 g). The birth weights, gender distribution, and multiplicity were similar between the iNO and no-iNO groups (data not shown). Fetal blood gases were similar between preterm lambs with and without PPHN (PaO_2 — 18.4 ± 7.2 and 17.5 ± 6.1 mmHg respectively) and between lambs ventilated with and without iNO (Figure 2).

   a. Preterm lambs without PPHN ventilated with 21% oxygen gradually increased their PaO_2 over the first 30 min. Ventilation with iNO significantly increased PaO_2 at 5 (39 ± 3 vs. 56 ± 11 mmHg) and 10 min (43 ± 3 vs. 63 ± 12 mmHg). There was no difference in PaO_2 with and without iNO by 30 min (Figure 2Ai). Ventilation with 50 and 100% oxygen significantly increased PaO_2 compared to 21% oxygen reaching supraphysiological levels by 5 min. However, addition of iNO did not increase PaO_2 when preterm lambs were ventilated with 50 and 100% oxygen (Figure 2A).

b. Preterm lambs with PPHN had low PaO_2 values compared to lambs without PPHN (Figure 2). Ventilation with 21% oxygen resulted in low PaO_2 values (30 ± 6 mmHg at 30 min). Increasing inspired oxygen from 21 to 50% significantly increased PaO_2 in lambs with PPHN (45 ± 13 mmHg at 30 min with 50% oxygen). However, further increase in inspired oxygen from 50 to 100% did not further increase PaO_2 (44.5 ± 20 mmHg at 30 min with 100% oxygen). Inhaled nitric oxide significantly increased PaO_2 with 21, 50 and 100% oxygen in lambs with PPHN. Three PPHN lambs were hydropic (one each in 21% oxygen, 21% oxygen + iNO, and 50% oxygen groups) with massive pleural effusions and ascites and were excluded, reducing the number of lambs in these groups to five.

II. **Hemodynamic studies**: Fifteen preterm lambs without PPHN and 15 lambs with PPHN underwent thoracotomy and placement of pressure and flow probes to measure PVR.

   a. Preterm lambs without PPHN were divided into three groups. The first group was ventilated with 21% O_2 (n = 5). A steady decline in PVR was measured with ventilation. The second group received titrated inspired oxygen adjusted every 5 min to maintain a PaO_2 between 45 and 80 mmHg (n = 5). This required increase in inspired oxygen to 41 ± 9% by 30 min. The decline in PVR in this group was similar to the 21% oxygen group. The third group received iNO at 20 ppm and inspired oxygen was titrated to maintain PaO_2 between 45 and 80 mmHg (n = 5). This group needed 21% oxygen throughout the 30 min period. The PaO_2 and PVR with 21% oxygen + iNO was significantly lower than the previous two groups (Figure 3A,B). The preductal SpO_2 value at 5 min was 66 ± 8, 63 ± 9 and 89 ± 11% in 21% O_2, titrated O_2 and 21% O_2 + iNO groups respectively. The corresponding values at 30 min were 86 ± 11, 87 ± 10 and 85 ± 13%.

   b. Preterm lambs with PPHN were also divided into 3 groups. The first was ventilated with 50% oxygen (n = 5). There was a modest decrease in PVR and increase in PaO_2 but some PPHN lambs remained hypoxemic with PaO_2 < 45 mmHg (Figure 4). The second group received titrated inspired oxygen starting at 50% and adjusted to maintain PaO_2 between 45 and 80 mmHg (n = 5). By 10 min, all lambs in this group were on 100% O_2. The reduction in PVR and increase in PaO_2 in this group was similar to the 50% oxygen group in spite of the significantly higher inspired oxygen. The third group was initially ventilated with 50% oxygen with iNO 20 ppm (n = 5). The PVR in this group was significantly lower and PaO_2 significantly higher than the other two. By 30 min, inspired oxygen could be weaned to 44 ± 2% (Figure 4). The preductal SpO_2 value at 5 min was 33 ± 14, 61 ± 11 and 71 ± 13% in 50% O_2, titrated O_2 and 50% O_2 + iNO groups respectively. The corresponding values at 30 min were 78 ± 13, 80 ± 14 and 92 ± 8%.

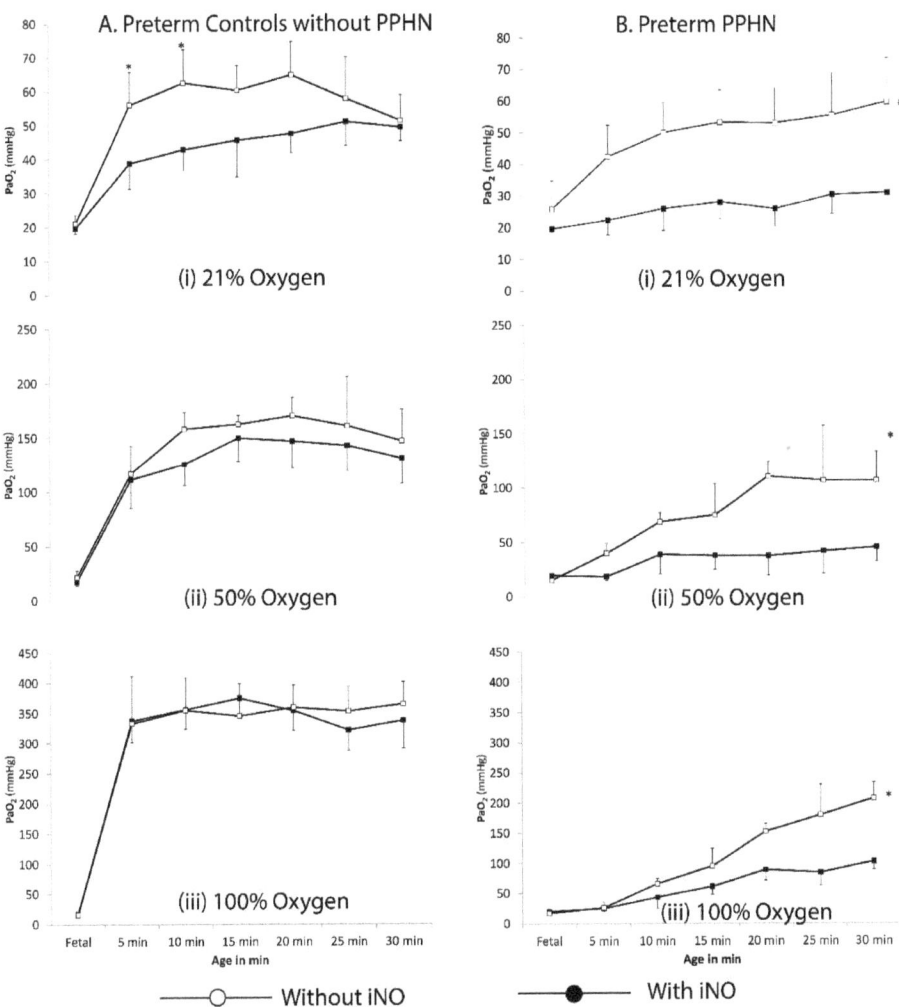

Figure 2. Changes in oxygenation with inhaled nitric oxide (iNO): PaO$_2$ in the first 30 min of life in (**A**) preterm lambs without persistent pulmonary hypertension of the newborn (PPHN) with exposure to 21, 50 and 100% oxygen with (open squares) and without iNO at 20 ppm (solid squares). (**B**) PaO$_2$ in the first 30 min of life in preterm lambs with PPHN on exposure to 21, 50 and 100% oxygen with (open squares) and without iNO (solid squares) at 20 ppm. * $p < 0.05$ compared to PaO$_2$ without iNO.

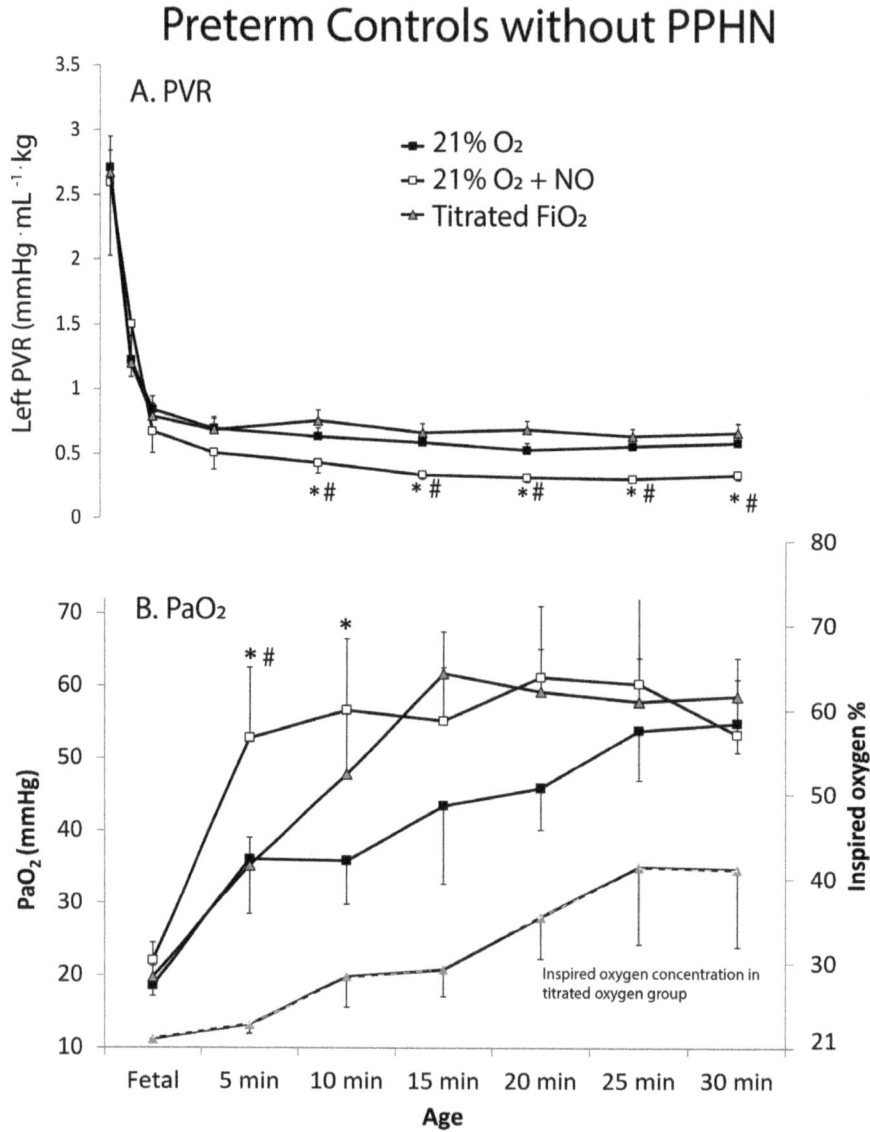

Figure 3. Changes in Pulmonary vascular resistance (PVR) in left lung (**A**) and PaO$_2$ (**B**) in preterm lambs exposed to 21% oxygen (solid squares) vs. 21% oxygen and iNO (open squares) and titrated oxygen (gray triangles). Inspired oxygen concentration needed in the titrated oxygen group to maintain PaO$_2$ between 45 to 80 mmHg is shown by a hyphenated line on the secondary y-axis (gray triangles). * $p < 0.05$ compared to 21% oxygen group; # $p < 0.05$ compared to titrated oxygen group.

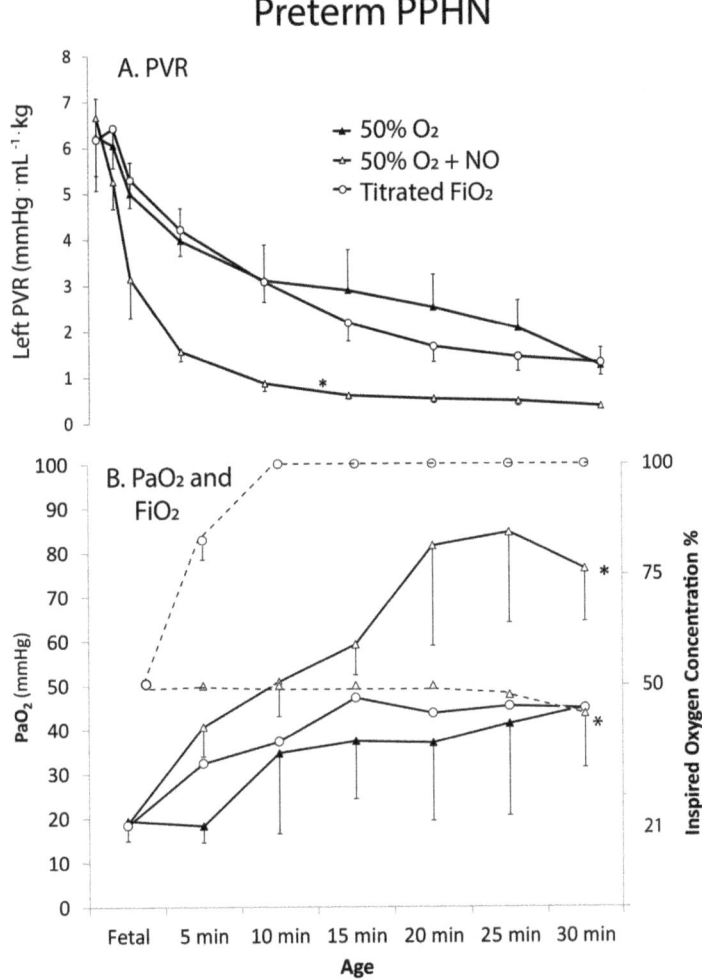

Figure 4. Changes in total pulmonary vascular resistance (PVR) in both lungs (**A**) and PaO$_2$ (**B**) in PPHN lambs exposed to 50% oxygen (solid triangles) vs initiation with 50% oxygen and iNO and titration (open triangles) and titrated oxygen (open circles). Inspired oxygen concentration in the titrated oxygen group (open circles) and titrated oxygen with iNO (open triangles) is represented by a hyphenated line (* $p < 0.05$ compared to corresponding value without iNO.

4. Discussion

In the current study, we demonstrated that supplementation with iNO during resuscitation at birth in preterm lambs with and without PPHN reduced PVR and inspired oxygen concentration necessary to achieve target PaO$_2$ levels. These findings have implications for delivery room resuscitation of preterm infants [10–12] and infants with PPHN [13].

The main goal of neonatal resuscitation is to achieve adequate ventilation of the lung and establishment of lung as the organ of gas exchange [5]. While 21% oxygen is effective for resuscitating term infants, the optimal oxygen concentration for resuscitation of preterm infants continues to be controversial [14], resulting in variations in clinical practice guidelines [15]. A comparison of low oxygen (initial oxygen concentration 21–30%) and high oxygen (60–100%) strategies has not demonstrated improvement in long-term outcomes in preterm infants. [3] Low-oxygen strategies are associated with reduced oxidative stress [16] and improved pulmonary outcomes in some studies [17]. However, not achieving a saturation of 80% by 5 min of postnatal age (whether due to inadequate oxygen supplementation or pulmonary or pulmonary vascular disease) is associated with adverse outcomes [12]. One approach to improving systemic oxygenation and promoting pulmonary vasodilation during transition at birth, while establishing the lung as the organ of gas exchange without excessive supplemental oxygen, is to use a selective pulmonary vasodilator such as iNO in the delivery room. In a recently published pilot double-blind randomized controlled trial on the use of inhaled nitric oxide in the delivery room resuscitation of extremely low birthweight preterm infants by Sekar et al., those who received 20 ppm iNO as an adjuvant in the resuscitation gas had a lower cumulative FiO_2 exposure and a lower rate of exposure to $FiO_2 > 0.6$ [18].

Inhaled NO improved PaO_2, and reduced the need for supplemental oxygen from 41 ± 9 to 21% in preterm lambs. PVR significantly decreased with the use of 21% oxygen with iNO. Studies in extremely preterm infants have suggested increased mortality in infants resuscitated in 21% [4,19] Although the physiological basis of the increased mortality is not fully understood, one plausible explanation is that infants who were resuscitated in 21% oxygen were exposed to hypoxia and inadequate pulmonary vasodilation in the immediate newborn period. Our study demonstrated improved oxygenation by 5 min and improved pulmonary vasodilation with the use of iNO at birth in preterm lambs.

During fetal life, adequate oxygen delivery is achieved by an umbilical venous pO_2 of 32–35 mmHg [20], and fetal PVR is high with physiologic pulmonary hypertension [21]. However, in the immediate postnatal period, similar PaO_2 values resulted in hypoxic pulmonary vasoconstriction [22]. Achieving a preductal PaO_2 of 45 mmHg (equivalent to 80% SpO_2) by 5 min [12] is an important goal and can be achieved with lower supplemental oxygen if iNO is started at birth in preterm infants (Figure 1). This PaO_2 of 45 mmHg is also the change point below which hypoxic pulmonary vasoconstriction was observed in newborn calves [22] and lambs [8,23]. Interestingly, the improvement in PaO_2 in preterm lambs with iNO was observed only in the 21% oxygen group, not in the 50 and 100% groups. We speculate that the increase in alveolar oxygen (PAO_2) and suprphysiological arterial oxygenation (PaO_2) achieved with 50 and 100% inspired oxygen in preterm lambs induced pulmonary vasodilation and the addition of iNO did not result in further pulmonary vasodilation. The administration of 21% oxygen with iNO results in low PVR with the benefit of avoiding hypoxia without increasing the risk of hyperoxia.

In the lambs with PPHN, resuscitation with supplemental oxygen alone (including 100% oxygen) did not achieve optimal PaO_2 levels by 5 and 10 min of postnatal age. Inhaled NO improves oxygenation at all levels of inspired oxygen (21, 50 and 100%). The use of iNO in the delivery room in infants with suspected PPHN may not be practical. In most cases, with the exception of congenital diaphragmatic hernia (CDH), PPHN is not diagnosed in the delivery room. In infants with CDH, iNO has not been effective in reducing the need for ECMO [24], and initial resuscitation with 50% oxygen is feasible and not associated with adverse events [13].

Preterm neonates have deficient antioxidant systems and are susceptible to oxygen toxicity [25]. Increased oxygen tension in the blood and tissues increases the risk of oxygen toxicity [26] by the formation of reactive oxygen species exceeding the antioxidant capability of the neonate [27]. The optimal inspired oxygen concentration should deliver an adequate amount of oxygen to the tissues at the lowest possible oxygen tension.

The use of high concentrations of oxygen or iNO at birth can have both short-term and long-term negative consequences. High concentration of oxygen during the resuscitation of an asphyxiated neonate can increase superoxide anions, [28] peroxynitrite and isoprostanes [9,29]. A combination of iNO and oxygen may have other unknown side effects (including potential epigenetic changes) [30,31]. The use of iNO in preterm infants with hypoxemic respiratory failure and pulmonary hypertension is controversial. [32–35] When used with high concentrations of oxygen, iNO can increase nitrosative stress. [9]

Using iNO adds a significant risk of generating toxic nitrosative derivatives such as nitrotyrosine, nitro-albumin and highly toxic perioynitrite. Nitric oxide scavenges superoxide anions by competing with superoxide dismutase. Superoxide anions are generated during the fetal-to-neonatal transition, especially when supplemental oxygen is provided [28]. Sequestration of superoxide by NO may lead to an apparent reduction in oxidative stress markers. [9] Simultaneous evaluation of nitrosative stress markers should be performed to avoid drawing erroneous conclusions. Inhaled NO use in the NICU has been associated with increased childhood malignancies [31,36]. Vento and Sanchez-Illana in a comment to the Sekar et al. trial recommend a long-term neurodevelopmental follow-up among preterm neonates exposed to iNO at birth [37].

There are several limitations to the current study. All preterm lambs were intubated during resuscitation. The effectiveness of iNO when administered through non-invasive ventilation in the delivery room is not known. However, in the pilot trial by Sekar et al., iNO was effective in reducing FiO_2 during resuscitation in the delivery room [18]. We monitored pulse oximetry but mainly relied on frequent preductal PaO_2 measurements for titrating inspired oxygen due to the variable relationship between SpO_2 and PaO_2 [38]. Such titration is not feasible in a clinical situation. Given the high concentration of fetal hemoglobin at birth, reliance on PaO_2 may result higher risk of hyperoxemia compared to titration using SpO_2. Preterm lambs were at 134 days gestation which corresponded approximately to late preterm infants at approximately 34 weeks gestation in late saccular stage. Lambs at 80 to 120 days of gestation corresponded to 17–27 weeks of human gestation and were in the canalicular stage of lung development [39]. This maturity at 134 days was older than the gestation of infants in the Sekar et al. trial (25–31 weeks) [18]. The ductal ligation model of PPHN did not have parenchymal lung disease. The results of this study may not be applicable to PPHN secondary to parenchymal diseases such as respiratory distress syndrome, meconium aspiration syndrome and pneumonia. Inhaled NO improved oxygenation in neonatal models of atelectasis [40], but its effectiveness in preventing hypoxic pulmonary vasoconstriction in such models is not known. It is possible that lower doses of iNO (<20 ppm) or other inhaled pulmonary vasodilators such as prostacyclin analogs may show similar results [41]. Presence of respiratory or metabolic acidosis may modify the lamb's response to hypoxia. We did not study the effect of pH and asphyxiation at birth on oxygenation and response to iNO [22,42]. There are substantial differences between animal models and controlled translational studies and human neonates in a hectic clinical setting. Recent studies have shown stark differences in the outcomes of translational and clinical studies, such as sustained inflation in preterm infants at birth [43]. Lastly, we did not measure oxidative or nitrosative stress.

5. Conclusions

We concluded that iNO is effective for improving oxygenation in both preterm lambs and lambs with PPHN without increasing inspired oxygen. Inhaled NO reduced PVR in the immediate newborn period in preterm neonatal lambs with normal lungs and with PPHN. A randomized controlled masked pilot study evaluating the use of iNO in preterm infants showed a reduced FiO_2 requirement with iNO use. Larger randomized studies with long-term follow-up and studies evaluating oxidative and nitrosative stress following short uses of iNO are warranted. The limited available information on the use of iNO in the delivery room precludes its use in neonatal resuscitation except in well-controlled trials.

Author Contributions: Conceptualization, S.L., K.S. and B.M.; Data curation, S.F.G. and J.N.; Methodology, S.L., S.F.G., S.W., C.K. and J.N.; Project administration, S.F.G.; Writing—original draft, S.L. and B.M.; Writing—review and editing, S.W., C.K. and J.N. All authors will be informed about each step of manuscript processing including submission, revision, revision reminders via emails from our system or the assigned assistant editor. All authors have read and agreed to the published version of the manuscript.

Funding: Funded by NIH 1 R01 HD072929 (SL); Inhaled nitric oxide was provided by Ikaria LLC, Hampton NJ, USA through an equipment grant. (currently Mallinckrodt Pharmaceuticals, Bedminster, NJ, USA).

Institutional Review Board Statement: This study was approved by the University at Buffalo Institutional Animal Care and Use Committee.

Data Availability Statement: Data provided on request.

Conflicts of Interest: S.L. was a speaker for Ikaria LLC from July 2011 to October 2014; Ikaria had no role in designing the study or analysis of the results or writing the manuscript.

References

1. Lakshminrusimha, S.; Steinhorn, R.H. Pulmonary vascular biology during neonatal transition. *Clin. Perinatol.* **1999**, *26*, 601–619. [CrossRef]
2. Wyckoff, M.H.; Wyllie, J.; Aziz, K.; de Almeida, M.F.; Fabres, J.; Fawke, J.; Guinsburg, R.; Hosono, S.; Isayama, T.; Kapadia, V.S.; et al. Neonatal Life Support: 2020 International Consensus on Cardiopulmonary Resuscitation and Emergency Cardiovascular Care Science With Treatment Recommendations. *Circulation* **2020**, *142*, S185–S221. [CrossRef] [PubMed]
3. Welsford, M.; Nishiyama, C.; Shortt, C.; Weiner, G.; Roehr, C.C.; Isayama, T.; Dawson, J.A.; Wyckoff, M.H.; Rabi, Y.; International Liaison Committee on Resuscitation Neonatal Life Support Task Force. Initial Oxygen Use for Preterm Newborn Resuscitation: A Systematic Review With Meta-analysis. *Pediatrics* **2019**, *143*. [CrossRef] [PubMed]
4. Oei, J.L.; Saugstad, O.D.; Lui, K.; Wright, I.M.; Smyth, J.P.; Craven, P.; Wang, Y.A.; McMullan, R.; Coates, E.; Ward, M.; et al. Targeted Oxygen in the Resuscitation of Preterm Infants, a Randomized Clinical Trial. *Pediatrics* **2017**, *139*. [CrossRef]
5. Wyckoff, M.H.; Aziz, K.; Escobedo, M.B.; Kapadia, V.S.; Kattwinkel, J.; Perlman, J.M.; Simon, W.M.; Weiner, G.M.; Zaichkin, J.G. Part 13: Neonatal Resuscitation: 2015 American Heart Association Guidelines Update for Cardiopulmonary Resuscitation and Emergency Cardiovascular Care (Reprint). *Pediatrics* **2015**. [CrossRef] [PubMed]
6. Perlman, J.M.; Wyllie, J.; Kattwinkel, J.; Wyckoff, M.H.; Aziz, K.; Guinsburg, R.; Kim, H.S.; Liley, H.G.; Mildenhall, L.; Simon, W.M.; et al. Part 7: Neonatal Resuscitation: 2015 International Consensus on Cardiopulmonary Resuscitation and Emergency Cardiovascular Care Science With Treatment Recommendations (Reprint). *Pediatrics* **2015**. [CrossRef]
7. Lakshminrusimha, S. Neonatal and Postneonatal Pulmonary Hypertension. *Children* **2021**, *8*, 131. [CrossRef]
8. Lakshminrusimha, S.; Swartz, D.D.; Gugino, S.F.; Ma, C.X.; Wynn, K.A.; Ryan, R.M.; Russell, J.A.; Steinhorn, R.H. Oxygen concentration and pulmonary hemodynamics in newborn lambs with pulmonary hypertension. *Pediatric Res.* **2009**, *66*, 539–544. [CrossRef]
9. Lakshminrusimha, S.; Russell, J.A.; Wedgwood, S.; Gugino, S.F.; Kazzaz, J.A.; Davis, J.M.; Steinhorn, R.H. Superoxide dismutase improves oxygenation and reduces oxidation in neonatal pulmonary hypertension. *Am. J. Respir. Crit. Care Med.* **2006**, *174*, 1370–1377. [CrossRef]
10. Kapadia, V.; Rabi, Y.; Oei, J.L. The Goldilocks principle. Oxygen in the delivery room: When is it too little, too much, and just right? *Semin. Fetal Neonatal Med.* **2018**, *23*, 347–354. [CrossRef] [PubMed]
11. Kapadia, V.; Wyckoff, M.H. Oxygen Therapy in the Delivery Room: What Is the Right Dose? *Clin. Perinatol.* **2018**, *45*, 293–306. [CrossRef]
12. Oei, J.L.; Finer, N.N.; Saugstad, O.D.; Wright, I.M.; Rabi, Y.; Tarnow-Mordi, W.; Rich, W.; Kapadia, V.; Rook, D.; Smyth, J.P.; et al. Outcomes of oxygen saturation targeting during delivery room stabilisation of preterm infants. *Arch. Dis. Child. Fetal Neonatal Ed.* **2018**, *103*, F446–F454. [CrossRef]
13. Riley, J.S.; Antiel, R.M.; Rintoul, N.E.; Ades, A.M.; Waqar, L.N.; Lin, N.; Herkert, L.M.; D'Agostino, J.A.; Hoffman, C.; Peranteau, W.H.; et al. Reduced oxygen concentration for the resuscitation of infants with congenital diaphragmatic hernia. *J. Perinatol.* **2018**, *38*, 834–843. [CrossRef]
14. Torres-Cuevas, I.; Cernada, M.; Nunez, A.; Escobar, J.; Kuligowski, J.; Chafer-Pericas, C.; Vento, M. Oxygen Supplementation to Stabilize Preterm Infants in the Fetal to Neonatal Transition: No Satisfactory Answer. *Front. Pediatr.* **2016**, *4*, 29. [CrossRef] [PubMed]
15. Wilson, A.; Vento, M.; Shah, P.S.; Saugstad, O.; Finer, N.; Rich, W.; Morton, R.L.; Rabi, Y.; Tarnow-Mordi, W.; Suzuki, K.; et al. A review of international clinical practice guidelines for the use of oxygen in the delivery room resuscitation of preterm infants. *Acta Paediatr.* **2018**, *107*, 20–27. [CrossRef] [PubMed]
16. Saugstad, O.D.; Lakshminrusimha, S.; Vento, M. Optimizing Oxygenation of the Extremely Premature Infant during the First Few Minutes of Life: Start Low or High? *J. Pediatrics* **2020**. [CrossRef]
17. Kapadia, V.S.; Chalak, L.F.; Sparks, J.E.; Allen, J.R.; Savani, R.C.; Wyckoff, M.H. Resuscitation of Preterm Neonates With Limited Versus High Oxygen Strategy. *Pediatrics* **2013**. [CrossRef]
18. Sekar, K.; Szyld, E.; McCoy, M.; Wlodaver, A.; Dannaway, D.; Helmbrecht, A.; Riley, J.; Manfredo, A.; Anderson, M.; Lakshminrusimha, S.; et al. Inhaled nitric oxide as an adjunct to neonatal resuscitation in premature infants: A pilot, double blind, randomized controlled trial. *Pediatric Res.* **2020**, *87*, 523–528. [CrossRef] [PubMed]

19. Rabi, Y.; Lodha, A.; Soraisham, A.; Singhal, N.; Barrington, K.; Shah, P.S. Outcomes of preterm infants following the introduction of room air resuscitation. *Resuscitation* **2015**, *96*, 252–259. [CrossRef]
20. Rudolph, A.M. *Congenital Diseases of the Heart: Clinical-Physiological Considerations*, 3rd ed.; John Wiley and Sons Ltd.: West Sussex, UK, 2009.
21. Vali, P.; Lakshminrusimha, S. The Fetus Can Teach Us: Oxygen and the Pulmonary Vasculature. *Children* **2017**, *4*, 67. [CrossRef]
22. Rudolph, A.M.; Yuan, S. Response of the pulmonary vasculature to hypoxia and H+ ion concentration changes. *J. Clin. Investig.* **1966**, *45*, 399–411. [CrossRef] [PubMed]
23. Lakshminrusimha, S.; Konduri, G.G.; Steinhorn, R.H. Considerations in the management of hypoxemic respiratory failure and persistent pulmonary hypertension in term and late preterm neonates. *J. Perinatol. Off. J. Calif. Perinat. Assoc.* **2016**, *36* (Suppl. 2), S12–S19. [CrossRef] [PubMed]
24. The Neonatal Inhaled Nitric Oxide Study Group, N. Inhaled nitric oxide and hypoxic respiratory failure in infants with congenital diaphragmatic hernia. The Neonatal Inhaled Nitric Oxide Study Group (NINOS). *Pediatrics* **1997**, *99*, 838–845.
25. Auten, R.L.; Davis, J.M. Oxygen toxicity and reactive oxygen species: The devil is in the details. *Pediatr. Res.* **2009**, *66*, 121–127. [CrossRef] [PubMed]
26. Richmond, S.; Goldsmith, J.P. Air or 100% oxygen in neonatal resuscitation? *Clin. Perinatol.* **2006**, *33*, 11–27. [CrossRef] [PubMed]
27. Buonocore, G.; Perrone, S.; Tataranno, M.L. Oxygen toxicity: Chemistry and biology of reactive oxygen species. *Semin. Fetal Neonatal Med.* **2010**, *15*, 186–190. [CrossRef]
28. Solberg, R.; Andresen, J.H.; Escrig, R.; Vento, M.; Saugstad, O.D. Resuscitation of hypoxic newborn piglets with oxygen induces a dose-dependent increase in markers of oxidation. *Pediatr. Res.* **2007**, *62*, 559–563. [CrossRef]
29. Lakshminrusimha, S.; Russell, J.A.; Steinhorn, R.H.; Ryan, R.M.; Gugino, S.F.; Morin, F.C., 3rd; Swartz, D.D.; Kumar, V.H. Pulmonary arterial contractility in neonatal lambs increases with 100% oxygen resuscitation. *Pediatr. Res.* **2006**, *59*, 137–141. [CrossRef]
30. Lorente-Pozo, S.; Parra-Llorca, A.; Lara-Canton, I.; Solaz, A.; Garcia-Jimenez, J.L.; Pallardo, F.V.; Vento, M. Oxygen in the neonatal period: Oxidative stress, oxygen load and epigenetic changes. *Semin. Fetal Neonatal Med.* **2020**, *25*, 101090. [CrossRef]
31. Vali, P.; Vento, M.; Underwood, M.; Lakshminrusimha, S. Free radical damage can cause serious long-lasting effects. *Acta Paediatr.* **2018**. [CrossRef]
32. Kumar, P. Use of inhaled nitric oxide in preterm infants. *Pediatrics* **2014**, *133*, 164–170. [CrossRef] [PubMed]
33. Finer, N.N.; Evans, N. Inhaled nitric oxide for the preterm infant: Evidence versus practice. *Pediatrics* **2015**, *135*, 754–756. [CrossRef] [PubMed]
34. Ellsworth, K.R.; Ellsworth, M.A.; Weaver, A.L.; Mara, K.C.; Clark, R.H.; Carey, W.A. Association of Early Inhaled Nitric Oxide With the Survival of Preterm Neonates With Pulmonary Hypoplasia. *JAMA Pediatr.* **2018**, *172*, e180761. [CrossRef] [PubMed]
35. Manja, V.; Guyatt, G.; Lakshminrusimha, S.; Jack, S.; Kirpalani, H.; Zupancic, J.A.F.; Dukhovny, D.; You, J.J.; Monteiro, S. Factors influencing decision making in neonatology: Inhaled nitric oxide in preterm infants. *J. Perinatol. Off. J. Calif. Perinat. Assoc.* **2018**. [CrossRef] [PubMed]
36. Dixon, F.; Ziegler, D.S.; Bajuk, B.; Wright, I.; Hilder, L.; Abdel Latif, M.E.; Somanathan, A.; Oei, J.L. Treatment with nitric oxide in the neonatal intensive care unit is associated with increased risk of childhood cancer. *Acta Paediatr.* **2018**, *107*, 2092–2098. [CrossRef]
37. Vento, M.; Sanchez-Illana, A. Nitric oxide and preterm resuscitation: Some words of caution. *Pediatr. Res.* **2020**, *87*, 438–440. [CrossRef]
38. Lakshminrusimha, S.; Manja, V.; Mathew, B.; Suresh, G.K. Oxygen targeting in preterm infants: A physiological interpretation. *J. Perinatol. Off. J. Calif. Perinat. Assoc.* **2015**, *35*, 8–15. [CrossRef]
39. Alcorn, D.G.; Adamson, T.M.; Maloney, J.E.; Robinson, P.M. A morphologic and morphometric analysis of fetal lung development in the sheep. *Anat. Rec.* **1981**, *201*, 655–667. [CrossRef]
40. Eyal, F.G.; Hachey, W.E.; Curtet-Eyal, N.L.; Kellum, F.E.; Alpan, G. Effect of modulators of hypoxic pulmonary vasoconstriction on the response to inhaled nitric oxide in a neonatal model of severe pulmonary atelectasis. *Semin. Perinatol.* **1996**, *20*, 186–193. [CrossRef]
41. Booke, M.; Bradford, D.W.; Hinder, F.; Harper, D.; Brauchle, R.W.; Traber, L.D.; Traber, D.L. Effects of inhaled nitric oxide and nebulized prostacyclin on hypoxic pulmonary vasoconstriction in anesthetized sheep. *Crit. Care Med.* **1996**, *24*, 1841–1848. [CrossRef]
42. Fike, C.D.; Hansen, T.N. The effect of alkalosis on hypoxia-induced pulmonary vasoconstriction in lungs of newborn rabbits. *Pediatr. Res.* **1989**, *25*, 383–388. [CrossRef] [PubMed]
43. Kirpalani, H.; Ratcliffe, S.J.; Keszler, M.; Davis, P.G.; Foglia, E.E.; Te Pas, A.; Fernando, M.; Chaudhary, A.; Localio, R.; van Kaam, A.H.; et al. Effect of Sustained Inflations vs Intermittent Positive Pressure Ventilation on Bronchopulmonary Dysplasia or Death Among Extremely Preterm Infants: The SAIL Randomized Clinical Trial. *JAMA J. Am. Med. Assoc.* **2019**, *321*, 1165–1175. [CrossRef] [PubMed]

Article

Mechanical Ventilation, Partial Pressure of Carbon Dioxide, Increased Fraction of Inspired Oxygen and the Increased Risk for Adverse Short-Term Outcomes in Cooled Asphyxiated Newborns

Stamatios Giannakis [1], Maria Ruhfus [2], Mona Markus [1], Anja Stein [2], Thomas Hoehn [1], Ursula Felderhoff-Mueser [2] and Hemmen Sabir [2,3,4,*]

[1] Department of General Pediatrics, Neonatology and Pediatric Cardiology, Faculty of Medicine, University Children's Hospital, Heinrich-Heine-University Duesseldorf, 40225 Düsseldorf, Germany; stamatios.giannakis@gmail.com (S.G.); mona.markus@hotmail.de (M.M.); Thomas.Hoehn@med.uni-duesseldorf.de (T.H.)

[2] Department of Pediatrics I/Neonatology, University Hospital Essen, University Duisburg Essen, 45147 Essen, Germany; maria.ruhfus@gmail.com (M.R.); Anja.Stein@uk-essen.de (A.S.); Ursula.Felderhoff@uk-essen.de (U.F.-M.)

[3] Department of Neonatology and Pediatric Intensive Care, Children's Hospital University of Bonn, 53127 Bonn, Germany

[4] German Centre for Neurodegenerative Diseases (DZNE), 53127 Bonn, Germany

* Correspondence: Hemmen.Sabir@ukbonn.de

Abstract: Neonates treated with therapeutic hypothermia (TH) following perinatal asphyxia (PA) suffer a considerable rate of disability and mortality. Several risk factors associated with adverse outcomes have been identified. Mechanical ventilation might increase the risk for hyperoxia and hypocapnia in cooled newborns. We carried out a retrospective study in 71 asphyxiated cooled newborns. We analyzed the association of ventilation status and adverse short-term outcomes and investigated the effect of the former on pCO_2 and oxygen delivery before, during and after TH. Death, abnormal findings on magnetic resonance imaging, and pathological amplitude-integrated electroencephalography traces were used to define short-term outcomes. The need for mechanical ventilation was significantly higher in the newborns with adverse outcomes (38% vs. 5.6%, $p = 0.001$). Compared to spontaneously breathing neonates, intubated newborns suffered from significantly more severe asphyxia, had significantly lower levels of mean minimum pCO_2 over the first 6 and 72 h of life (HOL) ($p = 0.03$ and $p = 0.01$, respectively) and increased supply of inspired oxygen, which was, in turn, significantly higher in the newborns with adverse outcomes ($p < 0.01$). Intubated newborns with adverse short-term outcomes had lower levels of pCO_2 over the first 36 HOL. In conclusion, need for mechanical ventilation was significantly higher in newborns with more severe asphyxia. In ventilated newborns, level of encephalopathy, lower pCO_2 levels, and increased oxygen supplementation were significantly higher in the adverse short-term outcomes group. Ventilatory parameters need to be carefully monitored in cooled asphyxiated newborns.

Keywords: perinatal asphyxia; hypoxic–ischemic encephalopathy; therapeutic hypothermia; outcome; hypocapnia; hyperoxia; mechanical ventilation

1. Introduction

Despite all advances in perinatal care, perinatal asphyxia (PA) remains a serious condition that can lead to hypoxic–ischemic encephalopathy (HIE) in preterm and term neonates. HIE is associated with early neurodevelopmental impairment (e.g., seizures, childhood epilepsy, cerebral palsy) and high mortality rates [1]. To date, therapeutic hypothermia (TH) remains the only established treatment improving neurodevelopmental outcomes in near-term and term infants with moderate to severe HIE, although around

30% of the cooled infants, included in recent randomized controlled trials, died or suffered from long-term neurodevelopmental impairment [2].

In acute phase of brain injury due to PA, brain homeostasis is impaired due to abrupt reduction of cerebral blood flow (CBF), which reduces the sufficient delivery of oxygen and high-energy metabolites to neurons, leading to cell depolarization and cytotoxic edema (primary cell death) [3]. The acute insult is followed by a reperfusion phase with normalization of CBF and recovery of cell swelling and cerebral oxidative metabolism [4]. A latent phase with slightly reduced CBF [5,6] lasting over about six hours may then be followed by a secondary deterioration (6–16 h) with secondary cell death, seizures, and failure of oxidative metabolism [7–9].

The reduction of cerebral metabolic rate due to brain impairment following HIE leads to a reduction of CBF and consecutively to a reduction of the endogenous carbon dioxide (CO_2)-production in the brain predisposing to hypocapnia [10]. Additionally, TH similarly reduces the cerebral metabolic rate and might as well predispose the asphyxiated newborn to hypocapnia [11]. The body's physiological response to severe acidosis is an increase of ventilatory rate, also predisposing to hypocapnia. However, it is not known yet whether this "physiological hypocapnia" is beneficial or should be avoided in cooled asphyxiated newborns. Furthermore, frequently observed symptoms in asphyxiated newborns, such as delayed initiation of spontaneous breathing, respiratory depression, pulmonary hypertension, and seizures often necessitate mechanical ventilation (in >60% of asphyxiated term newborns), increasing the risk of high oxygen supplementation and hyperventilation with subsequent hypocapnia [12–16]. This high incidence of hypocapnia among asphyxiated neonates has been associated with adverse neurodevelopmental outcomes both in non-cooled [17,18] and cooled near-term and term asphyxiated newborns with HIE [18,19]. However, it is unclear whether all cooled asphyxiated newborns do require mechanical ventilation in all instances.

Lower levels of carbon dioxide have the potential to exacerbate the brain injury caused by PA by further reducing CBF due to cerebral vasoconstriction and by decreasing the oxygen supply due to the leftward shift of the oxygen–hemoglobin dissociation curve [20]. While the decreased CBF can be tolerated by healthy term infants, it could harm the previously injured brain, causing cell death due to the diminished oxygen delivery [21]. In pre-clinical animal models of HIE, hypocapnia results also in DNA fragmentation and membrane lipid peroxidation in mitochondria of cerebral cortical neurons and may result in apoptotic cell death [22].

Furthermore, a brief exposure to hyperoxia depletes the glial progenitor pool and impairs functional recovery of the brain after hypoxia–ischemia by increasing the oxidative stress and the cerebral inflammatory response [23]. Resuscitation with room air has been shown to reduce mortality in preterm and term newborns compared to resuscitation using 100% oxygen, highlighting the importance of oxygen toxicity [24].

The aim of this current study was to describe the rate of mechanical ventilation in cooled asphyxiated newborns with HIE in association with short-term outcomes. Furthermore, we aimed to correlate the rates of partial pressure of carbon dioxide (pCO_2), it's differential pressures (ΔpCO_2) and the increased O_2-supply in ventilated cooled asphyxiated newborns in comparison to non-ventilated cooled asphyxiated newborns. Additionally, we evaluated the association of low and high pCO_2 and fraction of inspired oxygen (FiO_2) levels and adverse short-term outcomes during the first days of life in the ventilated cooled asphyxiated newborns. Moreover, we compared the short-term outcomes between the intubated cooled asphyxiated newborns with pCO_2 levels under 30 mmHg or $FiO_2 > 60\%$ and the rest of the cohort.

2. Materials and Methods

2.1. Data Collection

We performed a retrospective data analysis. Data of cooled asphyxiated newborns from two level I (highest level of care) neonatal intensive care units (NICUs) were collected.

Ethical approval was obtained from the local hospital ethic committees (19-8556-BO, 18-8191-BO, 2018-270-ProspDEuA, 2018-270-1). The infants were born between 2009 and 2018 and met the institutions' inclusion criteria for therapeutic hypothermia:

A. Gestational age $\geq 36^{+0}$ weeks, ≤ 6 h of life (HOL) AND
B. Cord/arterial pH ≤ 7.0 OR base excess ≤ -16 in the first sixty minutes of life OR APGAR-Score ≤ 5 AND/OR continued need for resuscitation at 10 min of life (criteria of perinatal asphyxia) AND
C. Evidence of moderate-to-severe encephalopathy [25] OR
D. Abnormalities on amplitude-integrated electroencephalography (aEEG) for at least 20 min or clinical and/or aEEG-defined seizures [26]

Seventy-one ($n = 71$) term newborns were assigned to whole-body hypothermia (core temperature of 33–34 °C) for 72 h starting within the first 6 HOL followed by a rewarming phase at a rate of 0.5 °C per hour. The treatment protocols of the two NICUs were similar. Twenty-three ($n = 23$) newborns were born at ($n = 14$) or transferred to ($n = 9$) the first NICU (University Hospital Duesseldorf, Germany) and forty-eight ($n = 48$) newborns were born at ($n = 29$) or transferred to ($n = 19$) the second NICU (University Hospital Essen, Germany). Demographic details and clinical data were collected for each newborn according to medical notes including birth weight, gender, gestational age, birth place (inborn/outborn), APGAR scores at 5 and 10 min, first pH, bases excess and lactate before initiation of TH, need for resuscitation at birth, Sarnat HIE grade, initial temperature before starting TH, aEEG time to normal trace, onset of clinical or subclinical seizures, signs of meconium aspiration, minimum blood glucose levels in the first 6 and 72 HOL, need for mechanical ventilation, cumulative morphine dose needed until discharge from hospital, survival, need for inotropic support before and during TH, duration of O_2-supplementation, and highest FiO_2 levels within the first 6 and 72 HOL.

Additionally, we collected data regarding respiratory monitoring before and after the initiation of TH until the end of rewarming. This included arterial, capillary, and venous blood gases, which were corrected for temperature during TH, lowest pCO_2 (minimum pCO_2), highest pCO_2 (maximum pCO_2) and ΔpCO_2 during the first 6 and 72 HOL as well as minimum and maximum pCO_2 levels every 6 h after initiation of TH until 6 h after rewarming. The mode of ventilation (intubated vs. not intubated), duration of mechanical ventilation, as well as average and maximal oxygen supplementation (measured as mean and maximum FiO_2 levels hourly) were also collected and analyzed. The indications for intubation and extubation were individually assessed from the neonatologists on duty and according to the International Liaison Committee on Resuscitation (ILCOR) recommendations for newborn resuscitation.

2.2. Outcome Definition

Adverse outcomes were defined as death or adverse magnetic resonance imaging (MRI) outcome. The original MRI-images (T1 and T2 weighted images) were evaluated by three independent individuals blinded to the clinical information. The basal ganglia/watershed score (BG/W score) developed by Barkovich defines MRI outcomes depending on severity and location of brain injury (1 = no injury, 2 = mild injury, 3 = moderate injury, 4 = severe injury) and discriminates accurately between asphyxiated newborns with good and poor neuromotor and cognitive outcomes at 3 and 12 months [27]. A recent study shows that this still holds true in the cooling-era with strong correlation of the BG/W score with long-term neurodevelopmental outcomes at 20–24 months of age [28]. For our study, the MRI outcomes were defined as good when the BG/W score was <2 and as adverse when the BG/W score was >2. MRI was available for 60/71 of the newborns in the cohort; 6 out of 9 newborns who died didn't have one before death. For the other 5 newborns without MRI scans, we used aEEG as an outcome predictor, which has been shown to be a good prognostic outcome parameter and correlates well with MRI outcomes in cooled asphyxiated newborns [29–31].

In both NICUs single-use needle electrodes (positions equal to C3-P3, C4-P4 of a standard EEG) were applied to record biparietal aEEG signal. Continuous recording was established after postnatal clinical stabilization and before initiation of TH until the end of the rewarming phase (Brainz or Olympic Brainz Monitor, Natus, San Carlos, CA, USA). Three independent individuals blinded to the clinical information evaluated the aEEG traces retrospectively. The aEEG background pattern was classified as previously described [32], with continuous normal voltage (CNV) and discontinuous normal voltage (DNV) as normal patterns and burst suppression (BS), low voltage (LV), and flat trace as pathological patterns. Normal aEEG was defined as a time of under 48 h taken to reach a normal aEEG trace after the initiation of TH [32], and aEEG was scored as pathological when seizures were detected.

2.3. Data Analysis

SPSS 26 (SPSS, Chicago, IL, USA) was used for statistical analysis. Mann–Whitney was used to compare non-parametric data between two groups (intubated versus non-intubated and good versus adverse short-term outcomes in the intubated group). Descriptive data are presented as median and interquartile range (IQR) for continuous variables and as frequency distributions for categorical variables. Categorical variables were compared using a Chi-square test. In the intubated cooled newborns, multivariate analysis using stepwise binary logistic regression was performed with good or adverse outcomes as the dependent variable. Independent variables were APGAR scores at 5 and 10 min, first pH, severity of encephalopathy, seizures (yes/no), aEEG time to normal trace, lowest pCO_2 (minimum pCO_2), highest pCO_2 (maximum pCO_2) and ΔpCO_2 during the first 6 and 72 HOL, and highest FiO_2 levels within the first 6 and 72 HOL.

To avoid calculating the high levels of pCO_2 in the cord gas and/or the first blood gases and the high oxygen supplementation during resuscitation, we used the trapezium rule to calculate the area under the curve (AUC) for pCO_2 and FiO_2 for the first HOL until the end of the rewarming phase [33]. $p \leq 0.05$ was considered significant. Parts of the results from this cohort have already been published [31].

3. Results

Seventy-one (n = 71) cooled asphyxiated newborns $\geq$36 + 0 weeks of gestation were included in our study; thirty-four (47.9%) were males and thirty-seven (52.1%) were females. Fifty-three (74.6%) had a good and eighteen (25.4%) had an adverse short-term outcome (defined as death (n = 9) or an adverse MRI outcome or pathological aEEG when MRI was not available) despite TH. As previously shown, there is a strong correlation between aEEG and MRI outcome in our cohort [31].

Fifty-three (74.6%) of the newborns were intubated and mechanically ventilated based on the neonatologist's discretion on duty. All of these newborns were intubated before initiation of TH within the first HOL and the mean ($\pm$SD) duration of mechanical ventilation was 91.8 ($\pm$86) h. The spontaneously breathing newborns (n = 18, 25.6%) were all respiratory-supported with continuous positive airway pressure (CPAP) or high-flow nasal cannula (HFNC). The need for mechanical ventilation was significantly correlated with adverse short-term outcomes (38% vs. 5.6%, p = 0.001).

Comparing the intubated and non-intubated cooled asphyxiated newborns, we found no significant differences between the two groups regarding birth weight, gestational age, first lactate level, time to initiation of therapeutic hypothermia, and time to target temperature. In our study neither lowest blood glucose levels within the first 72 HOL nor duration of morphine application impacted short-term outcomes (Table 1). However, we found that the APGAR scores at 5 and 10 min, as well as the cord or arterial pH and base excess values after birth were significantly lower in the intubated newborns who were treated with TH (p < 0.05). This is also reflected by the increased need for resuscitation in this group in comparison to the spontaneously breathing newborns (62.3% vs. 11.1%, p < 0.01). The first temperature measured after birth was significantly lower in newborns who needed mechanical ventilation ($p = 0.01$) and the severity of the Sarnat HIE grade was higher in the intubated group in comparison to the spontaneously breathing newborns ($p < 0.01$). We also found that the mechanically ventilated asphyxiated newborns had significantly lower levels of blood glucose in the first 6 HOL but these did not exceed the limits for hypoglycemia (<45 mg/dL). As expected, the need for ventilation required also significantly higher cumulative doses of morphine, and resulted in longer and higher oxygen supplementation ($p < 0.05$, Table 1). In addition, median (IQR) AUC mean and maximum FiO_2 values were higher in mechanically ventilated newborns (0.21 (0.21–0.24) vs. 0.21 (0.21–0.21)%, and 0.23 (0.21–0.29) vs. 0.21 (0.21–0.215)%, $p = 0.06$ and $p < 0.01$, respectively).

Table 1. Descriptive data of the analyzed cohort according to ventilation status (mechanically ventilated or not) before the start of therapeutic hypothermia (TH). Data are presented as median and interquartile range (IQR).

Clinical Characteristics	Intubated ($n = 53$)	Non-Intubated ($n = 18$)	p-Value
Birth weight (g), median (IQR)	3265 (2845–3840)	3070 (2722.5–3545)	0.09
Male gender, n (%)	30 (56.6%)	4 (22.2%)	<0.01
Gestational age in weeks, median (IQR)	39^{+6} (37^{+5}–40^{+4})	38^{+6} (37^{+1}–39^{+6})	0.12
APGAR score			
5 min, median (min, max)	4 (0–10)	5 (2–9)	0.03
10 min, median (min, max)	6 (0–10)	7 (4–10)	<0.01
First pH, median (IQR)	6.81 (6.68–6.93)	6.93 (6.85–6.98)	<0.01
First base excess (mmol/L), median (IQR)	22.15 (16.6–27)	18 (14.2–22)	<0.01
First lactate level (mmol/L), median (IQR)	12.7 (8.7–17)	10.95 (8.52–13.08)	0.11
HIE grade before cooling (n = mild, n = moderate, n = severe)	7, 22, 21	11, 5, 0	<0.01
Inborn, n (%)	29 (54.7%)	14 (77.8%)	0.03
Resuscitation at birth, n (%)	33 (62.3%)	2 (11.1%)	<0.01
Short-term adverse outcome	17 (32.1%)	1 (5.6%)	<0.01
Death, n (%)	9 (17.0%)	0 (0%)	<0.01
Initial temperature (°C) before start of TH, median (IQR)	35.5 (34.2–36.9)	36.1 (35.8–36.4)	0.01
Time (minutes) until start of TH, median (IQR)	37.5 (10–73.7)	30 (10–105)	0.50
Time (minutes) to target temperature, median (IQR)	120 (60–170)	120 (60–127.5)	0.37
EEG time (minutes) to normal trace, median (IQR)	13 (1–57)	1 (1–4.5)	<0.01
Lowest blood glucose levels (mg/dL)			
first 6 HOL, median (IQR)	81 (60–127)	68 (62.75–77.5)	0.04
first 72 HOL, median (IQR)	63 (48–77.5)	60 (48.5–68.5)	0.08
Morphine			
duration (hours), median (IQR)	72 (65–92)	72 (64–76)	0.09
cumulative dose (µg/kg/d), median (IQR)	0.6 (0.3–1.15)	0.25 (0.18–0.42)	<0.01
Inotropic support, n (%)	33 (62.3%)	4 (22.2%)	<0.01
Oxygen supplementation			
duration (minutes), median (IQR)	24 (8–102)	25 (0–3.25)	<0.01
highest FiO_2(%) × 100			
first 6 HOL, median (IQR)	80 (40–100)	21 (21–58)	0.01
first 72 HOL, median (IQR)	80 (48–100)	21 (21–58)	<0.01
Area under the curve (AUC) FiO_2(%) × 100 over 78 h			
maximum FiO_2, median (IQR)	23.6 (21.3–29.6)	21 (21–21.5)	<0.01
mean FiO_2, median (IQR)	21.6 (21–24)	21 (21–21)	0.06
AUC pCO_2 over 78 h			
maximum pCO_2, median (IQR)	42.6 (38.8–45.5)	45.7 (41.4–50.6)	0.03
minimum pCO_2, median (IQR)	46.7 (44.1–53.5)	47.5 (41.7–54.9)	0.29
ΔpCO_2 in mmHg			
first 6 HOL, median (IQR)	44.0 (15–74.3)	37.4 (27.7–58.75)	0.14
first 72 HOL, median (IQR)	55.1 (30.3–79.4)	43.7 (31.8–57.8)	0.03

We further analyzed the intubated group ($n = 53$) separately. We found that among cooled newborns who needed mechanical ventilation, the short-term outcomes were good in 36 (67.9%) vs. 17 (32.1%) with adverse outcomes. In intubated cooled newborns, the baseline characteristics (gender, gestational age, birth weight, birth place, first base excess and lactate levels, need for resuscitation at birth, meconium aspiration, initial temperature measured, as well as time to start TH and time to target temperature, lowest blood glucose levels at 6 and 72 HOL, cumulative dose of morphine, need for inotropes, duration of inspired oxygen and AUC mean and maximum FiO$_2$ values) were not significantly different between the groups with normal vs. adverse outcomes (Table 2). Intubated newborns with good short-term outcomes had significantly higher APGAR scores at the 5th and 10th minute and higher cord or arterial pH values ($p < 0.05$). The severity of hypoxic–ischemic encephalopathy was significantly lower in the intubated newborns with good short-term outcomes ($p < 0.001$). Seizures and longer time (minutes) to normal trace of the amplitude-integrated EEG (73 (2–300) vs. 12 (1–23)) were significantly different in newborns with adverse short-term outcomes ($p < 0.05$). Intubated newborns with adverse outcomes received higher maximum FiO$_2$ during the first 6 ($p = 0.01$) and 72 ($p = 0.05$) HOL.

Table 2. Descriptive data of the intubated cooled asphyxiated neonates according to short-term outcome. Data are presented as median and IQR.

Clinical Characteristics	Good Short-Term Outcomes ($n = 36$)	Adverse Short-Term Outcomes * ($n = 17$)	p-Value
Birth weight (g), median (IQR)	3212.5 (2827.5–3855)	3300 (2775–3827.5)	0.40
Male gender, n (%)	22 (61.1%)	8 (47.1%)	0.18
Gestational age (weeks), median (IQR)	38+6 (37 + 1–40 + 4)	40+2 (38 + 5–40 + 6)	0.07
APGAR score			
5 min, median (min, max)	5 (0–10)	2 (0–6)	<0.01
10 min, median (min, max)	7 (1–10)	4 (0–7)	<0.01
First pH, median (IQR)	6.85 (6.78–6.95)	6.8 (6.6–6.92)	0.03
First base excess (mmol/L), median (IQR)	21.8 (16.6–25.1)	23 (16.35–29.6)	0.27
First lactate level (mmol/L), median (IQR)	12.2 (7.65–17)	13.5 (11.2–19)	0.11
HIE grade before cooling (n = mild, n = moderate, n = severe)	7, 18, 9	0, 4, 12	<0.01
Inborn, n (%)	18 (50.0%)	11 (64.7%)	0.16
Resuscitation at birth, n (%)	20 (55.6%)	13 (76.5%)	0.08
Meconium aspiration, n (%)	8 (22.2%)	8 (47.1%)	0.15
Seizures, n (%)	15 (41.7%)	14 (82.4)	<0.01
Initial temperature (°C) before Start TH, median (IQR)	35.65 (34.1–37)	35.15 (34.3–36.5)	0.46
Time (minutes) until Start TH, median (IQR)	45 (10–77.5)	20 (10–71.3)	0.14
Time (minutes) to target temperature, median (IQR)	105 (52.5–150)	135 (60–183.5)	0.24
EEG time (minutes) to normal trace, median (IQR)	12 (1–23)	73 (2–300)	<0.01
Minimum blood glucose levels (mg/dL)			
first 6 HOL median (IQR)	77 (50–113)	86 (72–155)	0.25
first 72 HOL, median (IQR)	60 (45–79)	66 (50.3–74.8)	0.18
Morphine			
duration (hours), median (IQR)	79.5 (72–96)	67 (35–72)	<0.01
Cumulative dose (µg/kg/d), median (IQR)	0.61 (0.34–1.47)	0.42 (0.25–0.8)	0.43
Inotropic support, n (%)	22 (61.1%)	11 (64.7%)	0.39
Oxygen supplementation duration (minutes), median (IQR)	31.5 (3.75–106.5)	24 (11–88)	0.26
highest FiO$_2$(%) × 100			
first 6 HOL, median (IQR)	60 (30–100)	80 (30–100)	0.01
first 72 HOL, median (IQR)	95 (68–100)	90 (67–100)	0.05
Area under the curve (AUC) FiO$_2$(%) × 100 over 78 h			
maximum FiO$_2$, median (IQR)	22.6 (21.2–28.3)	26.2 (23.6–37.2)	0.46
mean FiO$_2$, median (IQR)	21.8 (21–23.9)	24.3 (21.6–32.8)	0.37
AUC pCO$_2$ (mmHg) over 78 h			
maximum pCO$_2$, median (IQR)	46.1 (43.6–50)	50 (45.5–55.9)	0.049
minimum pCO$_2$, median (IQR)	42.6 (39.6–45.5)	42.4 (37.1–46.0)	0.20
ΔpCO$_2$ in mmHg			
first 6 HOL, median (IQR)	25.9 (14.4–63.9)	70.2 (40.9–101.3)	<0.01
first 72 HOL, median (IQR)	41.0 (29.2–76.8)	66.3 (55.1–98.7)	0.01

* Adverse short-term outcomes defined as death ($n = 9$) or severe brain damage using magnetic resonance imaging (MRI, $n = 7$) or pathological amplitude-integrated EEG (aEEG) traces ($n = 1$) when MRI-data not available.

Evaluating significant differences of pCO$_2$ levels and short-term outcomes among all neonates included in the study, we found that the mean (±SD) minimum pCO$_2$ levels were lower within the first 6 and 72 HOL among newborns with adverse short-term outcomes (34.6 ± 12.6 vs. 31 ± 11.4 mmHg and 30.6 ± 9.3 vs. 26.4 ± 8.5 mmHg, $p = 0.15$ and $p = 0.05$, respectively) (Figure 1a). Interestingly, mean (±SD) maximum pCO$_2$ within the first 6 and

72 HOL (92.7 ± 36 vs. 69.7 ± 27.9 mmHg and 97.1 ± 30.1 vs. 78.1 ± 22.8 mmHg) was significantly higher ($p = 0.02$ and $p = 0.03$, respectively) in the adverse short-term outcome group (Figure 1a). In addition, higher median ΔpCO_2 (IQR), over the first 6 and 72 HOL was significantly associated with adverse short-term outcomes (31 (13.9–60.1) vs. 66.3 (39.9–98.7) mmHg and 41.0 (29.8–70.8) vs. 62.8 (44–97.6) mmHg), $p < 0.01$, respectively).

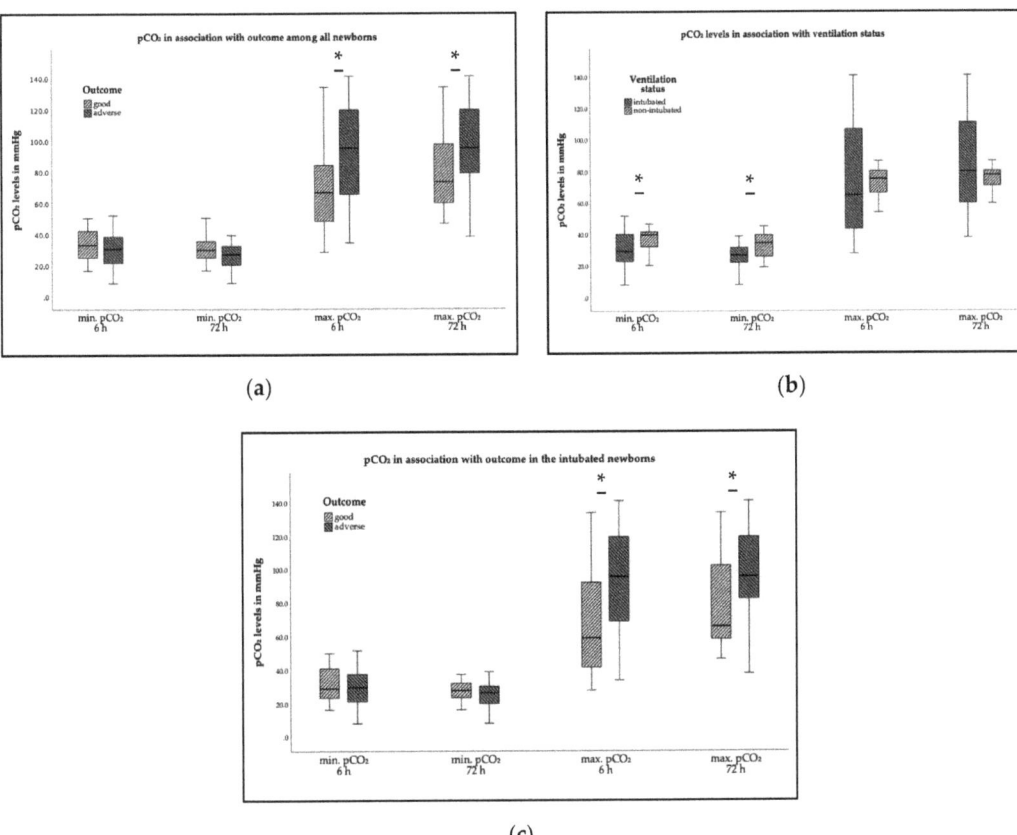

Figure 1. Box and whiskers plot representations. Minimum and maximum pCO_2 over the first 6 and 72 h of life (HOL): (a) in association with adverse outcomes among all included cooled asphyxiated neonates, (b) in association with ventilation status, and (c) in association with adverse outcomes in the group of intubated newborns. * $p < 0.05$.

Mean (±SD) minimum pCO_2 was significantly lower in intubated newborns during the first 6 and 72 HOL vs. spontaneously breathing neonates (32.3 ± 13.4 vs. 37.4 ± 8.3 mmHg and 28.1 ± 9.4 vs. 33.4 ± 7.9 mmHg, $p = 0.03$ and $p = 0.01$, respectively, Figure 1b). This also holds true when analyzing mean minimum pCO_2 every 6 h especially for the first 24 HOL (Figure 2a). Thirty ($n = 30$) intubated newborns had a pCO_2 level under 30 mmHg at least once over the first 72 h with the lowest level being 8.4 mmHg in comparison to the non-ventilated newborns, where only five ($n = 5$) had a pCO_2 under 30 mmHg with the lowest level being 19.4 mmHg. Intubated newborns with pCO_2 <30 mmHg were more likely to have adverse short-term outcomes compared to the rest of cohort ($p = 0.037$), while all the spontaneously breathing newborns with pCO_2 <30 mmHg had good short-term outcomes. Additionally, median AUC minimum pCO_2 was significantly lower ($p = 0.03$) in mechanically ventilated newborns vs. spontaneously breathing newborns (42.6 (38.8–45.5) vs. 45.7 (41.4–50.6) mmHg).

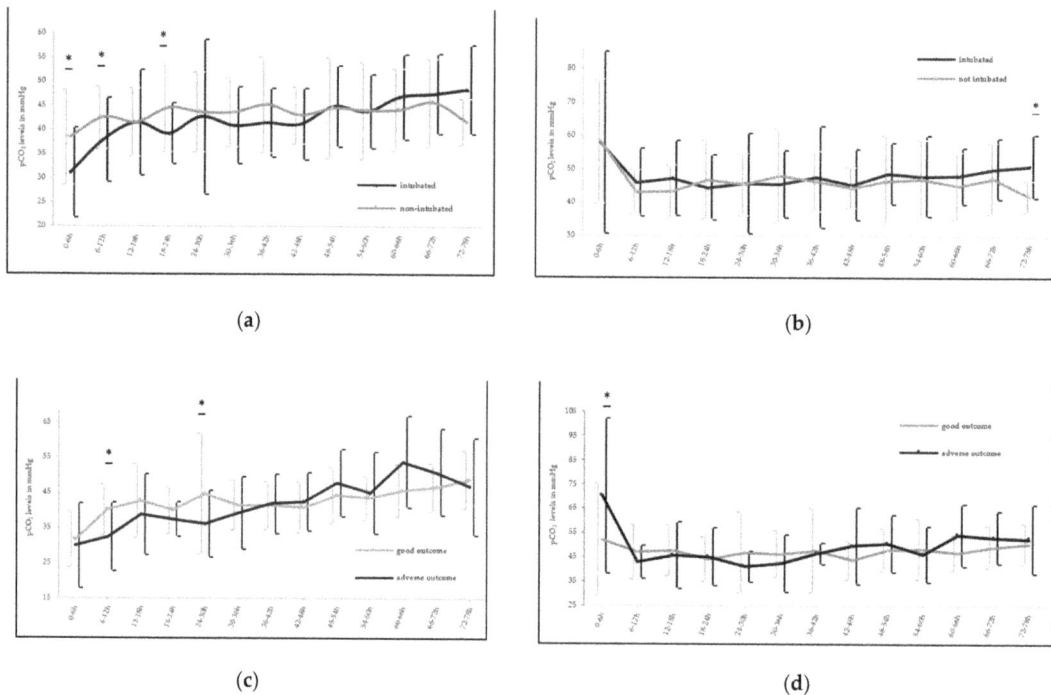

Figure 2. Significant differences between lowest and highest partial pressure of carbon dioxide (minimum and maximum pCO_2) correlated with outcome and ventilation status. Temporal course of minimum (**a**) and maximum pCO_2 (**b**) over the first 78 h after initiation of TH, examined every 6 h, in association with ventilation status and course of minimum (**c**) and maximum pCO_2 (**d**) over the first 78 h after initiation of therapeutic hypothermia (TH) compared to outcomes in the subgroup of intubated newborns. Values are represented as mean ± standard deviation (SD), * $p < 0.05$.

The maximum pCO_2 and AUC maximum pCO_2 during the 72 h of TH were not significantly different within the two groups, except for the first 6 h of the rewarming phase, where the mean (±SD) maximum pCO_2 levels were higher in the mechanically ventilated newborns (50.8 ± 9.4 vs. 41.7 ± 4.7 mmHg, $p < 0.01$, Figure 2b). Twenty-seven ($n = 27$) intubated cooled asphyxiated newborns had maximum pCO_2 levels over 70 mmHg with the maximum pCO_2 level being 140 mmHg during the first 72 HOL while only fourteen ($n = 14$) of the non-ventilated newborns had maximum pCO_2 levels above 70 mmHg, with the highest level being 110 mmHg. Mechanical ventilation was significantly related to higher ΔpCO_2 levels over the first 72 HOL (55.1 (30.3–79.4) vs. 43.7 (31.8–57.8), $p = 0.03$, Table 1). During the whole period of TH (including the 6 h of the rewarming phase) newborns who were intubated received significantly higher oxygen supplementation (measured as mean and maximum FiO_2, $p < 0.05$) as seen in Figure 3a,b. Higher FiO_2 within the first 6 and 72 HOL was also significantly different in the newborns with adverse short-term outcomes ($p < 0.05$, Figure 3e).

Comparing the short-term outcomes among ventilated newborns we found no significant association between mean (±SD) minimum pCO_2 levels in the first 6 and 72 HOL and adverse outcomes (33.1 ± 14.3 vs. 30.5 ± 11.6 and 29.1 ± 9.8 vs. 25.6 ± 8.1 mmHg, $p = 0.25$ and $p = 0.10$ respectively, Figure 1c). However, lower levels were observed over the first 36 HOL and adverse outcomes were significantly higher in the newborns with lower mean (±SD) minimum pCO_2 levels during the hours 6–12 (32.4 ± 9.8 vs. 40.2 ± 7.2 mmHg, $p < 0.01$) and 24–30 (36.2 ± 9.4 vs. 44.7 ± 17.2 mmHg) after initiating TH (Figure 2c). In this subgroup, we also found a significant difference of higher mean (±SD) maximum pCO$_2$ levels during the first 6 (93.6 ± 37.1 vs. 66.8 ± 31.4 mmHg, $p < 0.01$) and 72 HOL (98.3 ± 30.8 vs. 78.1 ± 25.9 mmHg, $p < 0.01$) and adverse short-term outcomes (Figure 1c).

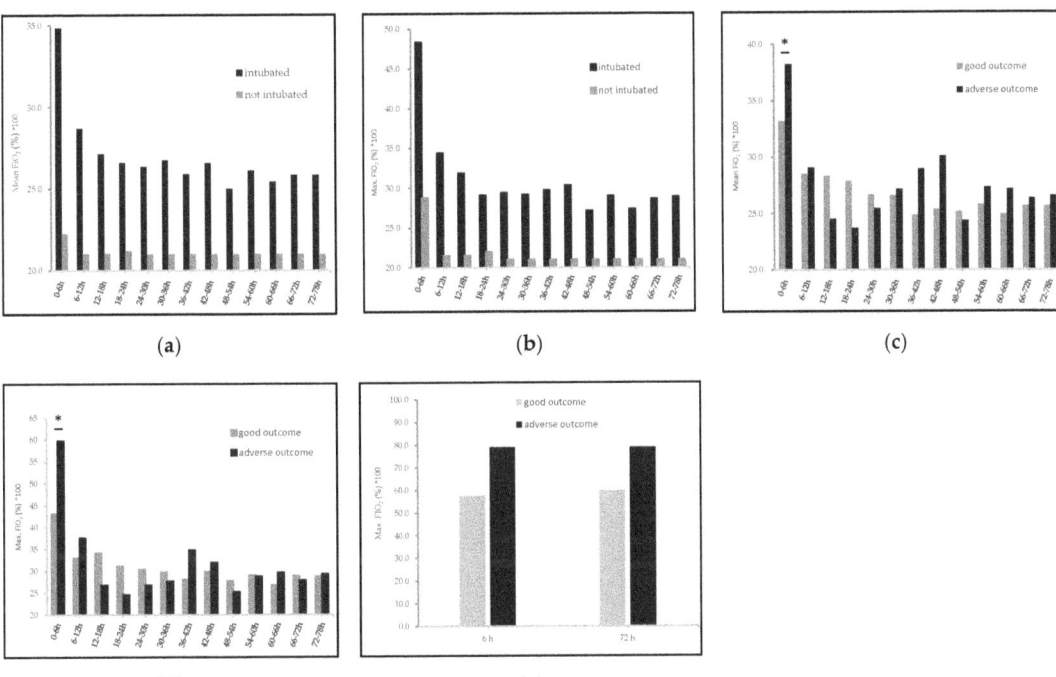

Figure 3. Significant differences of average and highest FiO$_2$ (mean and maximum FiO$_2$) with outcome and ventilation status. Maximum FiO$_2$ over the first 6 and 72 HOL was directly associated with adverse outcomes in the whole study group (e), $p < 0.05$. Mechanically ventilated neonates had significantly higher needs of inspired oxygen, mean (a) and maximum (b) FiO$_2$, during the whole period of TH, $p < 0.05$. Mean (c) and maximum (d) FiO$_2$ were in total not significantly associated with adverse outcomes in the group of intubated newborns after the initiation of TH. Values are represented as mean (±SD), * $p < 0.05$.

The result was strengthened from significantly higher median (IQR) AUC maximum pCO$_2$ levels among intubated newborns with adverse short-term outcomes [50 (45.5–55.9) vs. 46.1 (43.6–50) mmHg, $p < 0.05$]. Higher mean (±SD) maximum pCO$_2$ levels were significantly different in newborns with adverse outcomes only within the first 6 h after initiation of TH (70.2 ± 31.9 mmHg vs. 52.1 ± 23.1 mmHg, $p < 0.05$, Figure 2d). Comparing ΔpCO$_2$ levels over the first 6 and 72 HOL we found significantly larger differences in the group of the mechanical ventilated asphyxiated newborns with unfavorable short-term outcomes (Table 2).

Oxygen supplementation among intubated newborns was not significantly different except for higher FiO$_2$ levels in the first 6 HOL ($p = 0.01$, Table 2) and in the first 6 h after initiation of TH ($p = 0.04$, Figure 3c,d) in newborns with adverse short-term outcome. However, we found that for mechanically ventilated newborns with FiO$_2$ above 0.60 in the first 6 ($n = 30$) and 72 ($n = 33$) HOL adverse short-term outcomes were significantly more likely when compared to neonates with lower oxygen supply ($p < 0.05$).

Regression analysis did not show any significant differences between the good or adverse outcome groups in the ventilated cooled newborns.

4. Discussion

The current study was performed to compare ventilated and non-ventilated cooled asphyxiated newborns in two large NICUs in Germany. We found that there was a significant difference between cooled asphyxiated infants who needed mechanical ventilation after birth and adverse short-term outcomes, in comparison with infants who were not intubated. The need for mechanical ventilation was significantly higher in newborns with more severe asphyxia. In ventilated newborns, level of encephalopathy, lower pCO_2 levels within the first 24 h after birth and increased oxygen supplementation during the cooling period were significantly higher in the adverse short-term outcome group. In addition, higher maximum pCO_2 levels and consequently higher ΔpCO_2 levels were found in ventilated newborns with adverse short-term outcome.

Nadeem et al. showed in a small retrospective cohort study of cooled asphyxiated newborns that there was no association between pCO_2 values and adverse outcome, although only 6 out of 52 infants maintained normocapnia in the first 72 h of life. As in our study severe hypocapnia ($pCO_2 < 20$ mmHg) was documented only in ventilated infants [16]. We previously analyzed data from a cooling cohort in the UK, and also did not find an association between hypocapnia (defined as $pCO_2 < 30$ mmHg) and adverse outcomes in a retrospective study of 61 cooled asphyxiated newborns [34]. In the current study, comparing pCO_2 levels during the cooling period, we found that intubated newborns had significantly lower values of mean minimum pCO_2 during the first 6 and 72 h after birth in comparison to spontaneously breathing infants (Figure 1b). The mean minimum pCO_2 values were significantly lower in the intubated group, particularly in the first 12 HOL and at the end of the first day after initiation of TH (Figure 2a). Intubated newborns with adverse short-term outcomes had lower levels of mean minimum pCO_2 over the first 36 HOL and especially during the hours 6–12 and 24–30 after initiation of TH. Additionally, intubated newborns with pCO_2 levels under 30 mmHg had in general significantly more likely adverse short-term outcomes when compared to the rest of the cohort.

As mentioned in the introduction, the acute insult of PA with reduced CBF is followed by a reperfusion phase with restoration of cerebral circulation and (partial) recovery of the neuronal damage [3,4]. The latent phase is characterized by decreased metabolic rate and reduced CBF with increased tissue oxygenation [6], while the secondary deterioration correlates with an increase in CBF and metabolic demands due to the onset of seizures [5]. These frequent changes in the cerebral circulation highlight the importance of maintaining normocapnia, since CBF of the newborn is very sensitive to variations in pCO_2 levels with a close to exponential relationship. A reduction in pCO_2 of 1 kPa causes a reaction of 25–30% in CBF [35] and reduced CBF leads to cerebral cell death due to reduced cerebral oxygen supply [21]. In our study higher ΔpCO_2 was associated with adverse short-term outcomes and was more frequently noticed among newborns who were mechanically ventilated.

To date, there are several reports showing an association of lower levels of pCO_2 and adverse outcomes, mainly observed within the first HOL [15–19]. Klinger et al. first described the association between unfavorable outcomes and severe hypocapnia and/or severe hyperoxemia in the first 20 to 120 min after birth in non-cooled asphyxiated newborns [17]. Pappas et al. reported also that minimum pCO_2 and cumulative pCO_2 <35 mmHg over the first 12 h of life were significantly associated with unfavorable neurodevelopmental outcomes and higher risk of death, although in the subgroup of the infants treated with TH no significant association was documented [18]. The more recent study of Laporte et al., who evaluated pCO_2 levels over a longer period (0–96 h of life), reported a significant association of brain injury in MRI in term cooled asphyxiated newborns with lower minimum pCO_2 during the first 4 days of life and lower minimum pCO_2 averaged over days 1–4 of life. As also shown in our current study, there was also a significant association of brain impairment with intubation and mechanical ventilation [15].

Our study and the study of Laporte et al. highlight the potential association of mechanical ventilation with adverse outcomes and lower pCO_2 levels, suggesting close monitoring of ventilatory parameters and pCO_2 changes during TH. The tendency to lower pCO_2

levels is also enhanced by the impaired metabolism of the injured brain following perinatal asphyxia and also by the reduction of the metabolic rate with reduced carbon dioxide production in the brain due to TH [10]. Additionally, TH seems to be beneficial for lung mechanics, leading to increased tidal volume and minute ventilation [36,37], parameters that could lead to unintentional mechanical hyperventilation and consecutive hypocapnia. Hyperventilation is furthermore exacerbated by a strong respiratory drive to compensate for metabolic acidosis after asphyxia [38]. Although the spontaneously breathing newborns seem to compensate for lower pCO_2 levels as an effect of the high respiratory drive, we believe that mechanically supported hypocapnia has a risk of leading to adverse outcome. Thus, it is essential to monitor ventilatory settings carefully and maintain normal levels of pCO_2 during TH.

In our study, we found a significant difference of maximum pCO_2 levels during the first 6 and 72 HOL and adverse short-term outcomes among all newborns included in our study and in the subgroup of intubated infants. This could be partially explained by the increase of metabolic demands associated with the greater seizure burden during the secondary deterioration 3–16 days after PA [5]. Until now there have been controversial reports about the effects of hypercapnia on the hypoxic–ischemic brain. Vannucci et al. were the first to report in two experimental studies that mild hypercapnia in immature rats with cerebral hypoxia–ischemia could protect from brain damage [39,40]. However, in the following years they showed that extreme hypercapnia could have an aggravating effect on hypoxic–ischemic brain damage [41]. In the already mentioned studies, which examined the levels of pCO_2 in cooled asphyxiated newborns, only three studies compared the maximum levels of pCO_2 in association with adverse outcomes without statistically significant results. Our study is the first to describe this correlation.

The deleterious effects of oxygen in asphyxiated term and preterm infants are also well-established. We and others have previously shown that an FiO_2 above 0.40 within the first 6 HOL and severe hyperoxia ($paO_2 > 200$ mmHg) during the first 20–120 min of life were associated with adverse outcomes in cooled asphyxiated newborns [17,34]. In the current study we show that during the whole period of cooling treatment, newborns, who had higher and longer needs of O_2 supplementation, had significant worse short-term outcomes (Table 1 and Figure 3e). There were also significantly higher maximum levels of FiO_2 in the newborns that needed mechanical ventilation (Figure 3a). In the subgroup of intubated newborns, the ones with higher maximum FiO_2 over the first 6 and 72 HOL (Table 2) and especially during the first 6 h after initiation of TH (Figure 3c,d) had significantly more likely adverse short-term outcomes.

The observation mentioned above can probably be explained by the fact that the acute hypoxic–ischemic event, as well as the reperfusion/reoxygenation phase, are characterized by increased oxidative stress initiated through production of free radicals, leading to delayed cell death and neuronal loss [42–44]. Especially during reperfusion, the production of reactive oxygen species is proportional to oxygen concentration [43]. An additional exposure to hyperoxia, for example due to excessive oxygen delivery in the delivery room as seen in our cohort, might impair the functional recovery of the already compromised brain and lead to increased brain tissue damage due to induction of a cerebral proinflammatory response [23,45]. This is supported by Munkeby et al. who showed an increased brain damage in hypoxemic piglets after resuscitation with 100% oxygen in comparison with ambient air due to increased expression of matrix metalloproteinase (MMP) and production of extracellular glycerol [46]. Saugstad et al. showed later in a metanalysis a significant 31% reduction of neonatal mortality among term newborns resuscitated with room air rather than 100% O_2. Interestingly, there was also a trend of reduction of the grade of HIE severity in newborns who received only room air during resuscitation [47]. In addition to these results, Dalen et al. highlighted that resuscitation with 100% oxygen counteracts the neuroprotective effect of TH in neonatal rats [48]. Although most of the studies compared delivery of 100% oxygen versus room air and not milder differences, as observed in our study, the findings assume that supply of oxygen, especially during the vulnerable phase of reperfusion/reoxygenation, should be used restrictively and should be carefully monitored during resuscitation and the first hours and days of life after PA. Since increased O_2 supplementation is more likely to occur during mechanical ventilation, the routine application of the latter is once again critically questioned.

There are several limitations of this study. Blood-gas samples were a combination of arterial, capillary, and venous samples, since not every infant had an arterial line. This could probably underestimate the true degree of hypocapnia. Since our study was retrospective, we could not collect all desired data, such as partial pressure of oxygen and arterial oxygen saturation, mode of ventilation, ventilation frequencies and pressures, and definite cause or indications for intubation and extubation. These limitations could probably guide further prospective studies regarding respiratory support during therapeutic hypothermia. Additionally, blood gases were collected as clinically indicated and not at predefined times, so fluctuations of pCO_2 between the samples could have been missed. The need for continuous pCO_2 monitoring, as, for example, with transcutaneous CO_2 or end-tidal CO_2 monitoring, to better detect such fluctuations was highlighted by recent studies [15,49]. Technical difficulties and lack of systemic evaluation of these non-invasive techniques in cooled asphyxiated newborns remain unfortunately unsolved until now. Another limitation of this study is that we assessed the association of pCO_2 and FiO_2 levels with short-term outcomes and not with a standardized long-term outcome, such as the Bailey-Scales of infant development. The Barkovich MRI scoring is, however, an adequate scoring system, beside many others, which correlates well also with long-term outcomes until around 2 years of age [28]. Nevertheless, standardized long-term outcome assessments should be mandatory in all cooled asphyxiated newborns, as short-term assessments can never replace long-term neurodevelopmental outcome. Finally, our findings of low pCO_2 levels in intubated newborns with adverse short-term outcomes might also have been supported by the increased severity of acidosis and encephalopathy in this group. Whether the physiological tendency of hyperventilation following severe acidosis does impair brain injury in cooled asphyxiated newborns, or should be tolerated is not known. However, we believe that if newborns are ventilated, ventilatory settings should be carefully adjusted and hyperventilation should be avoided. Our study had a small sample size, which limits the statistical power to analyze subgroups. Unfortunately, the German Neonatal Hypothermia Registry does not register data regarding ventilatory status and blood-gas parameters in cooled asphyxiated newborns. Furthermore, we found in our online survey on routine clinical practices of cooled asphyxiated newborns in Germany, that there is also wide heterogeneity in treatment practices in German NICUs [50]. Therefore, we aimed to analyze data of two large university NICUs (both highest level of care) in Germany with similar treatment protocols of perinatal asphyxia and hypoxic–ischemic encephalopathy.

5. Conclusions

Lower pCO_2 levels and increased oxygen supply, which are well-known to be associated with adverse outcomes, were documented more frequently in intubated newborns in comparison to newborns without need of mechanical ventilation. Interestingly, mechanically ventilated newborns with lower pCO_2 values had worse short-term outcomes compared to spontaneously breathing newborns with lower pCO_2 values. Furthermore, higher ΔpCO_2 levels, which were observed more frequently in intubated newborns, were significantly higher in newborns with adverse short-term outcomes. Comparing outcomes among intubated newborns, there were no significant associations of pCO_2 and FiO_2 values with adverse short-term outcomes. However, we have shown that the combination of mechanical ventilation and $pCO_2 < 30$ mmHg or $FiO_2 > 0.60$ are significantly higher in newborns with adverse short-term outcomes, which may be also due to higher levels of encephalopathy in this group.

Mechanical ventilation in cooled asphyxiated newborns needs close monitoring to avoid hyperventilation and high ΔpCO_2 levels. Additionally, oxygen supplementation should be restricted as much as possible to prevent additional oxidative stress in this sensitive group of newborns.

Author Contributions: Conceptualization, S.G. and H.S.; Data curation, S.G., M.R., M.M., A.S. and H.S.; Formal analysis, S.G.; Methodology, S.G. and H.S.; Project administration, S.G. and H.S.; Resources, S.G., M.R., M.M., A.S. and H.S.; Software, S.G. and H.S.; Supervision, H.S.; Validation, S.G., M.R., M.M., A.S. and H.S.; Writing—original draft, S.G.; Writing—review & editing, S.G., A.S., T.H., U.F.-M. and H.S. All authors have read and agreed to the published version of the manuscript.

Funding: This research received no external funding.

Institutional Review Board Statement: The study was conducted according to the guidelines of the Declaration of Helsinki, and approved by the Institutional Ethics Committee of Heinrich Heine University Düsseldorf (protocol code 2018-270-ProspDEuA and 2018-270-1, date of approval 20 March 2019 and 5 August 2019, respectively) and of University Duisburg Essen (protocol code 18-8191-BO and 19-8556-BO, date of approval 7 June 2018 and 27 February 2019, respectively).

Informed Consent Statement: Patient consent was waived due to the retrospective design of the study.

Data Availability Statement: Data can be accessed and is available from the authors.

Conflicts of Interest: The authors declare no conflict of interest.

References

1. Kurinczuk, J.J.; White-Koning, M.; Badawi, N. Epidemiology of neonatal encephalopathy and hypoxic–ischaemic encephalopathy. *Early Hum. Dev.* **2010**, *86*, 329–338. [CrossRef] [PubMed]
2. Shankaran, S.; Laptook, A.R.; Pappas, A.; McDonald, S.A.; Das, A.; Tyson, J.E.; Poindexter, B.B.; Schibler, K.; Bell, E.F.; Heyne, R.J.; et al. Effect of Depth and Duration of Cooling on Death or Disability at Age 18 Months Among Neonates With Hypoxic-Ischemic Encephalopathy: A Randomized Clinical Trial. *JAMA* **2017**, *318*, 57–67. [CrossRef]
3. Tan, W.K.M.; Williams, C.E.; During, M.J.; Mallard, C.E.; Gunning, M.I.; Gunn, A.; Gluckman, P.D. Accumulation of Cytotoxins During the Development of Seizures and Edema after Hypoxic-Ischemic Injury in Late Gestation Fetal Sheep. *Pediatr. Res.* **1996**, *39*, 791–797. [CrossRef] [PubMed]
4. Williams, C.E.; Gunn, A.; Gluckman, P.D. Time course of intracellular edema and epileptiform activity following prenatal cerebral ischemia in sheep. *Stroke* **1991**, *22*, 516–521. [CrossRef] [PubMed]
5. Gunn, A.J.; Gunn, T.R.; De Haan, H.H.; Williams, C.E.; Gluckman, P.D. Dramatic neuronal rescue with prolonged selective head cooling after ischemia in fetal lambs. *J. Clin. Investig.* **1997**, *99*, 248–256. [CrossRef]
6. Jensen, E.C.; Bennet, L.; Hunter, C.J.; Power, G.C.; Gunn, A.J. Post-hypoxic hypoperfusion is associated with suppression of cerebral metabolism and increased tissue oxygenation in near-term fetal sheep. *J. Physiol.* **2006**, *572*, 131–139. [CrossRef]
7. Roth, S.C.; Edwards, A.D.; Cady, E.B.; Delpy, D.T.; Wyatt, J.S.; Azzopardi, D.; Baudin, J.; Townsend, J.; Stewart, A.L.; Reynolds, E.O.R. Relation between cerebral oxidative metabolism following birth asphyxia, and neurodevelopmental outcome and brain growth at one year. *Dev. Med. Child Neurol.* **2008**, *34*, 285–295. [CrossRef]
8. Roth, S.C.; Baudin, J.; Cady, E.; Johal, K.; Townsend, J.P.; Wyatt, J.S.; Reynolds, E.O.R.; Stewart, A.L. Relation of deranged neonatal cerebral oxidative metabolism with neurodevelopmental outcome and head circumference at 4 years. *Dev. Med. Child Neurol.* **2008**, *39*, 718–725. [CrossRef]
9. Lorek, A.; Takei, Y.; Cady, E.B.; Wyatt, J.S.; Penrice, J.; Edwards, A.D.; Peebles, D.; Wylezinska, M.; Owen-Reece, H.; Kirkbride, V.; et al. Delayed ("Secondary") Cerebral Energy Failure after Acute Hypoxia-Ischemia in the Newborn Piglet: Continuous 48-Hour Studies by Phosphorus Magnetic Resonance Spectroscopy. *Pediatr. Res.* **1994**, *36*, 699–706. [CrossRef]
10. Yenari, M.A.; Han, H.S. Neuroprotective mechanisms of hypothermia in brain ischaemia. *Nat. Rev. Neurosci.* **2012**, *13*, 267–278. [CrossRef]
11. Wood, T.; Thoresen, M. Physiological responses to hypothermia. *Semin. Fetal Neonatal Med.* **2015**, *20*, 87–96. [CrossRef] [PubMed]
12. Rainaldi, M.A.; Perlman, J.M. Pathophysiology of Birth Asphyxia. *Clin. Perinatol.* **2016**, *43*, 409–422. [CrossRef]
13. Morton, S.U.; Brodsky, D. Fetal Physiology and the Transition to Extrauterine Life. *Clin. Perinatol.* **2016**, *43*, 395–407. [CrossRef]
14. Lapointe, A.; Barrington, K.J. Pulmonary hypertension and the asphyxiated newborn. *J. Pediatr.* **2011**, *158* (Suppl. S2), e19–e24. [CrossRef] [PubMed]
15. Laporte, M.A.L.; Wang, H.; Sanon, P.-N.; Vargas, S.B.; Maluorni, J.; Rampakakis, E.; Wintermark, P. Association between hypocapnia and ventilation during the first days of life and brain injury in asphyxiated newborns treated with hypothermia. *J. Matern. Neonatal Med.* **2017**, *32*, 1312–1320. [CrossRef]
16. Nadeem, M.; Murray, D.; Boylan, G.; Dempsey, E.M.; Ryan, C.A. Blood Carbon Dioxide Levels and Adverse Outcome in Neonatal Hypoxic-Ischemic Encephalopathy. *Am. J. Perinatol.* **2009**, *27*, 361–365. [CrossRef] [PubMed]
17. Klinger, G.; Beyene, J.; Shah, P.; Perlman, M. Do hyperoxaemia and hypocapnia add to the risk of brain injury after intrapartum asphyxia? *Arch. Dis. Child. Fetal Neonatal Ed.* **2005**, *90*, F49–F52. [CrossRef]

18. Pappas, A.; Shankaran, S.; Laptook, A.R.; Langer, J.C.; Bara, R.; Ehrenkranz, R.A.; Goldberg, R.N.; Das, A.; Higgins, R.D.; Tyson, J.E.; et al. Hypocarbia and Adverse Outcome in Neonatal Hypoxic-Ischemic Encephalopathy. *J. Pediatr.* **2011**, *158*, 752–758.e1. [CrossRef]
19. Lingappan, K.; Kaiser, J.R.; Srinivasan, C.; Gunn, A.; on behalf of the CoolCap Study Group. Relationship between PCO_2 and unfavorable outcome in infants with moderate-to-severe hypoxic ischemic encephalopathy. *Pediatr. Res.* **2016**, *80*, 204–208. [CrossRef]
20. Laffey, J.G.; Kavanagh, B.P. Hypocapnia. *N. Engl. J. Med.* **2002**, *347*, 43–53. [CrossRef]
21. Victor, S.; Appleton, R.E.; Beirne, M.; Marson, A.G.; Weindling, A.M. Effect of carbon dioxide on background cerebral electrical activity and fractional oxygen extraction in very low birth weight infants just after birth. *Pediatr. Res.* **2005**, *58*, 579–585. [CrossRef] [PubMed]
22. Pirot, A.L.; Fritz, K.I.; Ashraf, Q.M.; Mishra, O.P.; Delivoria-Papadopoulos, M. Effects of Severe Hypocapnia on Expression of Bax and Bcl-2 Proteins, DNA Fragmentation, and Membrane Peroxidation Products in Cerebral Cortical Mitochondria of Newborn Piglets. *Neonatology* **2007**, *91*, 20–27. [CrossRef]
23. Koch, J.D.; Miles, D.K.; Gilley, J.A.; Yang, C.-P.; Kernie, S.G. Brief Exposure to Hyperoxia Depletes the Glial Progenitor Pool and Impairs Functional Recovery after Hypoxic-Ischemic Brain Injury. *Br. J. Pharmacol.* **2008**, *28*, 1294–1306. [CrossRef] [PubMed]
24. Davis, P.G.; Tan, A.; O'Donnell, C.P.; Schulze, A. Resuscitation of newborn infants with 100% oxygen or air: A systematic review and meta-analysis. *Lancet* **2004**, *364*, 1329–1333. [CrossRef]
25. Sarnat, H.B.; Sarnat, M.S. Neonatal encephalopathy following fetal distress. A clinical and electroencephalographic study. *Arch. Neurol.* **1976**, *33*, 696–705. [CrossRef] [PubMed]
26. Al Naqeeb, N.; Edwards, A.D.; Cowan, F.M.; Azzopardi, D. Assessment of Neonatal Encephalopathy by Amplitude-integrated Electroencephalography. *Pediatrics* **1999**, *103*, 1263–1271. [CrossRef] [PubMed]
27. Barkovich, A.J.; Hajnal, B.L.; Vigneron, D.; Sola, A.; Partridge, J.C.; Allen, F.; Ferriero, D.M. Prediction of neuromotor outcome in perinatal asphyxia: Evaluation of MR scoring systems. *Am. J. Neuroradiol.* **1998**, *19*, 143–149. [PubMed]
28. Al Amrani, F.; Marcovitz, J.; Sanon, P.-N.; Khairy, M.; Saint-Martin, C.; Shevell, M.; Wintermark, P. Prediction of outcome in asphyxiated newborns treated with hypothermia: Is a MRI scoring system described before the cooling era still useful? *Eur. J. Paediatr. Neurol.* **2018**, *22*, 387–395. [CrossRef] [PubMed]
29. Thoresen, M.; Hellström-Westas, L.; Liu, X.; De Vries, L.S. Effect of Hypothermia on Amplitude-Integrated Electroencephalogram in Infants With Asphyxia. *Pediatrics* **2010**, *126*, e131–e139. [CrossRef]
30. Sarkar, S.; Barks, J.D.; Donn, S.M. Should amplitude-integrated electroencephalography be used to identify infants suitable for hypothermic neuroprotection? *J. Perinatol.* **2008**, *28*, 117–122. [CrossRef]
31. Ruhfus, M.; Giannakis, S.; Markus, M.; Stein, A.; Hoehn, T.; Felderhoff-Mueser, U.; Sabir, H. Association of Routinely Measured Proinflammatory Biomarkers With Abnormal MRI Findings in Asphyxiated Neonates Undergoing Therapeutic Hypothermia. *Front. Pediatr.* **2021**, *9*. [CrossRef] [PubMed]
32. Toet, M.C.; Hellström-Westas, L.; Groenendaal, F.; Eken, P.; De Vries, L.S. Amplitude integrated EEG 3 and 6 hours after birth in full term neonates with hypoxic-ischaemic encephalopathy. *Arch. Dis. Child. Fetal Neonatal Ed.* **1999**, *81*, F19–F23. [CrossRef] [PubMed]
33. Reinhardt, F.; Soeder, H.; Falk, G. *DTV-Atlas zur Mathematik: Taf. u. Texte. Orig.-Ausg. Ed*; Deutscher Taschenbuch-Verlag: München, Germany, 1974.
34. Sabir, H.; Jary, S.; Tooley, J.; Liu, X.; Thoresen, M. Increased Inspired Oxygen in the First Hours of Life is Associated with Adverse Outcome in Newborns Treated for Perinatal Asphyxia with Therapeutic Hypothermia. *J. Pediatr.* **2012**, *161*, 409–416. [CrossRef]
35. Greisen, G. Autoregulation of cerebral blood flow in newborn babies. *Early Hum. Dev.* **2005**, *81*, 423–428. [CrossRef] [PubMed]
36. Cavallaro, G.; Filippi, L.; Cristofori, G.; Colnaghi, M.; Ramenghi, L.; Agazzani, E.; Ronchi, A.; Florini, P.; Mosca, F. Does pulmonary function change during whole-body deep hypothermia? *Arch. Dis. Child. Fetal Neonatal Ed.* **2011**, *96*, F374–F377. [CrossRef] [PubMed]
37. Dassios, T.; Austin, T. Respiratory function parameters in ventilated newborn infants undergoing whole body hypothermia. *Acta Paediatr.* **2014**, *103*, 157–161. [CrossRef] [PubMed]
38. Thoresen, M. Supportive care during neuroprotective hypothermia in the term newborn: Adverse effects and their prevention. *Clin. Perinatol.* **2008**, *35*, 749–763. [CrossRef] [PubMed]
39. Vannucci, R.C.; Towfighi, J.; Heitjan, D.F.; Brucklacher, R.M. Carbon dioxide protects the perinatal brain from hypoxic-ischemic damage: An experimental study in the immature rat. *Pediatrics* **1995**, *95*, 868–874. [PubMed]
40. Vannucci, R.C.; Brucklacher, R.M.; Vannucci, S.J. Effect of carbon dioxide on cerebral metabolism during hypoxia-ischemia in the immature rat. *Pediatr. Res.* **1997**, *42*, 24–29. [CrossRef] [PubMed]
41. Vannucci, R.C.; Towfighi, J.; Brucklacher, R.M.; Vannucci, S.J. Effect of Extreme Hypercapnia on Hypoxic-Ischemic Brain Damage in the Immature Rat. *Pediatr. Res.* **2001**, *49*, 799–803. [CrossRef] [PubMed]
42. Bracci, R.; Perrone, S.; Buonocore, G. Red blood cell involvement in fetal/neonatal hypoxia. *Biol. Neonate* **2001**, *79*, 210–212. [PubMed]
43. Saugstad, O.D.; Aasen, A.O. Plasma hypoxanthine concentrations in pigs. A prognostic aid in hypoxia. *Eur. Surg. Res.* **1980**, *12*, 123–129. [CrossRef] [PubMed]

44. Núnez, A.; Benavente, I.; Blanco, D.; Boix, H.; Cabañas, F.; Chaffanel, M.; Fernández-Colomer, B.; Fernández-Lorenzo, J.R.; Loureiro, B.; Moral, M.T.; et al. Oxidative stress in perinatal asphyxia and hypoxic-ischaemic encephalopathy. An. Pediatría 2018, 88, 228.e1–228.e9. [CrossRef]
45. Markus, T.; Hansson, S.; Amer-Wåhlin, I.; Hellström-Westas, L.; Saugstad, O.D.; Ley, D. Cerebral Inflammatory Response After Fetal Asphyxia and Hyperoxic Resuscitation in Newborn Sheep. Pediatr. Res. 2007, 62, 71–77. [CrossRef]
46. Munkeby, B.H.; Børke, W.B.; Bjørnland, K.; Sikkeland, L.I.B.; Borge, G.I.A.; Halvorsen, B.; Saugstad, O.D.; Oslash, B.W.B. Resuscitation with 100% O_2 increases cerebral injury in hypoxemic piglets. Pediatr. Res. 2004, 56, 783–790. [CrossRef]
47. Saugstad, O.D.; Ramji, S.; Soll, R.F.; Vento, M. Resuscitation of Newborn Infants with 21% or 100% Oxygen: An Updated Systematic Review and Meta-Analysis. Neonatology 2008, 94, 176–182. [CrossRef]
48. Dalen, M.L.; Liu, X.; Elstad, M.; Løberg, E.M.; Saugstad, O.D.; Rootwelt, T.; Thoresen, M. Resuscitation with 100% oxygen increases injury and counteracts the neuroprotective effect of therapeutic hypothermia in the neonatal rat. Pediatr. Res. 2012, 71, 247–252. [CrossRef]
49. Szakmar, E.; Jermendy, A.; El-Dib, M. Respiratory management during therapeutic hypothermia for hypoxic-ischemic encephalopathy. J. Perinatol. 2019, 39, 763–773. [CrossRef]
50. Giannakis, S.; Ruhfus, M.; Rüdiger, M.; Sabir, H.; Network, T.G.N.H.; Network, G.N.H. Hospital survey showed wide variations in therapeutic hypothermia for neonates in Germany. Acta Paediatr. 2019, 109, 200–201. [CrossRef]

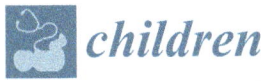 children

Review

Is Chest Compression Superimposed with Sustained Inflation during Cardiopulmonary Resuscitation an Alternative to 3:1 Compression to Ventilation Ratio in Newborn Infants?

Seung Yeon Kim [1,2,†], Gyu-Hong Shim [1,3,†] and Georg M. Schmölzer [1,4,5,*]

1 Centre for the Studies of Asphyxia and Resuscitation, Neonatal Research Unit, Royal Alexandra Hospital, Edmonton, AB T5H 3V9, Canada; dunggiduk@eulji.ac.kr (S.Y.K.); peddoc@paik.ac.kr (G.-H.S.)
2 Department of Pediatrics, Eulji University Hospital, Daejeon 35233, Korea
3 Department of Pediatrics, Inje University Sanggye Paik Hospital, Seoul 01757, Korea
4 Department of Pediatrics, Faculty of Medicine and Dentistry, University of Alberta, Edmonton, AB T6G 2R3, Canada
5 Division of Neonatology, Department of Pediatrics and Adolescent Medicine, Medical University of Graz, Graz 8036, Austria
* Correspondence: georg.schmoelzer@me.com; Tel.: +1-78-0735-5179; Fax: +1-78-0735-4072
† These authors contributed equally to this work.

Abstract: Approximately 0.1% for term and 10–15% of preterm infants receive chest compression (CC) in the delivery room, with high incidence of mortality and neurologic impairment. The poor prognosis associated with receiving CC in the delivery room has raised concerns as to whether specifically-tailored cardiopulmonary resuscitation methods are needed. The current neonatal resuscitation guidelines recommend a 3:1 compression:ventilation ratio; however, the most effective approach to deliver chest compression is unknown. We recently demonstrated that providing continuous chest compression superimposed with a high distending pressure or sustained inflation significantly reduced time to return of spontaneous circulation and mortality while improving respiratory and cardiovascular parameters in asphyxiated piglet and newborn infants. This review summarizes the current available evidence of continuous chest compression superimposed with a sustained inflation.

Keywords: newborn; neonatal resuscitation; chest compressions; sustained inflation

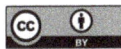

1. Introduction

Approximately 0.1% of term infants and 10–15% of preterm infants receive chest compressions (CC) in the delivery room (DR) [1–5]. Infants who receive CC have a high incidence of mortality and neurodevelopmental impairment [1–5]. Furthermore, newborns who received prolonged CC and epinephrine without signs of life at 10 min after birth have 83% mortality, with 93% of survivors suffering moderate-to-severe neurological disability [6,7]. The poor prognosis associated with receiving CC in the DR has raised concerns as to whether specifically-tailored cardiopulmonary resuscitation (CPR) methods could improve outcomes.

In newborn infants, bradycardia or cardiac arrest is mainly caused by hypoxia rather than a primary cardiac disease [8,9]. Therefore, the neonatal resuscitation guidelines put an emphasis on ventilation and adequate oxygen delivery. Current neonatal resuscitation guidelines recommend initiating CC if an infant's heart rate remains < 60 beats/min, despite adequate ventilation for at least 30 s [8,9]. CC should be delivered at a rate of 90/min in sequences of three CC followed by a pause to deliver 1 inflation at a rate of 30/min, which corresponds to a 3:1 compression:ventilation (C:V) ratio [8,9]. The 3:1 C:V ratio is recommended, as respiratory failure is the primary cause of bradycardia or asystole in newborn infants [8,9]. A 3:1 C:V ratio has a higher rate of inflations compared to the pediatric or adult C:V ratios, which will result in a higher oxygen delivery, hence improved ventilation [8,9]. While the current neonatal resuscitation guidelines recommend a 3:1 C:V ratio, the most effective C:V ratio in newborn infants remains controversial.

Several studies have compared various C:V ratios or continuous chest compression with asynchronized ventilation [10–14], however none of the studies reported any improved outcomes compared to the 3:1 C:V ratio. More recently, our group used a higher airway pressure or sustained inflation during continuous chest compression (CC + SI), which significantly improved time to return of spontaneous circulation (ROSC) and survival [15]. While the current available data is mostly limited to animal data, some human data are available. The aim of the review is to provide an in-depth analysis of CC + SI during neonatal CPR.

2. 3:1 Compression-to-Ventilation Ratio: Rationale and Evidence

Current resuscitation guidelines in newborns recommend a 3:1 C:V ratio [8,9], however this approach may not be optimizing coronary and cerebral perfusion while providing adequate ventilation to improve outcomes. Animal studies on cardiac arrest demonstrated that combining CC with ventilations, compared with ventilations or CC alone, improves ROSC and neurological outcome at 24 h in asphyxiated newborn piglets [16–18].

Solevåg et al. compared 9:3 C:V and 15:2 C:V to 3:1 C:V in asphyxiated newborn piglets with cardiac arrest and reported no significant differences in the time to ROSC [10,11]. These studies suggest that just using a higher C:V ratio does not improve outcome in asphyxiated newborn piglets. Alternatively, continuous CC with asynchronous ventilations (CCaV), where 90 CC are given continuously with 30 non-synchronized inflations, would potentially improve hemodynamics during CC as there are no interruptions. Indeed, a manikin study reported a significantly higher minute ventilation with CCaV compared to 3:1 C:V ratio (221 vs. 191 mL/kg/min, respectively) [19]. During CPR in asphyxiated newborn piglets, CCaV or 3:1 C:V had similar minute ventilation (387 vs. 275 mL/kg) and similar time to ROSC (114 and 143 s for CCaV and 3:1 C:V, respectively) and survival (3/8 and 6/8, respectively) between the two groups [12,13]. Furthermore, no differences in diastolic blood pressure or mean arterial blood pressure between CCaV and 3:1 C:V were observed [12,13]. These studies suggest that CCaV has no advantage compared to 3:1 C:V.

3. Chest Compression with Sustained Inflations (CC + SI)

Schmölzer et al. compared continuous CC superimposed with a high distending pressure (or sustained inflation = CC + SI) with 3:1 CV during CPR of asphyxiated newborn piglets and reported (i) significantly reduced time to ROSC (median (Interquartile range (IQR)) 38 (23–44) vs. 143 (84–303) s, respectively, (p = 0.0008), mortality (7/8 (87.5%) vs. 3/8 (37.5%), respectively, p = 0.038), epinephrine administration (0/8 vs. 7/8, respectively, $p < 0.0001$), and improved systemic and regional hemodynamic recovery; (ii) less infants received 100% oxygen (3/8 vs. 8/8, respectively, (p = 0.0042); (iii) minute ventilation (mean (SD) 936 (201) vs. 623 (116) mL/kg/min, respectively, p = 0.0080), and therefore alveolar oxygen delivery, was significantly increased with CC + SI; iv) compression of the chest during SI forced gas out of the chest and during passive chest recoil allowed air to be drawn back into the lungs [15].

During CC + SI, CCs are delivered continuously and superimposed by a constant high airway pressure or sustained inflation (SI). During CC + SI, a constant high airway pressure or SI is given for a set time (e.g., 30 s) with a set peak inflation pressure (e.g., 25 cm H_2O) while CCs are continuously delivered [20–24]. During compression and release phase, the distending pressure is fluctuating by ~1 cm H_2O. After the set time (i.e., 30 s), the SI is paused for 1 s while CCs are continued. The SI is then resumed for the same time frame (i.e., 30 s). Both CC and SI combined as CC + SI are continued until ROSC. While in all studies a 1 s pause between each SI was used, the optimal duration for the pause between each SI (e.g., 0.5, 1, 2 s) has never been examined.

Mechanism of CC + SI

Antegrade blood flow during CPR can be achieved by either direct cardiac compression between the sternum and vertebral column or increased intrathoracic pressure produced by CC [25]. Indeed, maneuvers that increase the intrathoracic pressure result in increased carotid blood flow during CPR, further augmenting antegrade blood flow [26,27]. Chandra et al. combined ventilation at high airway pressure while simultaneously performing CC in an animal model and demonstrated increased carotid flow, without compromising oxygenation [26,27]. Furthermore, providing continuous CC and lung inflation simultaneously substantially improved brain perfusion by enhancing cerebral perfusion pressure in a piglet model [28,29]. In addition, animal studies have demonstrated that an SI also increases intrathoracic pressure without impeding blood flow [30]. These data suggest that CC + SI might provide two maneuvers, which increase intrathoracic pressure and thereby improve blood flow.

4. Chest Compression Rate

The newborn infant normal respiratory rate and resting heart rate are 40–60 breaths/min and 120–160/min, respectively. In comparison, the current neonatal resuscitation guidelines recommend CC with 90 compressions and 30 inflations per minute [8,9], which is lower than the normal physiological parameters.

Schmölzer et al. compared CC + SI with a CC rate of 120/min with 3:1 C:V with a CC rate of 90/min in a newborn asphyxiated piglets experiment, and reported shorter time to ROSC (38 (23–44) vs. 143 (84–303) s; ($p = 0.0008$)) and survival to 4 h with 7/8 vs. 3/8, respectively [15]. Similarly, Vali et al. reported that CC + SI with CC rate of 120/min was as effective as CC with 90/min with a 3:1 C:V ratio in achieving ROSC [31]. Li et al. compared CC rates of 90/min and 120/min during CC + SI and reported a reduced time to ROSC (34 (28–156) vs. 99 (31–255) s $p = 0.29$), respectively [32]. Those studies suggest the 90/min CC rates in the CC + SI might be sufficient to deliver an adequate tidal volume and minute ventilation without impairing gas exchange. However, a mathematical model suggests that the most effective CC rate depends on body size and body weight, and CC rates of 180/min for term infants and even higher for preterm infants might improve survival [33]. The mathematical model calculated that the optimal systemic perfusion pressure occurs at CC rates of 180 and 250/min for infants weighing 3 and 1 kg, respectively [33]. In infants and newborns, there are fundamental physical and mathematical reasons including (i) effects of the mass of venous blood columns entering the chest pump, (ii) length, and (iii) area scale with body size [33]. However, these higher CC rates might be impossible during manual CPR as healthcare professionals will get fatigued more quickly, which conversely affects CC quality [34–36]. Using an automated CC machine might be the solution to achieving these high CC rates. While automated CC machines are routinely used in adults, no such device is currently available for newborn infants.

5. Peak Inflation Pressures

The optimal peak inflation pressure during CC + SI for adequate tidal volume delivery is unknown. While the current neonatal resuscitation guidelines recommend an initial distending pressure of 20–25 cm H_2O during positive pressure ventilation [8,9], the optimal peak inflation pressure remains unknown. During mask ventilation, a certain threshold peak inflation pressure is needed to move the liquid air interface downwards towards the alveoli [37,38]. Similarly, during CC + SI, a threshold sustained pressure is needed to deliver an adequate tidal volume. Solevåg et al. used manikins and cadaver piglets to establish the distending pressure required to achieve sufficient tidal volume delivery during CC + SI [39]. A distending pressure of 25 cm H_2O was required to achieve a tidal volume delivery of > 5 mL/kg [39]. Tidal volume increased with increasing distending pressure in all models, with an overall positive correlation ($r = 0.49$, $p < 0.001$) [39]. Shim et al. compared a peak inflation pressure of 10, 20, and 30 cm H_2O during CC + SI in asphyxiated newborn piglets and reported no difference in median (IQR) time to ROSC, with 75 (63–193), 94 (78–210), and 85 (70–90) s, respectively ($p = 0.56$) [22]. In addition, tidal volume was positively correlated with increasing pressure with a mean (SD) 7.3 (3.3), 10.3 (3.1), and 14.0 (3.3) mL/kg;($p = 0.0018$) with 10, 20, and 30 cm H_2O, respectively [22]. The higher tidal volume with a peak inflation pressure of 30 cm H_2O also showed increased concentrations of proinflammatory cytokines interleukin-1β and tumor necrosis factor-α in the frontoparietal cerebral cortex (both $p < 0.05$ vs. sham-operated controls). These data suggest that pressures of 20–25 cm H_2O might be sufficient to deliver an adequate tidal volume during CC + SI, and that higher pressures could lead to increases in lung inflammation markers.

6. Passive Ventilation

Tsui et al. applied a downward force of 0.16 kg per kg patient weight on the chest of infants undergoing surgery during general anesthesia and was able to deliver a tidal volume of 2.4 mL/kg or ~33% of an infant's physiological tidal volume [40]. This study suggests that chest recoil produces a distending pressure-dependent tidal volume, which achieves passive ventilation during CCs. In asphyxiated term piglets, the delivered tidal volume was 10–15 mL/kg with a constant distending pressure of 25–30 cm H_2O, and in preterm infants < 32 weeks' gestation, the tidal volume ranged between 0.6 to 4.4 mL/kg with a constant distending pressure of 24 cm H_2O [15,41]. These data demonstrate that passive ventilation is achieved when providing a constant high distending pressure during CC.

7. Tidal Volume

Providing adequate ventilation is a cornerstone of neonatal CPR. The main purpose of lung inflations during CCs is to provide an adequate tidal volume to facilitate oxygen delivery and gas exchange. However, during CPR with 3:1 C:V, Li et al. reported a cumulative loss of expiratory tidal volume of 4.5 mL/kg with each 3:1 C:V cycle [42], which could cause lung derecruitment and thereby interfere with oxygenation and ROSC. In comparison, during CC + SI, a constant lung recruitment and thereby gain in functional residual capacity was observed with a tidal volume gain of 2.4 mL/kg per CC + SI cycle [42]. This is supported by data from a human pilot trial comparing CC + SI with 3:1 C:V in the DR using a distending pressure of 24 cm H_2O (local hospital policy during neonatal resuscitation) in preterm infants < 32 weeks of gestation [41,43]. During CC + SI, a significantly higher tidal volume and minute ventilation was delivered, suggesting that CC + SI might improve ventilation and oxygenation during neonatal CPR. During CC + SI, adequate tidal volume delivery might lead to better alveolar oxygen delivery and lung aeration, hence faster ROSC compared to 3:1 C:V group.

8. Duration of Sustained Inflations

SI as initial respiratory support in the DR has been postulated to achieve a more unified lung aeration [44]. However, recent systematic reviews reported similar rates of bronchopulmonary dysplasia when SI was compared with intermittent positive pressure ventilation for initial respiratory support in the DR [45,46]. These reviews also reported that in a subgroup of <28 weeks' gestation, SI was associated with potential increased risk of death before discharge (risk ratio 2.42 (95% confidence interval = 1.15–5.09)) and increased risk of death within the first 2 days (risk ratio 1.38 (95% confidence interval = 1.00–1.91)), when compared to intermittent positive pressure ventilation [45,46]. However, the mechanism of how an initial SI could potentially increase risk of death is unknown.

Furthermore, the European resuscitation guidelines recommend five SIs of 3 s in asphyxiated term infants [47], though no human studies have examined this approach in newborn infants. However, a recent study in asphyxiated lambs reported that a 30 s SI will achieve lung aeration and hemodynamic stability, while five SIs of 3 s does not [48]. In the original study, we used a 30 s SI during CC + SI, which significantly reduces time to ROSC compared to 3:1 C:V ratio [15]. However, the optimal duration of SI to improve ROSC and reduce mortality during CC + SI remains unknown. Mustofa et al. compared CC + SI with either 20 s or 60 s in asphyxiated piglets and reported similar time to ROSC and survival, with no difference in tidal volume delivery [21]. In addition, there were no differences in markers of lung inflammation (IL-1ß, IL-6, IL-8, and TNF-α) and brain inflammation (IL-1ß, IL-6, and IL-8) between the groups [21]. This suggests that the duration of SI during CC + SI might be not the dependent factor, however further studies are needed to identify the optimal duration of SI during CC + SI.

9. Oxygen Concentration with CC + SI

The current neonatal resuscitation guidelines recommend 100% oxygen once CCs are initiated [8,9]. However, this is based on expert opinions and not supported by any clinical data. Several animal studies compared 21% or 100% oxygen during CC using the 3:1 C:V ratio in asphyxiated newborn piglets and reported no difference in time to ROSC or mortality. In addition, the cumulative alveolar oxygen exposure during resuscitation was significantly lower in the CC + SI group compared to the 3:1 C:V group, with mean (SD) 27,755 (4706) and 47,729 (6692) mmHg seconds, respectively ($p < 0.001$). Similar, a meta-analysis of these animal studies reported no difference in time to ROSC (mean difference of -3.8 (-29.7–22) s, $I^2 = 0\%$, $p = 0.77$) or mortality (risk ratio 1.04 (0.35, 3.08), $I^2 = 0\%$, $p = 0.94$) between 21% or 100% oxygen during CC with the 3:1 C:V ratio [49]. Recently, Hidalgo et al. compared 21% and 100% oxygen during CC + SI in term newborn asphyxiated piglets and reported similar time to ROSC (median (IQR) 80 (70–190) vs. 90 (70–324) s, respectively, $p = 0.56$), short-term survival (7/8 (88%) vs. 5/8 (63%), respectively, $p = 0.569$), and hemodynamic recovery [50]. In addition, there was no significant difference in injury markers in the left ventricle tissue or the frontoparietal cortex tissue. These data suggest that 21% oxygen during CPR might be efficient, however human data are needed.

10. Type of Cardiac Arrest

In 2015, the neonatal resuscitation guidelines added the use of an electrocardiograph to assess heart rate at birth [51,52]. This led to several reports of pulseless electrical activity during CPR in the DR [53,54]. In addition, rates of up to 50% of asphyxiated piglets displayed pulseless electrical activity during asphyxia-induced cardiac arrest [55–57]. Solevåg et al. reported that cardiac arrest due to pulseless electrical activity will result in lower rates of ROSC and lower 4 h survival, compared to asystole, in asphyxiated newborn piglets [56]. This suggests that the initial electrocardiograph algorithm might serve as an outcome predictor during neonatal CPR.

11. Inflammatory Markers

There are concerns that SI could adversely affect lung or brain injury. Lista et al. reported a pneumothorax rate of 6% compared to 1% with intermittent positive pressure in preterm infants with 25–28 weeks of gestation [58]. However, the mechanisms for an increased rate of pneumothorax during SI is unknown. Interestingly, none of the animal studies examining CC + SI reported pneumothoraxes during autopsy. There is also the concern that SI delivers an excessive large tidal volume, which could cause a pulmonary proinflammatory response and initiate systemic inflammatory cascade [59]. However, when SIs were given as initial respiratory support, no increase in lung injury marker has been reported [60,61]. Similar, during CPR with either CC + SI or 3:1 C:V, no difference in lung injury markers were observed.

The mechanism of brain injury is thought to be impaired venous return or secondary brain injury due to excessive tidal volume delivery. Sobotka et al. reported that a single 30 s SI followed by ventilation caused a blood–brain barrier disruption and cerebral vascular leakage, which may exacerbate brain injury in asphyxiated near-term lambs [62]. This injury might have occurred as a direct insult of the initial SI or due to the excessive tidal volume delivered during subsequent ventilation. Recently, Shim et al. reported that a peak inflation pressure of 30 cm H_2O delivered a significant higher tidal volume compared to peak inflation pressure of 20 cm H_2O, which was associated with significant increased cerebral tissue pro-inflammatory cytokines [22]. While CC + SI did not increase lung injury markers, markers of brain inflammation were increased, and therefore a peak inflation pressure of ≥ 25 cm H_2O should not be exceeded.

12. Clinical Studies

The animal data suggest that CC + SI might be an effective CC technique for newborn infants. A pilot trial compared CC + SI ($n = 5$) with 3:1 C:V ($n = 4$) in preterm infants < 32 weeks' gestation with a mean (SD) gestational age of 24.6 (1.3) and 25.6 (2.3) weeks [41]. There was a significantly shorter time to ROSC with CC + SI, compared to 3:1 C:V, with 31(9) vs. 138 (72) s, respectively ($p = 0.011$) [41]. In addition, CC + SI provided a higher minute ventilation and ventilation rate, while short-term outcomes, including intraventricular hemorrhages, air leak, retinopathy of prematurity, and chronic lung disease, were similar between groups [41]. Although mortality was higher in the CC + SI group with 2/5 vs. 0/4 in the 3:1 C:V group, this did not reach statistical significance, as the sample size was too small, and it was a very vulnerable patient population.

Currently, the Sustained Inflation and Chest Compression Versus 3:1 Chest Compression to Ventilation Ratio During Cardiopulmonary Resuscitation of Asphyxiated Newborns: A Randomized Controlled Trial (SURV1VE-trial) is recruiting term and preterm infants born > 28^{+0} weeks' gestational age requiring chest compression in the delivery room [63,64]. In this cluster trial, hospitals are randomized to either CC + SI or 3:1 C:V ratio for one year each [63,64]. The SURV1VE-trial has been approved by a human clinical research ethical committee at all participating sites, and a Data Safety Monitoring Committee is assessing the results of the trial at regular intervals to assure safety. The SURV1VE-trial hypothesis is that in newborn infants, CC + SI, compared to 3:1 C:V, during CPR will reduce the time needed to ROSC, and aims to recruit 218 participants (109 control group and 109 intervention group). The SURV1VE-trial aims to be completed by 2024.

13. Limitations

There are several limitations which prevent routine use of CC + SI in the DR. Most animal studies described in this review used piglets that have already undergone the fetal-to-neonatal transition. All experimental animals were sedated/anesthetized and intubated with a tightly sealed endotracheal tube to prevent any endotracheal tube leak, which may not occur in the delivery room as mask ventilation is frequently used [65].

Furthermore, sustained lung inflations have been postulated as a ventilation strategy immediately after birth [44]. Indeed, in intubated and sedated animals, SI improved lung aeration compared to intermittent positive pressure ventilation. However, several smaller randomized trials and meta-analyses were unable to identify any advantage or disadvantage for either SI or intermittent positive pressure ventilation [66]. Recently, the SAIL trial compared SI with intermittent positive pressure ventilation in < 28 weeks' gestation infants and reported an increased mortality within the first 48 h with SI [67]. Most recently, a meta-analysis from ILCOR raised concerns about the potential harm of SI for premature infants < 28 weeks' gestation [46]. These data raise some concerns about the use of SI during the initial respiratory support.

14. Conclusions

CC + SI reduces time to ROSC, improves mortality, and improves respiratory and hemodynamic parameters compared to 3:1 C:V ratio during neonatal CPR. CC + SI allows for passive lung ventilation and adequate tidal volume. Peak inflation pressures of 20–25 cm H_2O might be sufficient to deliver an adequate tidal volume during CC + SI, and higher pressures could lead to increases in lung inflammation markers. Furthermore, 21% oxygen had similar time to ROSC or mortality compared to 100% oxygen. However, more clinical data are needed before this can be routinely used in the delivery room during neonatal chest compression.

Author Contributions: Conception and design: S.Y.K., G.-H.S., and G.M.S. Collection and assembly of data: S.Y.K., G.-H.S., and G.M.S. Analysis and interpretation of the data: S.Y.K., G.-H.S., and G.M.S. Drafting of the article: S.Y.K., G.-H.S., and G.M.S. Critical revision of the article for important intellectual content: S.Y.K., G.-H.S., and G.M.S. Final approval of the article: S.Y.K., G.-H.S., and G.M.S. All authors have read and agreed to the published version of the manuscript.

Funding: We would like to thank the public for donating money to our funding agencies: GMS is a recipient of the Heart and Stroke Foundation/University of Alberta Professorship of Neonatal Resuscitation, a National New Investigator of the Heart and Stroke Foundation Canada and an Alberta New Investigator of the Heart and Stroke Foundation Alberta.

Institutional Review Board Statement: Not applicable.

Informed Consent Statement: Not applicable.

Data Availability Statement: All data are presented within the article.

Conflicts of Interest: The authors declare no conflict of interest.

Abbreviations

CC	chest compression
DR	delivery room
CPR	cardiopulmonary resuscitation
C:V	compression:ventilation
SI	sustained inflation
CC + SI	sustained inflation during chest compression
ROSC	return of spontaneous circulation
CCaV	continuous CC with asynchronous ventilations

References

1. Shah, P.S.; Shah, P.; Tai, K.F.Y.; Tai, K.F.Y. Chest compression and/or epinephrine at birth for preterm infants <32 weeks gestational age: Matched cohort study of neonatal outcomes. *J. Perinatol.* **2009**, *29*, 693–697.
2. Shah, P.K.; Narendran, V.; Kalpana, N. Aggressive posterior retinopathy of prematurity in large preterm babies in South India. *Arch. Dis. Child. Fetal Neonatal Ed.* **2012**, *97*, F371–F375. [CrossRef] [PubMed]
3. Wyckoff, M.H.; Perlman, J.M. Cardiopulmonary resuscitation in very low birth weight infants. *Pediatrics* **2000**, *106*, 618–620. [CrossRef] [PubMed]
4. Wyckoff, M.H.; Salhab, W.A.; Heyne, R.J.; Kendrick, D.E.; Stoll, B.; Laptook, A.R.; National Institute of Child Health and Human Development Neonatal Research Network. Outcome of extremely low birth weight infants who received delivery room cardiopulmonary resuscitation. *J. Pediatr.* **2012**, *160*, 239–244.e2. [CrossRef] [PubMed]
5. Soraisham, A.S.; Lodha, A.K.; Singhal, N.; Aziz, K.; Yang, J.; Lee, S.K.; Shah, P.S. On behalf of the Canadian Neonatal Network. Neonatal outcomes following extensive cardiopulmonary resuscitation in the delivery room for infants born at less than 33 weeks gestational age. *Resuscitation* **2014**, *85*, 238–243. [CrossRef]
6. Foglia, E.E.; Weiner, G.; de Almeida, M.F.B.; Wyllie, J.P.; Wyckoff, M.H.; Rabi, Y.; Guinsburg, R.; International Liaison Committee on Resuscitation Neonatal Life Support Task Force. Duration of Resuscitation at Birth, Mortality, and Neurodevelopment: A Systematic Review. *Pediatrics* **2020**, *146*, e20201449. [CrossRef]
7. Harrington, D.J.; Redman, C.W.; Redman, C.W.; Moulden, M.; Greenwood, C.E. The long-term outcome in surviving infants with Apgar zero at 10 minutes: A systematic review of the literature and hospital-based cohort. *Am. J. Obstet. Gynecol.* **2007**, *196*, 463.e1–463.e5. [CrossRef]
8. Wyckoff, M.H.; Wyllie, J.P.; Aziz, K.; de Almeida, M.F.; Fabres, J.; Fawke, J.; Guinsburg, R.; Hosono, S.; Isayama, T.; Kapadia, V.S.; et al. Neonatal Life Support: 2020 International Consensus on Cardiopulmonary Resuscitation and Emergency Cardiovascular Care Science with Treatment Recommendations. *Circulation* **2020**, *142*, S185–S221. [CrossRef]
9. Aziz, K.; Lee, H.C.; Escobedo, M.B.; Hoover, A.V.; Kamath-Rayne, B.D.; Kapadia, V.S.; Magid, D.J.; Niermeyer, S.; Schmölzer, G.M.; Szyld, E.G.; et al. Part 5: Neonatal Resuscitation: 2020 American Heart Association Guidelines for Cardiopulmonary Resuscitation and Emergency Cardiovascular Care. *Circulation* **2020**, *142*, S524–S550. [CrossRef]
10. Solevåg, A.; Dannevig, I.; Wyckoff, M.H.; Saugstad, O.D.; Nakstad, B. Extended series of cardiac compressions during CPR in a swine model of perinatal asphyxia. *Resuscitation* **2010**, *81*, 1571–1576. [CrossRef]
11. Solevåg, A.; Dannevig, I.; Wyckoff, M.H.; Saugstad, O.D.; Nakstad, B. Return of spontaneous circulation with a compression:ventilation ratio of 15:2 versus 3:1 in newborn pigs with cardiac arrest due to asphyxia. *Arch. Dis. Child. Fetal Neonatal Ed.* **2011**, *96*, F417–F421. [CrossRef] [PubMed]

12. Solevåg, A.; Schmölzer, G.M.; O'Reilly, M.; Lu, M.; Lee, T.-F.; Hornberger, L.K.; Nakstad, B.; Cheung, P.-Y. Myocardial perfusion and oxidative stress after 21% vs. 100% oxygen ventilation and uninterrupted chest compressions in severely asphyxiated piglets. *Resuscitation* **2016**, *106*, 7–13. [CrossRef] [PubMed]
13. Schmölzer, G.M.; O'Reilly, M.; LaBossiere, J.; Lee, T.-F.; Cowan, S.; Nicoll, J.; Bigam, D.L.; Cheung, P.-Y. 3:1 compression to ventilation ratio versus continuous chest compression with asynchronous ventilation in a porcine model of neonatal resuscitation. *Resuscitation* **2014**, *85*, 270–275. [CrossRef] [PubMed]
14. Pasquin, M.P.; Cheung, P.-Y.; Patel, S.; Lu, M.; Lee, T.-F.; Wagner, M.; O'Reilly, M.; Schmölzer, G.M. Comparison of Different Compression to Ventilation Ratios (2: 1, 3: 1, and 4: 1) during Cardiopulmonary Resuscitation in a Porcine Model of Neonatal Asphyxia. *Neonatology* **2018**, *114*, 37–45. [CrossRef] [PubMed]
15. Schmölzer, G.M.; O'Reilly, M.; LaBossiere, J.; Lee, T.-F.; Cowan, S.; Qin, S.; Bigam, D.L.; Cheung, P.-Y. Cardiopulmonary resuscitation with chest compressions during sustained inflations: A new technique of neonatal resuscitation that improves recovery and survival in a neonatal porcine model. *Circulation* **2013**, *128*, 2495–2503. [CrossRef]
16. Berg, R.A.; Kern, K.B.; Sanders, A.B.; Otto, C.W.; Hilwig, R.W.; Ewy, G.A. Bystander cardiopulmonary resuscitation. Is ventilation necessary? *Circulation* **1993**, *88*, 1907–1915. [CrossRef]
17. Berg, R.A.; Hilwig, R.W.; Kern, K.B.; Ewy, G.A. "Bystander" Chest Compressions and Assisted Ventilation Independently Improve Outcome From Piglet Asphyxial Pulseless "Cardiac Arrest". *Circulation* **2000**, *101*, 1743–1748. [CrossRef]
18. Berg, R.A.; Hilwig, R.W.; Kern, K.B.; Barbar, I.; Ewy, G.A. Simulated mouth-to-mouth ventilation and chest compressions (bystander cardiopulmonary resuscitation) improves outcome in a swine model of prehospital pediatric asphyxial cardiac arrest. *Crit. Care Med.* **1999**, *27*, 1893–1899. [CrossRef]
19. Boldingh, A.M.; Solevåg, A.; Aasen, E.; Nakstad, B. Resuscitators who compared four simulated infant cardiopulmonary resuscitation methods favoured the three-to-one compression-to-ventilation ratio. *Acta Paediatr.* **2016**, *105*, 910–916. [CrossRef]
20. Schmölzer, G.M.; Bhatia, R.; Davis, P.G.; Tingay, D.G. A comparison of different bedside techniques to determine endotracheal tube position in a neonatal piglet model. *Pediatr. Pulmonol.* **2013**, *48*, 138–145. [CrossRef]
21. Mustofa, J.; Cheung, P.-Y.; Patel, S.; Lee, T.-F.; Lu, M.; Pasquin, M.P.; O'Reilly, M.; Schmölzer, G.M. Effects of different durations of sustained inflation during cardiopulmonary resuscitation on return of spontaneous circulation and hemodynamic recovery in severely asphyxiated piglets. *Resuscitation* **2018**, *129*, 82–89. [PubMed]
22. Shim, G.-H.; Kim, S.Y.; Cheung, P.-Y.; Lee, T.-F.; O'Reilly, M.; Schmölzer, G.M. Effects of sustained inflation pressure during neonatal cardiopulmonary resuscitation of asphyxiated piglets. *PLoS ONE* **2020**, *15*, e0228693. [CrossRef] [PubMed]
23. La Garde, R.P.; Cheung, P.-Y.; Yaskina, M.; Lee, T.-F.; O'Reilly, M.; Schmölzer, G.M. Sex Differences Between Female and Male Newborn Piglets During Asphyxia, Resuscitation, and Recovery. *Front. Pediatr.* **2019**, *7*. [CrossRef] [PubMed]
24. Kim, S.Y.; Shim, G.-H.; O'Reilly, M.; Cheung, P.-Y.; Lee, T.-F.; Schmölzer, G.M. Asphyxiated Female and Male Newborn Piglets Have Similar Outcomes with Different Cardiopulmonary Resuscitation Interventions. *Front. Pediatr.* **2020**, *8*. [CrossRef]
25. Rudikoff, M.; Maughan, W.L.; Effron, M.; Fresson, J.; Weisfeldt, M.L. Mechanisms of blood flow during cardiopulmonary resuscitation. *Circulation* **1980**, *61*, 345–352. [CrossRef]
26. Chandra, N.; Weisfeldt, M.L.; Tsitlik, J.; Vaghaiwalla, F.; Snyder, L.D.; Hoffecker, M.; Rudikoff, M. Augmentation of carotid flow during cardiopulmonary resuscitation by ventilation at high airway pressure simultaneous with chest compression. *Am. J. Cardiol.* **1981**, *48*, 1053–1063. [CrossRef]
27. Chandra, N.; Rudikoff, M.; Weisfeldt, M.L. Simultaneous chest compression and ventilation at high airway pressure during cardiopulmonary resuscitation. *Lancet* **1980**, *315*, 175–178. [CrossRef]
28. Koehler, R.C.; Tsitlik, J.; Chandra, N.; Guerci, A.D.; Rogers, M.C.; Weisfeldt, M.L. Augmentation of cerebral perfusion by simultaneous chest compression and lung inflation with abdominal binding after cardiac arrest in dogs. *Circulation* **1983**, *67*, 266–275. [CrossRef]
29. Berkowitz, I.D.; Chantarojanasiri, T.; Koehler, R.C.; Schleien, C.L.; Dean, J.M.; Michael, J.R.; Rogers, M.C.; Traystman, R.J. Blood Flow during Cardiopulmonary Resuscitation with Simultaneous Compression and Ventilation in Infant Pigs. *Pediatr. Res.* **1989**, *26*, 558–559. [CrossRef]
30. Sobotka, K.; Hooper, S.B.; Allison, B.J.; Davis, P.G.; Morley, C.J.; Moss, T.J.M. An initial sustained inflation improves the respiratory and cardiovascular transition at birth in preterm lambs. *Pediatr. Res.* **2011**, *70*, 56–60. [CrossRef]
31. Vali, P.; Chandrasekharan, P.K.; Rawat, M.; Gugino, S.F.; Koenigsknecht, C.; Helman, J.; Mathew, B.; Berkelhamer, S.; Nair, J.; Lakshminrusimha, S. Continuous Chest Compressions During Sustained Inflations in a Perinatal Asphyxial Cardiac Arrest Lamb Model. *Pediatr. Crit. Care Med.* **2017**, *18*, e370–e377. [CrossRef] [PubMed]
32. Li, E.S.; Görens, I.; Cheung, P.Y.; Lee, T.F.; Lu, M.; O'Reilly, M.; Schmölzer, G.M. Chest Compressions during Sustained Inflations Improve Recovery When Compared to a 3:1 Compression:Ventilation Ratio during Cardiopulmonary Resuscitation in a Neonatal Porcine Model of Asphyxia. *Neonatology* **2017**, *112*, 337–346. [CrossRef] [PubMed]
33. Babbs, C.; Meyer, A.; Nadkarni, V. Neonatal CPR: Room at the top—A mathematical study of optimal chest compression frequency versus body size. *Resuscitation* **2009**, *80*, 1280–1284. [CrossRef] [PubMed]
34. Solevåg, A.; Cheung, P.-Y.; Li, E.S.-S.; Xue, S.Z.; O'Reilly, M.; Fu, B.; Zheng, B.; Schmölzer, G.M. Chest Compression Quality in a Newborn Manikin: A Randomized Crossover Trial (August 2016). *IEEE J. Transl. Eng. Health Med.* **2018**, *6*, 1–5. [CrossRef]
35. Enriquez, D.; Meritano, J.; Shah, B.A.; Song, C.; Szyld, E. Fatigue during Chest Compression Using a Neonatal Patient Simulator. *Amer. J. Perinatol.* **2018**, *35*, 796–800. [CrossRef]

36. Haque, I.U.; Udassi, J.P.; Udassi, S.; Theriaque, D.W.; Shuster, J.J.; Zaritsky, A.L. Chest compression quality and rescuer fatigue with increased compression to ventilation ratio during single rescuer pediatric CPR. *Resuscitation* **2008**, *79*, 82–89. [CrossRef]
37. Te Pas, A.B.; Davis, P.G.; Hooper, S.B.; Morley, C.J. From liquid to air: Breathing after birth. *J. Pediatr.* **2008**, *152*, 607–611. [CrossRef]
38. Hooper, S.B.; Te Pas, A.B.; Kitchen, M. Respiratory transition in the newborn: A three-phase process. *Arch. Dis. Child. Fetal Neonatal Ed.* **2016**, *101*, F266–F271.
39. Solevåg, A.; Lee, T.-F.; Lu, M.; Schmölzer, G.M.; Cheung, P.-Y. Tidal volume delivery during continuous chest compressions and sustained inflation. *Arch. Dis. Child. Fetal Neonatal Ed.* **2017**, *102*, F85–F87. [CrossRef]
40. Tsui, B.C.H.; Horne, S.; Tsui, J.; Corry, G.N. Generation of tidal volume via gentle chest pressure in children over one year old. *Resuscitation* **2015**, *92*, 148–153. [CrossRef]
41. Schmölzer, G.M.; O'Reilly, M.; Fray, C.; van Os, S.; Cheung, P.-Y. Chest compression during sustained inflation versus 3:1 chest compression:ventilation ratio during neonatal cardiopulmonary resuscitation: A randomised feasibility trial. *Arch. Dis. Child. Fetal Neonatal Ed.* **2018**, *103*, F455–F460. [CrossRef] [PubMed]
42. Li, E.S.-S.; Cheung, P.-Y.; O'Reilly, M.; Schmölzer, G.M. Change in tidal volume during cardiopulmonary resuscitation in newborn piglets. *Arch. Dis. Child. Fetal Neonatal Ed.* **2015**, *100*, F530–F533. [CrossRef] [PubMed]
43. Li, E.S.-S.; Cheung, P.-Y.; Pichler, G.; Aziz, K.; Schmölzer, G.M. Respiratory function and near infrared spectroscopy recording during cardiopulmonary resuscitation in an extremely preterm newborn. *Neonatology* **2014**, *105*, 200–204. [CrossRef]
44. Foglia, E.E.; Te Pas, A.B. Sustained Lung Inflation: Physiology and Practice. *Clin. Perinatol.* **2016**, *43*, 633–646. [CrossRef] [PubMed]
45. Foglia, E.E.; Te Pas, A.B.; Kirpalani, H.M.; Davis, P.G.; Owen, L.; van Kaam, A.H.; Onland, W.; Keszler, M.; Schmölzer, G.M.; Hummler, H.D.; et al. Sustained Inflation vs Standard Resuscitation for Preterm Infants. *JAMA Pediatr.* **2020**, *174*. [CrossRef]
46. Kapadia, V.S.; Urlesberger, B.; Soraisham, A.S.; Liley, H.G.; Schmölzer, G.M.; Rabi, Y.; Wyllie, J.P.; Wyckoff, M.H. On behalf of the International Liaison Committee on Resuscitation Neonatal Life Support Task Force. Sustained Lung Inflations During Neonatal Resuscitation at Birth: A Meta-analysis. *Pediatrics* **2021**, *147*. [CrossRef]
47. Wyllie, J.P.; Bruinenberg, J.; Roehr, C.-C.; Rüdiger, M.; Trevisanuto, D.; Urlesberger, B. European Resuscitation Council Guidelines for Resuscitation 2015: Section 7. Resuscitation and support of transition of babies at birth. *Resuscitation* **2015**, *95*, 249–263. [CrossRef]
48. Klingenberg, C.; Sobotka, K.; Ong, T.; Allison, B.J.; Schmölzer, G.M.; Moss, T.J.M.; Polglase, G.R.; Dawson, J.A.; Davis, P.G.; Hooper, S.B. Effect of sustained inflation duration; resuscitation of near-term asphyxiated lambs. *Arch. Dis. Child. Fetal Neonatal Ed.* **2013**, *98*, F222–F227. [CrossRef]
49. Garcia-Hidalgo, C.; Cheung, P.-Y.; Vento, M.; O'Reilly, M.; Schmölzer, G.M. A Review of Oxygen Use During Chest Compressions in Newborns—A Meta-Analysis of Animal Data. *Front. Pediatr.* **2018**, *6*, 400. [CrossRef]
50. Garcia-Hidalgo, C.; Solevåg, A.; Kim, S.Y.; Shim, G.-H.; Cheung, P.-Y.; Lee, T.-F.; O'Reilly, M.; Schmölzer, G.M. Sustained inflation with 21% versus 100% oxygen during cardiopulmonary resuscitation of asphyxiated newborn piglets—A randomized controlled animal study. *Resuscitation* **2020**, *155*, 39–47. [CrossRef]
51. Perlman, J.M.; Wyllie, J.P.; Kattwinkel, J.; Wyckoff, M.H.; Aziz, K.; Guinsburg, R.; Kim, H.-S.; Liley, H.G.; Mildenhall, L.F.J.; Simon, W.M.; et al. Neonatal Resuscitation Chapter Collaborators Part 7: Neonatal Resuscitation: 2015 International Consensus on Cardiopulmonary Resuscitation and Emergency Cardiovascular Care Science with Treatment Recommendations (Reprint). *Pediatrics* **2015**, *136*, S120–S166. [CrossRef] [PubMed]
52. Wyckoff, M.H.; Aziz, K.; Escobedo, M.B.; Kapadia, V.S.; Kattwinkel, J.; Perlman, J.M.; Simon, W.M.; Weiner, G.M.; Zaichkin, J.G. Part 13: Neonatal Resuscitation: 2015 American Heart Association Guidelines Update for Cardiopulmonary Resuscitation and Emergency Cardiovascular Care (Reprint). *Pediatrics* **2015**, *136*, S196–S218. [CrossRef] [PubMed]
53. Luong, D.H.; Cheung, P.-Y.; Barrington, K.J.; Davis, P.G.; Unrau, J.; Dakshinamurti, S.; Schmölzer, G.M. Cardiac arrest with pulseless electrical activity rhythm in newborn infants: A case series. *Arch. Dis. Child. Fetal Neonatal Ed.* **2019**, *104*, F572–F574. [CrossRef] [PubMed]
54. Sillers, L.; Handley, S.C.; James, J.R. Pulseless Electrical Activity Complicating Neonatal Resuscitation. *Neonatology* **2018**, *115*, 95–98. [CrossRef] [PubMed]
55. Patel, S.; Cheung, P.-Y.; Solevåg, A.; Barrington, K.J.; Kamlin, C.O.F.; Davis, P.G.; Schmölzer, G.M. Pulseless electrical activity: A misdiagnosed entity during asphyxia in newborn infants? *Arch. Dis. Child. Fetal Neonatal Ed.* **2019**, *104*, F215–F217. [CrossRef] [PubMed]
56. Solevåg, A.L.; Luong, D.; Lee, T.F.; O'Reilly, M.; Cheung, P.Y.; Schmölzer, G.M. Non-perfusing cardiac rhythms in asphyxiated newborn piglets. *PLoS ONE* **2019**, *14*. [CrossRef]
57. Luong, D.H.; Cheung, P.-Y.; O'Reilly, M.; Lee, T.-F.; Schmölzer, G.M. Electrocardiography vs. Auscultation to Assess Heart Rate During Cardiac Arrest with Pulseless Electrical Activity in Newborn Infants. *Front. Pediatr.* **2018**, *6*, 366. [CrossRef] [PubMed]
58. Lista, G.; Boni, L.; Scopesi, F.; Mosca, F.; Trevisanuto, D.; Messner, H.; Vento, G.; Magaldi, R.; Del Vecchio, A.; Agosti, M.; et al. SLI Trial Investigators Sustained lung inflation at birth for preterm infants: A randomized clinical trial. *Pediatrics* **2015**, *135*, e457–e464. [CrossRef]

59. Polglase, G.R.; Miller, S.L.; Barton, S.K.; Baburamani, A.A.; Wong, F.Y.; Aridas, J.D.S.; Gill, A.W.; Moss, T.J.M.; Tolcos, M.; Kluckow, M.; et al. Initiation of resuscitation with high tidal volumes causes cerebral hemodynamic disturbance, brain inflammation and injury in preterm lambs. *PLoS ONE* **2012**, *7*, e39535. [CrossRef]
60. La Verde, A.; Franchini, S.; Lapergola, G.; Lista, G.; Barbagallo, I.; Livolti, G.; Gazzolo, D. Effects of Sustained Inflation or Positive Pressure Ventilation on the Release of Adrenomedullin in Preterm Infants with Respiratory Failure at Birth. *Amer. J. Perinatol.* **2019**, *36*, S110–S114. [CrossRef]
61. Harling, A.E.; Beresford, M.W.; Vince, G.S.; Bates, M.; Yoxall, C.W. Does sustained lung inflation at resuscitation reduce lung injury in the preterm infant? *Arch. Dis. Child. Fetal Neonatal Ed.* **2005**, *90*, F406–F410. [CrossRef] [PubMed]
62. Sobotka, K.; Hooper, S.B.; Crossley, K.J.; Ong, T.; Schmölzer, G.M.; Barton, S.K.; McDougall, A.R.A.; Miller, S.L.; Tolcos, M.; Klingenberg, C.; et al. Single Sustained Inflation followed by Ventilation Leads to Rapid Cardiorespiratory Recovery but Causes Cerebral Vascular Leakage in Asphyxiated Near-Term Lambs. *PLoS ONE* **2016**, *11*, e0146574.
63. Schmölzer, G.M. Chest Compressions During Sustained Inflation During Cardiopulmonary Resuscitation in Newborn Infants Translating Evidence From Animal & Bench Studies to the Bedside. *JACC Basic Transl. Sci.* **2019**, *4*, 116–121. [PubMed]
64. Schmölzer, G.M.; Pichler, G.; Solevåg, A.; Fray, C.; van Os, S.; Cheung, P.-Y. The SURV1VE trial—Sustained inflation and chest compression versus 3:1 chest compression-to-ventilation ratio during cardiopulmonary resuscitation of asphyxiated newborns: Study protocol for a cluster randomized controlled trial. *Trials* **2019**, *20*, 39. [CrossRef] [PubMed]
65. Aziz, K.; Chadwick, M.; Baker, M.; Andrews, W. Ante- and intra-partum factors that predict increased need for neonatal resuscitation. *Resuscitation* **2008**, *79*, 444–452. [CrossRef]
66. Schmölzer, G.M.; Kumar, M.; Aziz, K.; Pichler, G.; O'Reilly, M.; Lista, G.; Cheung, P.Y. Sustained inflation versus positive pressure ventilation at birth: A systematic review and meta-analysis. *Arch. Dis. Child. Fetal Neonatal Ed.* **2015**, *100*, F361–F368. [CrossRef]
67. Kirpalani, H.M.; Ratcliffe, S.J.; Keszler, M.; Davis, P.G.; Foglia, E.E.; Te Pas, A.B.; Fernando, M.; Chaudhary, A.; Localio, R.; van Kaam, A.H.; et al. Effect of Sustained Inflations vs Intermittent Positive Pressure Ventilation on Bronchopulmonary Dysplasia or Death Among Extremely Preterm Infants. *JAMA* **2019**, *321*, 1165–1175. [CrossRef]

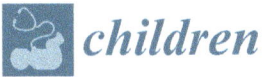

Article

The Use of a Disposable Umbilical Clamp to Secure an Umbilical Venous Catheter in Neonatal Emergencies—An Experimental Feasibility Study

Bernhard Schwaberger [1,2,*], Christoph Schlatzer [1], Daniel Freidorfer [2], Marlies Bruckner [1], Christina H. Wolfsberger [1], Lukas P. Mileder [1], Gerhard Pichler [1] and Berndt Urlesberger [1]

[1] Division of Neonatology, Department of Pediatrics and Adolescent Medicine, Medical University of Graz, 8036 Graz, Austria; christoph.schlatzer@stud.medunigraz.at (C.S.); marlies.bruckner@medunigraz.at (M.B.); christina.wolfsberger@medunigraz.at (C.H.W.); lukas.mileder@medunigraz.at (L.P.M.); gerhard.pichler@medunigraz.at (G.P.); berndt.urlesberger@medunigraz.at (B.U.)

[2] Medizinercorps Graz, Austrian Red Cross Federal Association Styria, 8010 Graz, Austria; Daniel.Freidorfer@st.roteskreuz.at

* Correspondence: bernhard.schwaberger@medunigraz.at; Tel.: +43-316-3853-0018

Citation: Schwaberger, B.; Schlatzer, C.; Freidorfer, D.; Bruckner, M.; Wolfsberger, C.H.; Mileder, L.P.; Pichler, G.; Urlesberger, B. The Use of a Disposable Umbilical Clamp to Secure an Umbilical Venous Catheter in Neonatal Emergencies—An Experimental Feasibility Study. Children 2021, 8, 1093. https://doi.org/10.3390/children8121093

Academic Editor: Joaquim M. B. Pinheiro

Received: 2 November 2021
Accepted: 24 November 2021
Published: 26 November 2021

Publisher's Note: MDPI stays neutral with regard to jurisdictional claims in published maps and institutional affiliations.

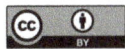

Copyright: © 2021 by the authors. Licensee MDPI, Basel, Switzerland. This article is an open access article distributed under the terms and conditions of the Creative Commons Attribution (CC BY) license (https://creativecommons.org/licenses/by/4.0/).

Abstract: Recent guidelines recommend the umbilical venous catheter (UVC) as the optimal vascular access method during neonatal resuscitation. In emergencies the UVC securement may be challenging and time-consuming. This experimental study was designed to test the feasibility of new concepts for the UVC securement. Umbilical cord remnants were catheterized with peripheral catheters and secured with disposable umbilical clamps. Three different securement techniques were investigated. Secure 1: the disposable umbilical clamp was closed at the level of the inserted catheter. Secure 2: the clamp was closed at the junction of the catheter and plastic wings. Secure 3: the setting of Secure 2 was combined with an umbilical tape. The main outcomes were the feasibility of fluid administration and the maximum force to release the securement. This study shows that inserting peripheral catheters into the umbilical vein and securing them with disposable umbilical clamps is feasible. Rates of lumen obstruction and the effectiveness of the securement were superior with Secure 2 and 3 compared to Secure 1. This new approach may be a rewarding option for umbilical venous catheterization and securement particularly in low-resource settings and for staff with limited experience in neonatal emergencies. However, although promising, these results need to be confirmed in clinical trials before being introduced into clinical practice.

Keywords: (secure method for) umbilical venous catheter (UVC); UVC securement technique; neonatal resuscitation; neonatal emergency; disposable umbilical clamp; vascular access; newborn

1. Introduction

The umbilical venous catheter (UVC) is considered "the most quickly accessible direct intravenous route" into the newborn [1,2]. Thus, recent guidelines recommend the UVC as the optimal vascular access method for drug administration during neonatal resuscitations [3–5]. Despite its frequent use, there is still a lack of knowledge on the best technique for this catheterization and UVC securement in emergency situations. The proper position of a centrally positioned UVC should be confirmed sonographically or radiographically, although this might be challenging during an actual resuscitation [6–8]. In the case of UVC malpositioning, there is the risk of adverse events including infusing drugs directly into the liver veins, potentially resulting in hepatic injuries [9–12], and furthermore, cardiac complications such as arrhythmias or cardiac tamponades [13,14]. Therefore, in neonatal emergencies it is recommended to insert the UVC only two to five cm below the skin (and even less for premature infants) until the blood can be aspirated gently via a syringe [1,2,15]. For the UVC securement, in the 7th edition of the *Textbook of Neonatal Resuscitation* a combination of suturing and taping of the UVC, or, alternatively, the use of a clear adhesive dressing is recommended. Nevertheless, both techniques require some time and may not be easily realized during emergencies [1]. However, due to a considerable risk of the accidental dislocation of the UVC during resuscitation, there is the need for an effective securement method.

In July 2018, a physician-staffed Emergency Medical Service (EMS) was faced with an unplanned out-of-hospital delivery of an extremely low-birth-weight infant of 27 weeks' gestation weighing approximately 900 g in the urban area of Graz, Austria [16]. During the neonatal resuscitation, epinephrine and a fluid administration was required, and an umbilical venous catheterization using a 22-gauge peripheral catheter was successfully performed. For the securement of the UVC, the EMS staff spontaneously used a disposable umbilical clamp. Epinephrine and a fluid bolus administration was feasible, and the securement was deemed very effective.

To investigate this concept of umbilical venous catheterization using a standard peripheral catheter and securement with a disposable umbilical clamp, we decided to perform this experimental feasibility study. The feasibility of the fluid administration and the force needed to release the securement was measured to detect relevant obstructions of the catheter lumen caused by the securement technique and to evaluate the effectiveness of the securement. The aim was to find a feasible and effective technique for neonatal emergencies, which could be performed even in low-resource settings (e.g., the out-of-hospital setting) using standard equipment.

2. Materials and Methods

This experimental feasibility study was conducted at the Division of Neonatology, Department of Paediatrics and Adolescent Medicine, Medical University of Graz, from July to August 2019. Human umbilical cords, which were already separated from the newborn infants, were used for this study. We included umbilical cord remnants from both premature and full-term infants, without a predefined number of umbilical cord remnants from premature and full-term infants.

Immediately after their separation from the newborn infant, the umbilical cord remnants were perpendicularly cut with a scalpel. The cut surface was cleaned using saline solution to identify the umbilical vein. Any visible clots at the meatus of the vein were gently removed. The umbilical vein was then catheterized with a standard peripheral catheter (B. Braun, Melsungen, Germany), using an 18-gauge catheter for full-term infants and a 20-gauge catheter for premature infants with <37 + 0 weeks' gestation. Whenever the catheterization with an 18-gauge catheter was not feasible, another attempt was made using a 20-gauge catheter. The catheter was inserted into the umbilical vein as far as possible until the plastic wings of the catheter adjoined the cut surface of the umbilical cord.

For the securement of the inserted catheter a disposable umbilical clamp (pfm medical, Cologne, Germany) was used. Three different securement techniques were investigated and compared: Secure 1, Secure 2 and Secure 3. We randomly assigned the umbilical cord remnants to one of the securement techniques and aimed for 20 successful catheterizations with each technique. For the random assignment we did not stratify for premature and full-term infants.

Secure 1: The disposable umbilical clamp was closed at the level of the inserted transparent catheter (Figures 1A and 2A).

Secure 2: The disposable umbilical clamp was closed at the junction of the transparent catheter and the colored plastic wings (Figure 1A,B and Figure 2B).

Secure 3: The disposable umbilical clamp was used identically to that in Secure 2, but additionally an "umbilical tape" (Medi-Loop Sterile Surgical Vessel Loops, Medline Industries, Warrington, United Kingdom) was placed around the umbilical cord at the level of the transparent catheter (Figure 1A,B and Figure 2C).

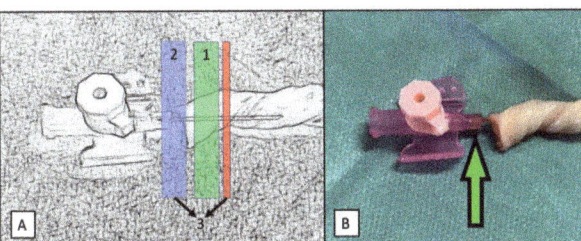

Figure 1. (**A**): Graphic illustration of the three different securement techniques (Secure 1–3): a human umbilical cord remnant was catheterized with a peripheral catheter. For Secure 1, a disposable umbilical clamp was closed in the area of the green box (1) at the level of the inserted transparent part of the catheter. For Secure 2 and Secure 3, a disposable umbilical clamp was closed in the area of the blue box (2) at the junction of the transparent catheter and the plastic wings. For Secure 3, an umbilical tape was additionally placed around the umbilical cord in the area of the red box at the level of the transparent catheter (3). (**B**): The green arrow indicates the junction of the transparent catheter and the colored plastic wings of a 20-gauge peripheral catheter. The disposable umbilical clamp was closed at the level of this junction in Secure 2 and Secure 3.

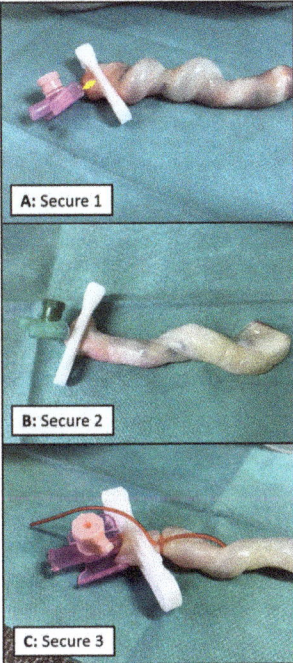

Figure 2. (**A**): Secure 1: a 20-gauge peripheral catheter inserted into the umbilical vein secured by a disposable umbilical clamp closed at the level of the transparent catheter. The yellow arrows indicate the distance between the colored plastic wings and the disposable umbilical clamp, which is longer in Secure 1 compared to Secure 2 and Secure 3. (**B**): Secure 2: an 18-gauge peripheral catheter inserted into the umbilical vein secured by a disposable umbilical clamp closed at the junction of the transparent catheter and the colored plastic wings. (**C**): Secure 3: a 20-gauge peripheral catheter inserted into the umbilical vein secured by a disposable umbilical clamp closed at the junction of the transparent catheter and the colored plastic wings, and by an additional umbilical tape placed around the umbilical cord at the level of the transparent catheter.

The main outcomes of this study were (i) the feasibility of the fluid administration and (ii) the effectiveness of the three UVC securement techniques.

To test the feasibility of the fluid administration, a predefined bolus of 10 mL 0.9% saline solution per kg of the body weight of the corresponding newborn infant was continuously administered by hand via the inserted catheter using disposable syringes (Chirana T. Injecta, Stará Turá, Slovakia). We aimed at infusing the entire fluid bolus within one minute. The free end of the umbilical cord remnant was positioned in a measuring cup, and the infused fluid was thereby collected (Figure 3A). The other end of the umbilical cord remnant with the inserted catheter and the connected syringe was held outside of the measuring cup beneath the level of its opening to prevent retrogradely leaking fluid to drip into the measuring cup. To record the fluid level in the measuring cup, the umbilical cord remnant was removed after the one-minute administration and held in position to allow the fluid to drip off into the cup for another 30 s (Figure 3B). The ratio of the within-one-minute actually administered fluid volume to the predefined volume was calculated afterward to evaluate the feasibility of the fluid administration. There were two factors that might have affected the feasibility of the fluid administration: obstruction and leakage. Failing to purge any fluid from the syringes was defined as a complete obstruction of the catheter lumen due to the securement technique. A fluid amount (that was not equal to the entire predefined volume) that remained in the syringes after the one-minute fluid administration indicated a partial obstruction. Leakage was defined by the fluid amount from the predefined bolus that was not collected in the measuring cup and that did not remain in the syringes after the one-minute fluid administration.

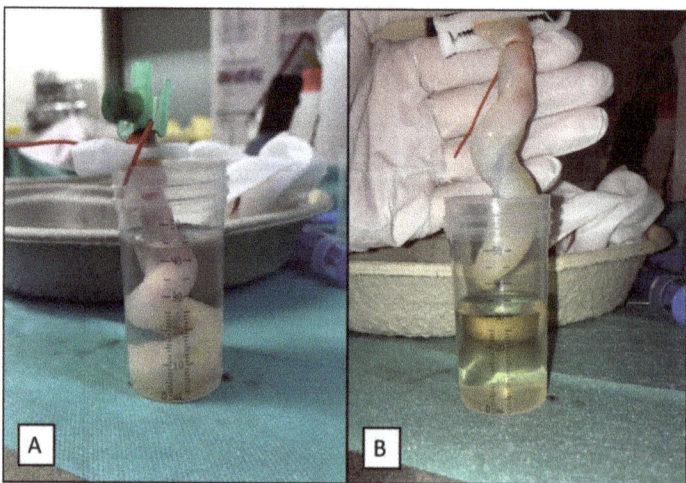

Figure 3. (**A**): The predefined fluid bolus of 0.9% saline solution was administered over one minute via the inserted and secured catheter. The free end of the umbilical cord remnant was positioned into a measuring cup, and the infused fluid was thereby collected. (**B**): To record the fluid level in the measuring cup, the umbilical cord remnant was removed and held in position to allow the fluid to drip off into the cup for another 30 s.

To measure the effectiveness of the three UVC securement techniques, an electronic spring scale (Dr. Meter, United Kingdom) was connected to a prepared disposable syringe and to the catheter via a Luer lock connection. By slowly pulling the disposable umbilical clamp, the force to release the securement was measured (Figure 4). To determine the maximum force value on the spring scale's display, the display was filmed with a digital camera and the maximum force value was identified retrospectively in a slow-motion video analysis.

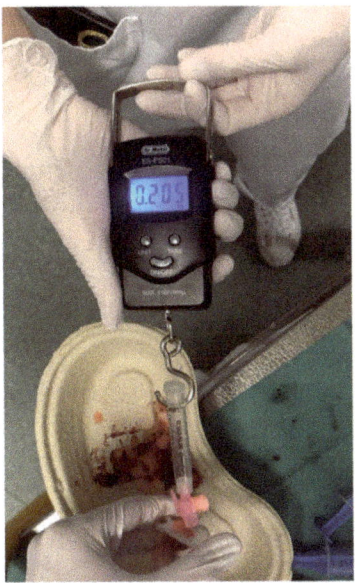

Figure 4. An electronic spring scale was connected to a prepared disposable syringe and to the catheter via a Luer lock connection. By slowly pulling the disposable umbilical clamp, the force to release the securement was measured.

Data collected included: the actually infused fluid volume; complete obstruction of the catheter lumen; remaining fluid amounts in the syringes after the one-minute fluid administration; leakage; maximum force required to release the securement; size of the peripheral catheter (20 or 18 gauge); and demographic data, including the gestational age and birth weight of the corresponding newborn infant. The parameters are presented as mean ± standard deviation (SD), median and interquartile range (IQR) or count (proportion), as appropriate. For the gestational age and birth weight the range is provided additionally to highlight the broad spectrum of newborn infants whose umbilical cord remnants were used. Data analysis was conducted with SPSS 26.0.0.1 (IBM, Armonk, NY, USA). Comparisons between the securement techniques were made using the chi-square test, Student's *t*-test or Mann–Whitney U-test, as appropriate. A *p*-value < 0.05 was considered statistically significant.

3. Results

A total of 65 umbilical cord remnants were prepared for umbilical venous catheterization. Five had to be excluded: in four of them the UVC could not be inserted far enough into the umbilical vein and thus a securement was not feasible. Another one was excluded due to the extravasation of the infused fluid bolus into the Wharton jelly. Thus, data on 20 umbilical cord remnants per securement technique were finally analyzed.

Umbilical cord remnants from 40 (67%) full-term infants and 20 (33%) premature infants with <37 + 0 weeks' gestation were included. The mean (SD) birth weight of the corresponding newborn infants was 2.86 (0.85) kg (range 0.35–4.42), and the median gestational age was 36.9 (IQR 33.9–39.9) weeks (range 26.1–40.6).

3.1. Size of Catheter

In only 58% (23 of 40 cases) of the umbilical cord remnants from full-term infants it was feasible to insert an 18-gauge catheter into the umbilical vein. There was no significant difference in the ratio of the actually administered fluid to the predefined volume depending on the size of the peripheral catheter: 100% (IQR 83–100) with the 18-gauge catheter and 93% (IQR 71–100) with the 20-gauge catheter ($p = 0.64$).

3.2. Feasibility of Fluid Administration

A complete obstruction of the UVC lumen was observed six times (30%) with Secure 1, never (0%) with Secure 2 and once (5%) with Secure 3 (Secure 1 vs. 2, $p < 0.01$; Secure 1 vs. 3, $p = 0.04$; Secure 2 vs. 3, $p = 0.31$). A partial obstruction was observed twice (10%) with Secure 1, never (0%) with Secure 2 and twice (10%) with Secure 3 (Secure 1 vs. 2, $p = 0.15$; Secure 1 vs. 3, $p = 1.00$; Secure 2 vs. 3, $p = 0.15$).

The ratio of the within-one-minute actually administered fluid volume to the predefined volume was 97% (IQR 0–100%) with Secure 1, compared to 90% (IQR 69–100%) with Secure 2 and 95% (IQR 89–100%) with Secure 3. There were no significant differences between these three securement techniques (Secure 1 vs. 2, $p = 0.27$; Secure 1 vs. 3, $p = 0.21$; Secure 2 vs. 3, $p = 0.71$).

The leakage was calculated to be 0 (IQR 0–0) mL with Secure 1, compared to 1.5 (IQR 0–3.0) mL with Secure 2 and 3.0 (IQR 0–7.5) mL with Secure 3 (Secure 1 vs. 2, $p = 0.05$; Secure 1 vs. 3, $p < 0.01$; Secure 2 vs. 3, $p = 0.27$).

3.3. Effectiveness of the Securement

The maximal force required to release the securement was 4.6 N (IQR 3.9–6.0) with Secure 1, 50.1 N (IQR 38.9–70.6) with Secure 2 and 65.9 N (IQR 56.5–68.9) with Secure 3 (Secure 1 vs.2, $p < 0.01$; Secure 1 vs.3, $p < 0.01$; Secure 2 vs. 3, $p = 0.22$).

4. Discussion

This experimental feasibility study was designed to test a new method for gaining vascular access in neonatal emergencies by inserting a standard peripheral catheter into the umbilical vein and securing it with a disposable umbilical clamp. The study demonstrates that using a disposable umbilical clamp for a UVC securement is feasible and effective. In our experience, this approach is simple and can be performed quickly. Thus, it may be a rewarding option, particularly for staff with limited experience in neonatal resuscitation.

In this study three different UVC securement techniques using disposable umbilical clamps were compared. The feasibility of the fluid administration was not different between the three techniques. However, the fluid administration was impeded by both obstructions and leakages, and concerning these factors, we observed relevant differences between the three securement techniques.

A catheter obstruction may be caused by closing the disposable umbilical clamp and thereby compressing the catheter lumen. A complete lumen obstruction can be distinguished from a partial lumen obstruction as defined in the methods section. The rate of complete catheter obstruction was significantly higher with Secure 1 compared to Secure 2 and Secure 3, which is clinically most relevant, since in cases of a complete catheter obstruction neither epinephrine nor fluids could be administered successfully during neonatal resuscitation. For Secure 1, the disposable umbilical clamp was closed at the level of the inserted transparent catheter. The transparent part of the catheter is obviously more flexible and, thus, compressible compared to the junction of the transparent catheter and the colored plastic wings, which is the position of the closed umbilical clamp in Secure 2 and Secure 3. Furthermore, we observed cases of partial obstruction not only with Secure 1 but also with Secure 3, which may impede the quick application of a fluid bolus. However, despite a partial obstruction, administering epinephrine, including a fluid flush of 1–2 mL, is still feasible within seconds, and a fluid bolus administration may also be possible even though slower infusion rates must be accepted. Based on these findings, the use of both Secure 2 and Secure 3 seem to be reasonable for UVC securements.

The leakage was significantly lower with Secure 1 compared to Secure 2 and Secure 3, which explains why the overall feasibility of the fluid administration was not different between the three techniques, despite higher obstruction rates with Secure 1. Leakages mainly occurred during the first seconds of the one-minute fluid administration with high purging pressures at the beginning. As soon as the umbilical vein was free from obstructions over its entire length and the purging pressure could be reduced, there was no retrogradely leaking fluid in most cases. Therefore, we speculate that the measured leakage was artificially high with Secure 2 and Secure 3 and probably caused by the experimental set-up of the study. Furthermore, the leakage was per definition zero in cases of complete obstruction, and due to the high complete obstruction rate the median leakage was probably underestimated with Secure 1. Hence, in our opinion the observed median leakage may not provide sufficient information to assess the effectiveness of the bleeding control. To answer this question, clinical studies are certainly needed.

The effectiveness of the UVC securement (measured by the maximal force required to release the securement) was significantly higher with Secure 2 and Secure 3 compared to Secure 1. In our experience, the maximal forces needed were rather high, especially with Secure 2 and Secure 3, compared to other previously described securement techniques [17]. However, there are no data available that would allow a direct numerical comparison with our data. Indeed, the effectiveness of the securement technique may be particularly relevant during neonatal transport and in low-resource settings, in which the patients frequently need to be transferred and/or repositioned. Therefore, Secure 2 or Secure 3 should be considered for UVC securement especially in such circumstances.

Different techniques for UVC securement have been described before, which use tapes, other adhesive materials or sutures [17]. However, immediately after birth the newborn's skin may be wet and covered with vernix, and tapes and adhesive materials may not adhere properly. Using suture needles in such situations is accompanied by a related risk of needlestick injuries, and may be difficult to perform in particular if chest compressions are required or during out-of-hospital situations. In addition, traditional techniques for UVC securement are technically challenging and relatively time-consuming during neonatal emergencies. A simulation-based study has shown that UVC placements and securements during neonatal resuscitations take approximately six minutes, and thus may severely delay the intravenous administration of epinephrine [18]. However, it is recommended that one person should hold the successfully inserted UVC in place, while another person administers the first dose of epinephrine and/or a fluid bolus during resuscitation [1]. The securement of the UVC for continued vascular access should be performed only after the first emergency drugs have been successfully administered [1]. Based on our experience, the newly introduced securement techniques can be performed quickly and with ease, although we did not measure time intervals, since our study was not a simulation-based study but an experimental feasibility study. Nonetheless, this new approach may be a rewarding option for UVC securement particularly during neonatal resuscitations.

Recent guidelines [3–5] recommend the UVC for drug administration during neonatal resuscitations, which is rarely performed (required in only 0.12% of all deliveries), requires significant skill and may be further impeded by space constraints for the resuscitation team [19]. Alternatively, vascular access may be achieved via a peripheral vein [20] or intraosseously [21,22]. Outside of the delivery room setting, the intraosseous access is being used more frequently by health care providers with limited experience and training in neonatal resuscitation, but with experience with intraosseous needle placement (i.e., EMS staff) [3]. With the herein presented new approach to umbilical venous catheterization and securement, which can be performed easily and quickly with standard equipment, the UVC might gain significance also in the abovementioned settings. Non-neonatologist health care providers might benefit from the introduction of the new technique and the potentially increased utilization of the UVC in the future, since adverse effect rates attributable to emergency umbilical venous catheterization might be lower compared to the intraosseous access. Further, a UVC can be achieved even in extremely low-birth-weight infants, while most of the available devices for intraosseous access have a higher minimum weight limit [21]. Indeed, personnel should be trained in umbilical venous catheterization periodically, even with the simple new approach for securement, ideally with real umbilical cords due to the higher physical and functional fidelity [23,24].

Limitations and Disadvantages

The main limitation of this study is its experimental character, which implies that some clinical research questions (e.g., the effectiveness of bleeding control) cannot be resolved. Although the feasibility of the new securement techniques was demonstrated experimentally, clinical studies are required to confirm our results, before this approach can be introduced safely into clinical practice. Furthermore, future research should include red blood cell transfusions, since in our study 0.9% saline solution was administered through the UVC, and different viscosities may have an impact on the feasibility of the new approach.

One disadvantage of the newly introduced securement techniques is the risk of catheter obstructions caused by the disposable umbilical clamp. Once the disposable umbilical clamp is closed, it may irreversibly compress the lumen of the peripheral plastic catheter. Using a metal cannula (e.g., a bulb-headed probe) instead of the flexible peripheral catheter could help preventing such lumen obstructions. Alternatively, reusable plastic clamps that spring open again when released could be used. However, we aimed to test the concept of using peripheral catheters in combination with disposable umbilical clamps for UVC securement, since these devices are generally available even in low-resource settings and belong to the standard equipment (e.g., in ambulance vehicles).

Considering a recent animal study, in which a higher flush volume after the first dose of epinephrine was shown to be beneficial during neonatal resuscitation [25], there is likely need for an even higher volume of saline flush following epinephrine with the new UVC techniques compared to the centrally placed UVC, because of the additional length of the umbilical vein to be flushed.

Another disadvantage is that the integrity of the umbilical arteries will likely be compromised following the placement of the umbilical clamp, and the umbilical arterial access and placement of a long-term umbilical venous catheter would need to be performed distal to the clamp placement. Therefore, there should be enough umbilical cord remaining between the clamp and the umbilicus to ensure that future access to the umbilical vessels will be possible.

5. Conclusions

Inserting a standard peripheral catheter (18 or 20 gauge) into the umbilical vein and securing it by using a disposable umbilical clamp was feasible with all three investigated securement techniques (Secure 1–3). Rates of complete catheter lumen obstruction and the effectiveness of securement was superior with Secure 2 and 3 compared to Secure 1. Still, these results need to be confirmed in clinical trials before being introduced into clinical routines. During neonatal resuscitations, the new approach may be a rewarding option for umbilical venous catheterizations and UVC securements, particularly in low-resource settings and for staff with limited experience in neonatal emergencies.

Author Contributions: Conceptualization, B.S. and D.F.; methodology, B.S., C.S. and B.U.; software, B.S. and C.S.; validation, B.S., C.S. and B.U.; formal analysis, B.S. and C.S.; investigation, B.S. and C.S., M.B. and C.H.W.; resources, B.S., G.P. and B.U.; data curation, B.S., C.S. and B.U.; writing—original draft preparation, B.S. and C.S.; writing—review and editing, B.S., C.S., D.F., M.B., C.H.W., L.P.M., G.P. and B.U.; supervision, B.S, G.P. and B.U.; project administration, B.S. All authors have read and agreed to the published version of the manuscript.

Funding: This research received no external funding.

Institutional Review Board Statement: The study protocol was approved by the Regional Committee on Biomedical Research Ethics (No. 31-548 ex 18/19), approval date is 24 October 2019.

Informed Consent Statement: Written informed consent was obtained from the parents prior to study inclusion.

Data Availability Statement: The data presented in this study are available in this article.

Conflicts of Interest: The authors declare no conflict of interest.

References

1. American Academy of Pediatrics; American Heart Association. *Textbook of Neonatal Resuscitation*, 7th ed.; American Academy of Pediatrics: Healdsburg, CA, USA, 2016.
2. Anderson, J.; Leonard, D.; Braner, D.A.V.; Lai, S.; Tegtmeyer, K. Umbilical vascular catheterization. *N. Engl. J. Med.* **2008**, *359*, e18. [CrossRef]
3. Wyckoff, M.H.; Wyllie, J.; Aziz, K.; de Almeida, M.F.; Fabres, J.W.; Fawke, J.; Guinsburg, R.; Hosono, S.; Isayama, T.; Kapadia, V.S.; et al. Neonatal life support 2020 international consensus on cardiopulmonary resuscitation and emergency cardiovascular care science with treatment recommendations. *Resuscitation* **2020**, *156*, A156–A187. [CrossRef]
4. Madar, J.; Roehr, C.C.; Ainsworth, S.; Ersdal, H.; Morley, C.; Rudiger, M.; Skare, C.; Szczapa, T.; Te Pas, A.; Trevisanuto, D.; et al. European resuscitation council guidelines 2021: Newborn resuscitation and support of transition of infants at birth. *Resuscitation* **2021**, *161*, 291–326. [CrossRef]
5. Aziz, K.; Lee, C.H.C.; Escobedo, M.B.; Hoover, A.V.; Kamath-Rayne, B.D.; Kapadia, V.S.; Magid, D.J.; Niermeyer, S.; Schmolzer, G.M.; Szyld, E.; et al. Part 5: Neonatal resuscitation 2020 american heart association guidelines for cardiopulmonary resuscitation and emergency cardiovascular care. *Pediatrics* **2021**, *147*, e2020038505E. [CrossRef]
6. Greenberg, M.; Movahed, H.; Peterson, B.; Bejar, R. Placement of umbilical venous catheters with use of bedside real-time ultrasonography. *J. Pediatr.* **1995**, *126*, 633–635. [CrossRef]
7. Michel, F.; Brevaut-Malaty, V.; Pasquali, R.; Thomachot, L.; Vialet, R.; Hassid, S.; Nicaise, C.; Martin, C.; Panuel, M. Comparison of ultrasound and X-ray in determining the position of umbilical venous catheters. *Resuscitation* **2012**, *83*, 705–709. [CrossRef] [PubMed]
8. Fleming, S.E.; Kim, J.H. Ultrasound-guided umbilical catheter insertion in neonates. *J. Perinatol.* **2011**, *31*, 344–349. [CrossRef] [PubMed]
9. Derinkuyu, B.E.; Boyunaga, O.L.; Damar, C.; Unal, S.; Ergenekon, E.; Alimli, A.G.; Oztunali, C.; Turkyilmaz, C. Hepatic complications of umbilical venous catheters in the neonatal period: The ultrasound spectrum. *J. Ultrasound Med.* **2018**, *37*, 1335–1344. [CrossRef] [PubMed]
10. Chen, H.J.; Chao, H.C.; Chiang, M.C.; Chu, S.M. Hepatic extravasation complicated by umbilical venous catheterization in neonates: A 5-year, single-center experience. *Pediatr. Neonatol.* **2020**, *61*, 16–24. [CrossRef]
11. Mutlu, M.; Aslan, Y.; Kul, S.; Yilmaz, G. Umbilical venous catheter complications in newborns: A 6-year single-center experience. *J. Matern. Fetal. Neonatal. Med.* **2016**, *29*, 2817–2822. [CrossRef]
12. Grizelj, R.; Vukovic, J.; Bojanic, K.; Loncarevic, D.; Stern-Padovan, R.; Filipovic-Grcic, B.; Weingarten, T.N.; Sprung, J. Severe liver injury while using umbilical venous catheter: Case series and literature review. *Am. J. Perinatol.* **2014**, *31*, 965–974. [CrossRef]
13. Traen, M.; Schepens, E.; Laroche, S.; van Overmeire, B. Cardiac tamponade and pericardial effusion due to venous catheterization. *Acta Paediatr.* **2005**, *94*, 626–628. [CrossRef]
14. Sheta, A.; Al-Awad, E.; Soraisham, A. Supraventricular tachycardia associated with umbilical venous catherterization in neonates. *J. Clin. Neonatol.* **2018**, *7*, 166–169.
15. Schwaberger, B.; Eichinger, M.; Martensen, J.; Baik-Schneditz, N.; Pocivalnik, M.; Urlesberger, B. Regional recommendations for the stabilisation of preterm infants in the pre-hospital setting in styria. *Notarzt* **2019**, *35*, 314–322.
16. Schwaberger, B.; Schörghuber, M.; Schober, L.; Eichinger, M.; Urlesberger, B. Out-of-hospital resuscitation of an extremly premature infant at the limit of viability—Case report. *Notarzt* **2019**, *35*, 137–140.
17. Elser, H.E. Options for securing umbilical catheters. *Adv. Neonatal. Care* **2013**, *13*, 426–429. [CrossRef]
18. McKinsey, S.; Perlman, J.M. Resuscitative interventions during simulated asystole deviate from the recommended timeline. *Arch. Dis. Child. Fetal Neonatal Ed.* **2016**, *101*, F244–F247. [CrossRef] [PubMed]
19. Rajani, A.K.; Chitkara, R.; Oehlert, J.; Halamek, L.P. Comparison of umbilical venous and intraosseous access during simulated neonatal resuscitation. *Pediatrics* **2011**, *128*, e954–e958. [CrossRef]
20. Baik-Schneditz, N.; Pichler, G.; Schwaberger, B.; Mileder, L.; Avian, A.; Urlesberger, B. Peripheral intravenous access in preterm neonates during postnatal stabilization: Feasibility and safety. *Front. Pediatr.* **2017**, *5*, 171. [CrossRef] [PubMed]
21. Scrivens, A.; Reynolds, P.R.; Emery, F.E.; Roberts, C.T.; Polglase, G.R.; Hooper, S.B.; Roehr, C.C. Use of intraosseous needles in neonates: A systematic review. *Neonatology* **2019**, *116*, 305–314. [CrossRef]
22. Mileder, L.P.; Urlesberger, B.; Schwaberger, B. Use of intraosseous vascular access during neonatal resuscitation at a tertiary center. *Front. Pediatr.* **2020**, *8*, 571285. [CrossRef]
23. Sawyer, T.; Starr, M.; Jones, M.; Hendrickson, M.; Bosque, E.; McPhillips, H.; Batra, M. Real vs. simulated umbilical cords for emergency umbilical catheterization training: A randomized crossover study. *J. Perinatol.* **2017**, *37*, 177–181. [CrossRef] [PubMed]
24. Mileder, L.P.; Pocivalnik, M.; Schwaberger, B.; Pansy, J.; Urlesberger, B.; Baik-Schneditz, N. Practice of umbilical venous catheterization using a resource-efficient 'blended' training model. *Resuscitation* **2018**, *122*, e21–e22. [CrossRef] [PubMed]
25. Sankaran, D.; Vali, P.; Chandrasekharan, P.; Chen, P.; Gugino, S.F.; Koenigsknecht, C.; Helman, J.; Nair, J.; Mathew, B.; Rawat, M.; et al. Effect of a Larger Flush Volume on Bioavailability and Efficacy of Umbilical Venous Epinephrine during Neonatal Resuscitation in Ovine Asphyxial Arrest. *Children* **2021**, *8*, 464. [CrossRef] [PubMed]

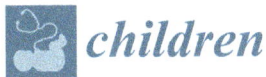

Article

Effect of a Larger Flush Volume on Bioavailability and Efficacy of Umbilical Venous Epinephrine during Neonatal Resuscitation in Ovine Asphyxial Arrest

Deepika Sankaran [1,*], Payam Vali [1], Praveen Chandrasekharan [2], Peggy Chen [1], Sylvia F. Gugino [2], Carmon Koenigsknecht [2], Justin Helman [2], Jayasree Nair [2], Bobby Mathew [2], Munmun Rawat [2], Lori Nielsen [2], Amy L. Lesneski [3], Morgan E. Hardie [1], Ziad Alhassen [1], Houssam M. Joudi [1], Evan M. Giusto [1], Lida Zeinali [2], Heather K. Knych [4], Gary M. Weiner [5] and Satyan Lakshminrusimha [1]

1. Department of Pediatrics, University of California, Davis, Sacramento, CA 95817, USA; pvali@ucdavis.edu (P.V.); pegchen@ucdavis.edu (P.C.); mehardie@ucdavis.edu (M.E.H.); zalhassen@ucdavis.edu (Z.A.); hmjoudi@ucdavis.edu (H.M.J.); egiusto@ucdavis.edu (E.M.G.); slakshmi@ucdavis.edu (S.L.)
2. Department of Pediatrics, University at Buffalo, Buffalo, NY 14203, USA; pkchandr@buffalo.edu (P.C.); sfgugino@buffalo.edu (S.F.G.); carmonko@buffalo.edu (C.K.); jhelman@buffalo.edu (J.H.); jnair@upa.chob.edu (J.N.); bmathew@upa.chob.edu (B.M.); mrawat@buffalo.edu (M.R.); lnielsen@buffalo.edu (L.N.); lizeinali@ucdavis.edu (L.Z.)
3. Department of Stem Cell Research, University of California, Davis, Sacramento, CA 95817, USA; allesneski@ucdavis.edu
4. Department of Molecular Biosciences, Davis School of Veterinary Medicine, University of California, Davis, CA 95616, USA; hkknych@ucdavis.edu
5. Department of Pediatrics, University of Michigan, Ann Arbor, MI 48109, USA; gweiner@med.umich.edu
* Correspondence: dsankaran@ucdavis.edu

Abstract: The 7th edition of the *Textbook of Neonatal Resuscitation* recommends administration of epinephrine via an umbilical venous catheter (UVC) inserted 2–4 cm below the skin, followed by a 0.5-mL to 1-mL flush for severe bradycardia despite effective ventilation and chest compressions (CC). This volume of flush may not be adequate to push epinephrine to the right atrium in the absence of intrinsic cardiac activity during CC. The objective of our study was to evaluate the effect of 1-mL and 2.5-mL flush volumes after UVC epinephrine administration on the incidence and time to achieve return of spontaneous circulation (ROSC) in a near-term ovine model of perinatal asphyxia induced cardiac arrest. After 5 min of asystole, lambs were resuscitated per Neonatal Resuscitation Program (NRP) guidelines. During resuscitation, lambs received epinephrine through a UVC followed by 1-mL or 2.5-mL normal saline flush. Hemodynamics and plasma epinephrine concentrations were monitored. Three out of seven (43%) and 12/15 (80%) lambs achieved ROSC after the first dose of epinephrine with 1-mL and 2.5-mL flush respectively ($p = 0.08$). Median time to ROSC and cumulative epinephrine dose required were not different. Plasma epinephrine concentrations at 1 min after epinephrine administration were not different. From our pilot study, higher flush volume after first dose of epinephrine may be of benefit during neonatal resuscitation. More translational and clinical trials are needed.

Keywords: epinephrine; flush volume; neonatal resuscitation; chest compressions; asphyxia; cardiac arrest; epinephrine concentrations

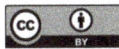

1. Introduction

The International Liaison Committee on Resuscitation (ILCOR) advocates use of epinephrine in neonates with severe bradycardia (heart rate < 60 beats per minute [bpm]) despite effective positive pressure ventilation (PPV) and chest compressions (CC) if return of spontaneous circulation (ROSC) is not achieved [1,2]. Intravenous (IV) route is the preferred route for epinephrine administration due to greater efficacy and plasma epinephrine concentrations when compared to the endotracheal route [3–5]. In the delivery room, an umbilical venous catheter (UVC) can be inserted to 2–4 cm below the skin to allow quick administration of epinephrine. The 7th edition of the *Textbook of Neonatal Resuscitation* recommends 0.5-mL to 1-mL flush following IV epinephrine (0.01 to 0.03 mg/kg dose) via a low-lying UVC [6]. Although this flush volume may be sufficient in the setting of spontaneous cardiac activity (i.e., bradycardia), the recommended flush volume may only clear a 5 Fr UVC (internal volume = 0.55 mL) that is placed for term neonates and may not be sufficient to drive epinephrine to the heart and the circulating blood in the setting of cardiac arrest and CC [7]. Earlier ROSC following effective and quick delivery of an epinephrine dose by a route with maximum bioavailability may potentially improve survival and outcomes [8,9].

Recently, use of a 3-mL flush following IV or intraosseous (IO) epinephrine has been proposed by the American Academy of Pediatrics/American Heart Association (AAP/AHA) Neonatal Resuscitation Program (NRP) guidelines [10]. This recommendation is based on expert opinion and not based on robust scientific evidence. Our objective was to evaluate and compare the effect of different flush volumes of 1-mL and 2.5-mL following a 0.03 mg/kg epinephrine dose through a low UVC on the incidence of ROSC, and the incidence of ROSC after the first dose of epinephrine. We also evaluated the secondary outcomes of time to achieve successful ROSC and plasma epinephrine concentrations.

2. Materials and Methods

The current study protocol was approved by the Institutional Animal Care and Use Committee (IACUC) at the State University of New York, Buffalo, NY, USA (protocol PED10085N) and University of California Davis, Davis, CA, USA (protocol 20734). The experiments were performed in compliance with animal ethical guidelines (the ARRIVE guidelines) [11]. Time-dated healthy pregnant ewes from May Family Enterprises (Buffalo Mills, PA, USA) and Van Laningham Farms (Arbuckle, CA, USA) were fasted overnight and underwent cesarean section after endotracheal intubation under general anesthesia with IV diazepam and ketamine, and inhaled 2% isoflurane, as previously described [12,13].

2.1. Fetal Instrumentation

The fetal lamb was partially exteriorized for instrumentation while still attached to placental circulation. The lamb's airway was intubated and the endotracheal tube was occluded. Carotid arterial and jugular venous catheters were inserted on the right sided blood vessels for preductal arterial blood draws, invasive blood pressure and heart rate monitoring, and IV access respectively. A flow probe (Transonics, Ithaca, New York, NY, USA) was placed around the left carotid artery to continuously measure blood flow.

2.2. Asphyxial Arrest and Resuscitation

The umbilical cord was compressed and occluded to induce asphyxia and cardiac arrest. Electrocardiogram leads (3- lead EKG) were applied. The lambs were resuscitated after 5 min of cardiac arrest (flat line on carotid arterial tracing and pulseless electrical activity of <20 bpm on EKG) per NRP guidelines. PPV was initiated with peak inflation pressures of 30–35 cm H_2O, positive end expiratory pressure (PEEP) of 5 cm H_2O and rate of 40 breaths per minute using 21% oxygen [14]. If the lambs did not achieve ROSC with effective PPV, then CC were initiated at 3:1 compression-to-ventilation ratio and supplemental oxygen was simultaneously increased to 100%. The lambs that did not have ROSC with PPV and CC alone and required IV epinephrine were included in the study. IV epinephrine (0.03 mg/kg/dose) was administered every 3 min via a low-lying UVC placed to a depth of 2–4 cm from the skin until ROSC was achieved. The epinephrine dose was followed by a flush volume of either 1-mL or 2.5-mL normal saline. The resuscitators were not blinded to the flush volumes. ROSC was defined as sustained spontaneous heart rate of >100 bpm along with a systolic blood pressure > 40 mm Hg. If ROSC was not achieved, cardiopulmonary resuscitation was continued for a total of 20 min with IV epinephrine repeated every 3 min for a maximum of 4 doses. Lambs were euthanized using IV pentobarbital (Fatal-Plus, Vortech Pharmaceuticals, Dearborn, MI, USA).

Arterial blood samples were obtained at the start of PPV and at 1 min after epinephrine and flush administration (since we anticipate peak plasma epinephrine concentrations at this time point). Plasma samples were frozen at −80 °C until analysis for epinephrine concentrations by ELISA (Eagle Biosciences, New York, NY, USA).

2.3. Primary and Secondary Outcomes

Primary outcome measures were incidence of ROSC and incidence of ROSC with the first dose of epinephrine.

Secondary outcome measures included time to achieve ROSC from time of epinephrine and flush, and plasma epinephrine concentration at 1 min after epinephrine and flush administration.

2.4. Data Collection and Statistical Analysis

Hemodynamic variables were continuously monitored during asphyxia, resuscitation and after ROSC, and recorded using BIOPAC systems (Goleta, CA, USA) software version-4.3.1. Categorical data were analyzed by chi-squared test with Fisher's exact test as required, non-parametric continuous variables by Mann–Whitney U test, and parametric continuous variables by unpaired t-test. Data were analyzed using Statview 5.0.1 (SAS Institute Inc., New York, NY, USA). Probability of <5% was used for statistical significance. Some of the data included in this manuscript were previously published [9,12].

Power calculation: Power was calculated for the parameter: incidence of ROSC with the first dose of epinephrine. We planned a study of 15 experimental subjects and 7 control subjects. Prior data indicate that the ROSC rate among controls is 0.40. If the true ROSC rate for experimental subjects is 0.80, we can reject the null hypothesis that the ROSC rates for experimental and control subjects are equal with probability (power) 0.47. The type I error probability associated with this test of this null hypothesis is 0.05.

3. Results

Twenty-two near-term lambs were asphyxiated until cardiac arrest by umbilical cord occlusion. Birth characteristics such as gestational age, birth weight, sex, and time to cardiac arrest from the time of umbilical cord occlusion were not different between the two study groups (Table 1).

Table 1. Comparison of characteristics between lambs that received 1-mL and 2.5-mL flush volumes after 0.03 mg/kg low UVC epinephrine.

Flush Volume	1-mL Flush $n = 7$	2.5-mL Flush $n = 15$	p-Value
Gestational age (days)	142 (2)	140 (1)	0.97
Weight (kg)	4.45 (1.3)	3.6 (0.8)	0.07
Sex distribution n (%)	4 females (57%)	6 females (40%)	0.45
Time to cardiac arrest (min)	14.7 (3.6)	15.6 (4.6)	0.89
ROSC incidence with the 1st dose of epinephrine n (%)	3 (42.8%)	12 (80%)	0.08
ROSC incidence n (%)	5 (71.4%)	13 (86.6%)	0.38
Median time to ROSC from time of epinephrine and flush (s)	95 (60–120)	72 (56–111)	0.71
Cumulative dose of epinephrine (mg/kg) median (interquartile range)	0.06 (0.03–0.075)	0.03 (0.03–0.03)	0.26
Mean blood pressure at 10 min after ROSC (mmHg)	64 (25)	65 (15)	0.26 0.96
Heart rate at 10 min after ROSC (beats per minute)	195 (14)	194 (13)	0.88
Left Carotid artery blood flow at 10 min after ROSC (ml/kg/min)	26 (6)	31 (13)	0.47

Data presented as mean (standard deviation) or median (interquartile range) as specified. Parameters were not different between the groups. Categorical data were analyzed by chi-squared test with Fisher's exact test as required, non-parametric continuous variables by Mann–Whitney U test, and parametric continuous variables by unpaired t-test. UVC: umbilical venous catheter. ROSC: return of spontaneous circulation.

3.1. Incidence of ROSC and Time to Achieve ROSC

Three out of seven (43%) and twelve out of fifteen (80%) lambs had ROSC after the first dose of epinephrine with 1-mL and 2.5-mL flush respectively (p = 0.08, Table 1). The time to achieve ROSC from the time of epinephrine administration was not different (p = 0.71, Table 1).

3.2. Cumulative Dose of Epinephrine and Epinephrine Concentrations in Plasma

The cumulative epinephrine dose required to achieve ROSC was not different with use of 1-mL and 2.5-mL flush volumes following the epinephrine dose (Table 1). Plasma epinephrine concentrations at 1 min after epinephrine and flush administration were also not different (Table 2).

Table 2. Comparison of peak plasma epinephrine pharmacokinetics at 1 min following 1st dose of low UVC epinephrine at 0.03 mg/kg.

Parameter	1-mL Flush	2.5-mL Flush	p-Value
Plasma epinephrine concentration at 1 min after epinephrine dose among all the lambs studied (ng/mL).	494 (171)	519 (140)	0.92
Plasma epinephrine concentration at 1 min after epinephrine and flush among lambs that achieved ROSC with 1st dose (ng/mL)	572 (50)	545 (165)	0.94

Data are presented as mean (standard error of mean). Data not different by unpaired t-test.

3.3. Post-ROSC Hemodynamics

Heart rates, arterial blood pressures, and carotid blood flows at 10 min after ROSC were similar between the lambs that received 1-mL and 2.5-mL flush volumes after epinephrine via low UVC (Table 1).

4. Discussion

Perinatal asphyxia requiring extensive resuscitation including CC and epinephrine administration is associated with poor neurodevelopmental outcomes in neonates. Clinical measures to increase the incidence and hasten ROSC may potentially improve outcomes. The current study reports that larger flush volume of 2.5-mL normal saline following epinephrine at a dose of 0.03 mg/kg is associated with 80% incidence of ROSC, following the first dose of IV epinephrine, compared to 42% with the use of 1-mL flush.

The 7th edition AAP–NRP *Textbook of Neonatal Resuscitation* recommended 0.5-mL to 1-mL of saline flush following epinephrine administration through a low umbilical venous route [6]. Due to lack of valves in the ductus venosus and high resistance in the ductus venosus during CC, epinephrine may be deposited in the umbilical vein and not reach the heart with 0.5 mL to 1 mL flush. Furthermore, epinephrine may increase the portal venous resistance, thus barricading the epinephrine within the portal venous system (Figure 1) [7]. A larger flush volume following low UVC epinephrine may maintain the patency of the ductus venosus and propel epinephrine into the right atrium. Contrast studies and angiography using a low UVC (inserted ~6 cm in a term newborn) in 1961 showed opacification of the left atrium and ventricle with contrast within seconds of injection [15]. We speculate that with adequate flush, epinephrine is propelled across the patent foramen ovale (PFO) to the left heart and systemic circulation (Figure 1). The AAP- NRP in the 8th edition of the Textbook of Neonatal Resuscitation have changed the recommendation and increased the flush volume to 3-mL following epinephrine [9,10].

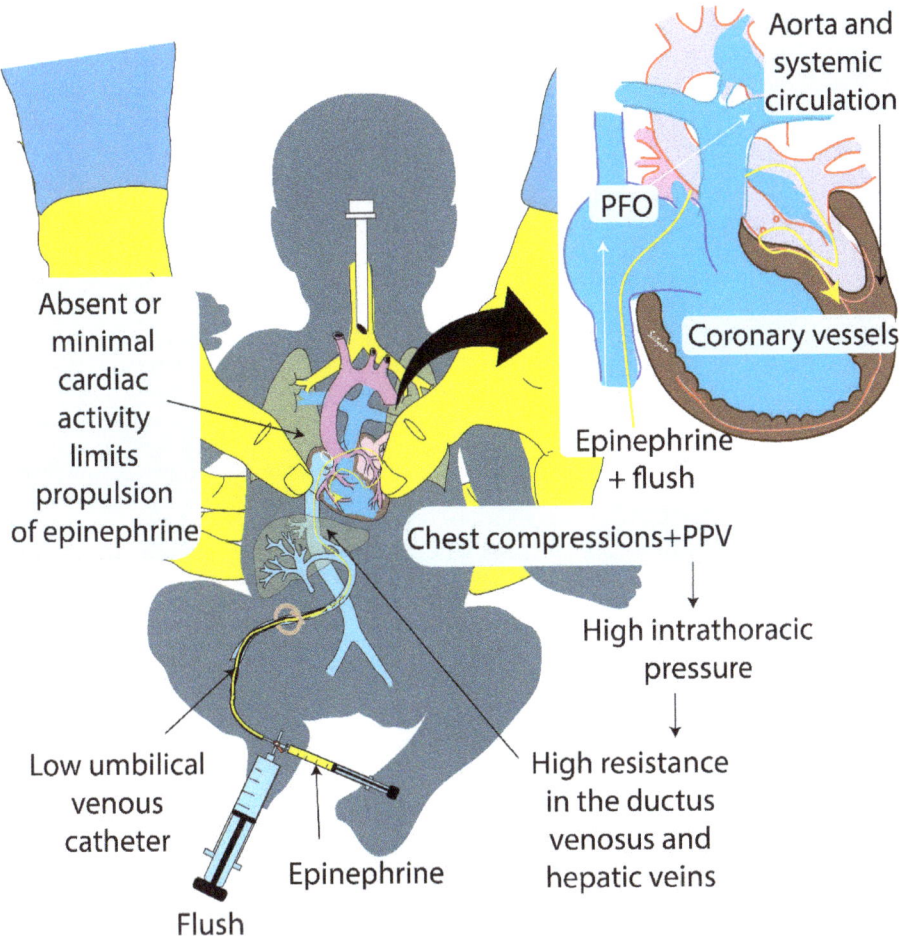

Figure 1. Schematic showing the speculative mechanism of larger flush volume following low umbilical venous catheter (UVC) epinephrine in term newborns. During cardiac arrest (absence of spontaneous cardiac activity) and during chest compressions and positive pressure ventilation (PPV) that increase the intrathoracic pressure and cause back pressure in the inferior vena cava, the epinephrine injected via a low umbilical venous catheter followed by a low flush volume of 0.5 mL to 1 mL may not be delivered to the right atrium. The epinephrine may be deposited in the umbilical vein or hepatic veins. The use of a higher flush volume may propel the epinephrine to the right atrium and across the patent foramen ovale (PFO) to left heart, aorta, systemic circulation, and coronary arteries increasing the chances of return of spontaneous circulation (ROSC). Inset shows a magnified view of the heart and coronary vessels. The yellow line represents the path of epinephrine and flush in the figure and the inset. Copyright Satyan Lakshminrusimha.

We have previously compared the effect of flush volumes of 1-mL and ~10-mL after low UVC epinephrine in a term ovine model of perinatal cardiac arrest [12]. Larger flush volume of ~10-mL resulted in quicker ROSC when compared to 1-mL flush after the first epinephrine dose. However, use of flush volumes as high as ~10 mL may not be preferred by neonatal providers in the delivery room due to two reasons. Firstly, perinatal asphyxia can lead to myocardial dysfunction (systolic and diastolic) [16,17]. Excess volume administration during resuscitation may pose a strain on the already compromised heart, further increasing myocardial workload and oxygen demand [18,19]. Secondly, after prolonged asphyxia, hypercapnia and rapid increase in cerebral blood flow follows [20]. In this setting, further increases in cerebral blood flow due to excessive volume use during resuscitation may potentially worsen reperfusion injury. In extremely preterm infants, high flush volumes administered rapidly can lead to fluctuations in cerebral blood flow with a potential for severe intraventricular hemorrhage. In our previous experiment, we limited the larger flush volume to the first epinephrine dose. In contrast, in the current study, we used a 2.5-mL flush volume following subsequent doses of epinephrine as well.

Use of 1-mL flush had a trend towards lower incidence of ROSC following the first dose of epinephrine. Achieving early ROSC with the minimum required epinephrine doses may improve outcomes and avoid post-ROSC adverse effects of epinephrine including tachycardia, hypertension, and increased myocardial oxygen demand [21]. The current study did not demonstrate a difference in hemodynamic parameters of heart rate, arterial blood pressure, or carotid arterial blood flow at 10 min after ROSC when 1-mL and 2.5-mL flush volumes were used after the epinephrine dose. In addition to increasing efficacy of IV epinephrine, a larger flush volume may potentially decrease adverse effects by lowering the cumulative epinephrine dose required prior to achieving ROSC and warrants adequately powered clinical trials.

There are several limitations to this study. The included lambs were not randomized and the resuscitators were not blinded to the intervention. Furthermore, our study was underpowered to demonstrate a difference between the groups, and we may have seen a statistically significant difference if we had a larger sample size. We evaluated the effect of flush volume following low UVC epinephrine administration in a term large mammalian model of perinatal asphyxial arrest but did not evaluate preterm or bradycardia models. We have not evaluated the effect of flush volume following IO epinephrine. Species differences may result in different effects of flush volume in human neonates. Long-term cardiovascular and neurological outcomes were not evaluated. Real time physiological monitoring and epinephrine pharmacokinetics with plasma epinephrine concentrations are the strengths of this study. Furthermore, this is the first report evaluating the effects of using a 2.5-mL flush volume following a low UVC epinephrine in neonatal asphyxial arrest.

Data from our previously published study evaluating 3 mL/kg flush volume (approximately 10-mL in term lambs) resulted in ROSC in 8/9 lambs with the first dose of epinephrine at 0.03 mg/kg (88%). In one lamb that did not achieve ROSC with the first dose, a subsequent dose of epinephrine 0.03 mg/kg with 1-mL flush led to ROSC. A graphic summary combining results from the current paper and our previous publication [12] of 3 doses of flush (1-mL, 2.5-mL, and 10-mL) is shown in Figure 2.

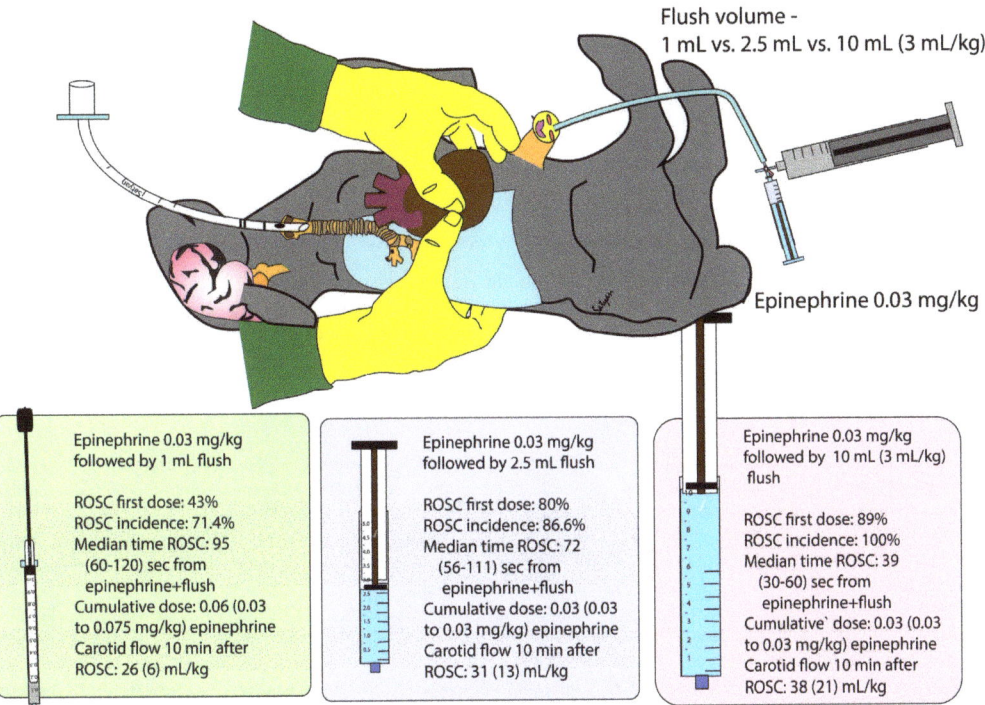

Figure 2. Graphic abstract of data from current study and Sankaran et al. [12] comparing 1-mL, 2.5-mL, and 3 mL/kg (~10 mL) flush in term lambs with asphyxial arrest induced by umbilical cord occlusion. In lambs receiving 10-mL flush, only the first dose of epinephrine was associated with high volume flush. (Copyright Satyan Lakshminrusimha).

5. Conclusions

Larger flush volume following low UVC epinephrine may increase the incidence of ROSC with the first dose of epinephrine. Adequately powered clinical trials are warranted to study the effect of a larger flush volume following UVC epinephrine on survival and long-term cardiovascular and neurodevelopmental outcomes.

Author Contributions: Conceptualization, D.S. and S.L.; methodology, D.S., P.V., P.C. (Praveen Chandrasekharan), P.C. (Peggy Chen), S.F.G., C.K., J.H., J.N., B.M., M.R., L.N., A.L.L., M.E.H., E.M.G., Z.A., H.M.J., L.Z., H.K.K., G.M.W., S.L.; software: D.S., C.K., J.N., M.E.H., H.M.J.; investigation, D.S., P.V., P.C. (Praveen Chandrasekharan), P.C. (Peggy Chen), S.F.G., C.K., J.H., J.N., B.M., M.R., L.N., A.L.L., M.E.H., E.M.G., Z.A., H.M.J., L.Z., H.K.K., G.M.W., S.L.; validation, D.S., S.L.; formal analysis, D.S.; resources, S.L.; data curation, D.S., C.K., J.N., M.E.H., H.M.J.; writing- original draft preparation, D.S., S.L.; writing- review and editing- D.S., P.V., P.C. (Praveen Chandrasekharan), P.C. (Peggy Chen), S.F.G., C.K., J.H., J.N., B.M., M.R., L.N., A.L.L., M.E.H., E.M.G., Z.A., H.M.J., L.Z., H.K.K., G.M.W., S.L.; visualization, D.S., S.L.; supervision, S.F.G., S.L., P.C. (Praveen Chandrasekharan); project administration, D.S., P.V., P.C. (Praveen Chandrasekharan), P.C. (Peggy Chen), S.F.G., C.K., J.H., J.N., B.M., M.R., L.N., A.L.L., M.E.H., E.M.G., Z.A., H.M.J., L.Z., H.K.K., G.M.W., S.L.; Funding acquisition, S.L., P.C. (Praveen Chandrasekharan). All authors have read and agreed to the published version of the manuscript.

Funding: This research was funded by American Academy of Pediatrics–Neonatal Resuscitation Program Research Grant (S.L. P.C.) and the Eunice Kennedy Shriver National Institute of Child Health and Human Development (NICHD) 5R01 HD072929 (S.L.), Children's Miracle Network at University of California, Davis, First Tech Federal Credit Union and UC Davis Pediatrics, Canadian Pediatric Society NRP research grant (D.S.), National Institutes of Health (NIH)/National Heart Lung and Blood Institute (NHLBI) K12 HL138052 (P.C.), NICHD R03HD096510 (P.C.) and National Center for Advancing Translational Sciences of the National Institutes of Health under award number UL1TR001412 (P.C.) to the University at Buffalo.

Institutional Review Board Statement: The study was conducted according to the guidelines of the Declaration of Helsinki, and approved by the Institutional Animal Care and Use Committee (IACUC) at the State University of New York, Buffalo, NY, USA (protocol PED10085N) and University of California Davis, Davis, CA, USA (protocol 20734).

Informed Consent Statement: Not applicable.

Data Availability Statement: The data presented in this study are available in this article.

Conflicts of Interest: The authors declare no conflict of interest. G.W. and S.L. are members of the AAP NRP steering committee. The views expressed in this article are their own and do not represent the official position of AAP or NRP. The funders had no role in the design of the study; in the collection, analyses, or interpretation of data; in the writing of the manuscript, or in the decision to publish the results.

References

1. Wyckoff, M.H.; Wyllie, J.; Aziz, K.; De Almeida, M.F.; Fabres, J.; Fawke, J.; Guinsburg, R.; Hosono, S.; Isayama, T.; Kapadia, V.S.; et al. Neonatal life support: 2020 international consensus on cardiopulmonary resuscitation and emergency cardiovascular care science with treatment recommendations. *Circulation* **2020**, *142*, S185–S221. [CrossRef] [PubMed]
2. Isayama, T.; Mildenhall, L.; Schmölzer, G.M.; Kim, H.-S.; Rabi, Y.; Ziegler, C.; Liley, H.G. International Liaison Committee on Resuscitation Newborn Life Support Task Force The route, dose, and interval of epinephrine for neonatal resuscitation: A systematic review. *Pediatrics* **2020**, *146*, e20200586. [CrossRef] [PubMed]
3. Vali, P.; Chandrasekharan, P.; Rawat, M.; Gugino, S.; Koenigsknecht, C.; Helman, J.; Jusko, W.J.; Mathew, B.; Berkelhamer, S.; Nair, J.; et al. Evaluation of timing and route of epinephrine in a neonatal model of asphyxial arrest. *J. Am. Heart. Assoc.* **2017**, *6*, e004402. [CrossRef] [PubMed]
4. Nair, J.; Vali, P.; Gugino, S.F.; Koenigsknecht, C.; Helman, J.; Nielsen, L.C.; Chandrasekharan, P.; Rawat, M.; Berkelhamer, S.; Mathew, B.; et al. Bioavailability of endotracheal epinephrine in an ovine model of neonatal resuscitation. *Early Hum. Dev.* **2019**, *130*, 27–32. [CrossRef] [PubMed]
5. Aziz, K.; Lee, H.C.; Escobedo, M.B.; Hoover, A.V.; Kamath-Rayne, B.D.; Kapadia, V.S.; Magid, D.J.; Niermeyer, S.; Schmölzer, G.M.; Szyld, E.; et al. Part 5: Neonatal resuscitation: 2020 american heart association guidelines for cardiopulmonary resuscitation and emergency cardiovascular care. *Circulation* **2020**, *142*, S524–S550. [CrossRef] [PubMed]
6. American Academy of Pediatrics; American Heart Association. *Textbook of Neonatal Resuscitation*, 7th ed.; American Academy of Pediatrics: Healdsburg, CA, USA, 2016.
7. Vali, P.; Sankaran, D.; Rawat, M.; Berkelhamer, S.; Lakshminrusimha, S. Epinephrine in neonatal resuscitation. *Children* **2019**, *6*, 51. [CrossRef] [PubMed]
8. Foglia, E.E.; Weiner, G.; De Almeida, M.F.B.; Wyllie, J.; Wyckoff, M.H.; Rabi, Y.; Guinsburg, R. International liaison committee on resuscitation neonatal life support task force duration of resuscitation at birth, mortality, and neurodevelopment: A systematic review. *Pediatrics* **2020**, *146*, e20201449. [CrossRef] [PubMed]
9. Vali, P.; Weiner, G.M.; Sankaran, D.; Lakshminrusimha, S. What is the optimal initial dose of epinephrine during neonatal resuscitation in the delivery room? *J. Perinatol.* **2021**, 1–5. [CrossRef]
10. NRP 8th Edition Busy People Update. 2021. Available online: https://downloads.aap.org/AAP/PDF/NRP%208th%20Edition%20Busy%20People%20Update%20(1).pdf (accessed on 1 March 2021).
11. Kilkenny, C.; Browne, W.J.; Cuthill, I.C.; Emerson, M.; Altman, D.G. Improving bioscience research reporting: The arrive guidelines for reporting animal research. *PLoS Biol.* **2010**, *8*, e1000412. [CrossRef] [PubMed]
12. Sankaran, D.; Chandrasekharan, P.K.; Gugino, S.F.; Koenigsknecht, C.; Helman, J.; Nair, J.; Mathew, B.; Rawat, M.; Vali, P.; Nielsen, L.; et al. Randomised trial of epinephrine dose and flush volume in term newborn lambs. *Arch. Dis. Child. Fetal Neonatal Ed.* **2021**. [CrossRef] [PubMed]
13. Vali, P.; Gugino, S.; Koenigsknecht, C.; Helman, J.; Chandrasekharan, P.; Rawat, M.; Lakshminrusimha, S.; Nair, J. The perinatal asphyxiated lamb model: A model for newborn resuscitation. *J. Vis. Exp.* **2018**, *2018*, e57353. [CrossRef] [PubMed]
14. Sankaran, D.; Chen, P.; Alhassen, Z.; Lesneski, A.; Hardie, M.; Lakshminrusimha, S.; Vali, P. Optimal inspired oxygen weaning strategy following return of spontaneous circulation after perinatal asphyxial arrest. *Sect. Neonatal Perinat. Med. Program* **2021**, *147*, 757–759. [CrossRef]

15. Hirvonen, L.; Peltonen, T.; Ruokola, M. Angiocardiography of the newborn with contrast injected into the umbilical vein. *Ann. Paediatr. Fenn.* **1961**, *7*, 124–130. [PubMed]
16. Bhasin, H.; Kohli, C. Myocardial dysfunction as a predictor of the severity and mortality of hypoxic ischaemic encephalopathy in severe perinatal asphyxia: A case-control study. *Paediatr. Int. Child Health* **2019**, *39*, 259–264. [CrossRef] [PubMed]
17. Rajakumar, P.; Bhat, B.V.; Sridhar, M.; Balachander, J.; Konar, B.; Narayanan, P.; Chetan, G. Cardiac enzyme levels in myocardial dysfunction in newborns with perinatal asphyxia. *Indian J. Pediatr.* **2008**, *75*, 1223–1225. [CrossRef] [PubMed]
18. Popescu, M.R.; Panaitescu, A.M.; Pavel, B.; Zagrean, L.; Peltecu, G.; Zagrean, A.-M. Getting an early start in understanding perinatal asphyxia impact on the cardiovascular system. *Front. Pediatr.* **2020**, *8*. [CrossRef] [PubMed]
19. Wyckoff, M.H.; Perlman, J.M.; Laptook, A.R. Use of volume expansion during delivery room resuscitation in near-term and term infants. *Pediatric* **2005**, *115*, 950–955. [CrossRef] [PubMed]
20. Kasdorf, E.; Perlman, J.M. Strategies to prevent reperfusion injury to the brain following intrapartum hypoxia-ischemia. *Semin. Fetal Neonatal Med.* **2013**, *18*, 379–384. [CrossRef] [PubMed]
21. Berg, R.A.; Otto, C.W.; Kern, K.B.; Hilwig, R.W.; Sanders, A.B.; Henry, C.P.; Ewy, G.A. A randomized, blinded trial of high-dose epinephrine versus standard-dose epinephrine in a swine model of pediatric asphyxial cardiac arrest. *Crit. Care Med.* **1996**, *24*, 1695–1700. [CrossRef] [PubMed]

Article

Iatrogenic Blood Loss in Very Low Birth Weight Infants and Transfusion of Packed Red Blood Cells in a Tertiary Care Neonatal Intensive Care Unit

Ahmed Aboalqez, Philipp Deindl, Chinedu Ulrich Ebenebe, Dominique Singer and Martin Ernst Blohm *

Division of Neonatology and Pediatric Intensive Care Medicine, University Children's Hospital, University Medical Center Hamburg-Eppendorf, Martinistr. 52, 20246 Hamburg, Germany; a.aboalqez@uke.de (A.A.); p.deindl@uke.de (P.D.); c.ebenebe@uke.de (C.U.E.); d.singer@uke.de (D.S.)
* Correspondence: m.blohm@uke.de

Abstract: An adequate blood volume is important for neonatal adaptation. The study objective was to quantify the cumulative iatrogenic blood loss in very low birth weight (VLBW) infants by blood sampling and the necessity of packed red cell transfusions from birth to discharge from the hospital. In total, 132 consecutive VLBW infants were treated in 2019 and 2020 with a median birth weight of 1180 g (range 370–1495 g) and a median length of stay of 54 days (range 0–154 days) were included. During the initial four weeks of life, the median absolute amount of blood sampling was 16.5 mL (IQR 12.3–21.1 mL), sampling volume was different with 14.0 mL (IQR 12.1–16.2 mL) for non-transfused infants and 21.6 mL (IQR 17.5–29.4 mL) for transfused infants. During the entire length of stay, 31.8% of the patients had at least one transfusion. In a generalized logistic regression model, the cumulative amount of blood sampling ($p < 0.01$) and lower hematocrit at birth ($p = 0.02$) were independent predictors for the necessity of blood transfusion. Therefore, optimized patient blood management in VLBW neonates should include sparse blood sampling to avoid iatrogenic blood loss.

Keywords: VLBW neonate; blood sampling; blood transfusion; iatrogenic blood loss

1. Introduction

An adequate circulatory volume is essential in perinatal transition and during the neonatal period [1]. During a regular physiological vaginal delivery, a placental blood transfusion to the newborn occurs in the period after the birth of the child, before the umbilical cord is clamped.

At delivery of a mature neonate, 70 mL/kg blood, referring to the infant's body weight, are in the infant, and 35 mL/kg in the placenta [2]. With delayed cord clamping, placental blood is shifted to the newly born infant resulting in a blood volume of approximately 93 mL/kg body weight after three minutes [2]. This perinatal auto-transfusion of placental blood into the neonate appears to be a biologically useful mechanism to help perinatal adaptation [1–5], particularly for premature infants with their physiologically low absolute amount of blood volume.

Neonatal blood volume can be preserved by sparse blood sampling for diagnostic purposes. Iatrogenic neonatal blood loss in association with blood sampling [6–13] has been an issue for decades. Several studies have actually quantified the iatrogenic blood loss in VLBW neonates [6–11]. The amount of blood taken from ELBW and VLBW infants during the first 28 days of life has been reported as 31 mL/kg body weight in 1981 [6], 50.3 mL/kg body weight [7] in 1988, and 24.2 mL/kg body weight in 2019 [8]. In a recent study published in 2020, the average cumulative 28 d blood loss in ELBW neonates with an umbilical artery catheter (UAC) in place was 69 mL (108 mL/kg) while the average cumulative blood loss without UAC in place was 32 mL (43 mL/kg) [9]. Different studies quantifying iatrogenic neonatal blood loss have in common, that smaller neonates (ELBW and VLBW) have a relatively higher amount of blood sampling in mL/kg body weight than larger neonates [6–11]. Still, iatrogenic blood loss by blood sampling is one of the main factors for anemia in VLBW infants, leading to the necessity of packed red cell transfusions. Even in recent publications, approximately 50% of VLBW neonates with a normal hematocrit at birth require at least one transfusion during their hospital stay [14]. This study aimed to quantify cumulative iatrogenic blood losses in VLBW neonates and correlate them to demographic and clinical outcome parameters and to blood transfusions. With this study, we want to raise awareness for good neonatal patient blood management [15] by preserving blood volume, starting at initial stabilization or resuscitation and then throughout the entire length of hospital stay of this patient population.

2. Materials and Methods

This observational study was conducted as a retrospective single-center study at a tertiary referral center (University Hamburg-Eppendorf Medical Center, Hamburg, Germany). We included VLBW and ELBW infants born in the University Medical Center Hamburg-Eppendorf during 2019 and 2020 into the analysis. Transfusion triggers for packed red cells were restrictive [16–18], based on the national guidelines, generally following the restrictive arm of the ETTNO trial [18]. Neonatal outcome parameters were defined as follows: Bronchopulmonary dysplasia (BPD) as additional oxygen demand at a corrected age of 36 weeks, intraventricular hemorrhage (IVH) in cases with IVH grade 3 or 4, necrotizing enterocolitis (NEC) as Bell stage 2 and 3, retinopathy of prematurity (ROP) was defined by the necessity of intraocular vascular endothelial growth inhibitor (VEGF-inhibitor) administration or laser treatment. Blood sampling, transfusion, and clinical and outcome data were extracted from the electronic patient data management system (PDMS ICM, Dräger, Lübeck, Germany). For individual types of laboratory tests (e.g., full blood count, clinical chemistry, drug level monitoring, clotting studies, blood gas analysis, blood samples for crossmatching packed red cells, neonatal metabolic screening, genetic testing) the amount of blood typically required in the setting of the neonatal intensive care unit (NICU) and blood losses in association with vascular access were defined as follows: blood gas analysis 100 µL, newborn screening 250 µL, full blood count 750 µL, infection screen including IL6 and CRP 750 µL, extended blood tests including liver and renal function tests 1000 µL, blood culture 500 µL, drug levels 750 µL, clotting studies 1300 µL, blood losses with the establishment of venous or arterial access 750 µL. The cumulative volume of all blood samples and losses for each patient during the entire hospital stay was then calculated based on the laboratory results in the PDMS. In total, 164 patients were eligible. Patients transferred to other hospitals or in-house wards not equipped with the electronic PDMS before discharge at home were excluded. Subsequently, 132 VLBW neonates were included in the analysis.

For statistical analysis with appropriate tests (Chi-Square test statistics and Fisher's exact test, pairwise Pearson correlation, t-test, generalized logistic regression model) R (Version 4.0.3, R Core Team, 2020) and SPSS (version 20, IBM Inc., Chicago, IL, USA) were used. Data collection and anonymized data handling were in concordance with the local Review Board (Ethik-Kommission Ärztekammer Hamburg, Germany, WF-075/21, 29 March 2021).

3. Results

3.1. Patients

Data from 132 VLBW infants were included. Table 1 shows the demographic and outcome parameters of the studied sample cohort.

Table 1. Demographic and clinical characteristics of the study population sample.

	Study Population (n = 132)
Birth weight [g, median, IQR, range]	1180 (IQR 903–1360, range 370–1495)
Gestational age [weeks, median, IQR, range]	29 + 5 (IQR 27 + 5 to 31 + 2; range 23 + 5 to 36 + 5)
LOS [days, median, IQR, range]	54 (IQR 35–74; range 0–154)
Multiple gestation [n; %]	66 (50%)
Female sex [n; %]	63 (47.7%)
Delivery mode C-section	121 (91.7%)
Sepsis/Infection [n; %]	39 (29.5%)
IVH [n; %]	6 (4.5%)
BPD [n; %]	6 (4.5%)
ROP [n; %]	6 (4.5%)
NEC [n; %]	4 (3.0%)
PDA treated medically	28 (21.2%)
PDA treated operatively [n; %]	4 (3.0%)
Fatal outcome [n; %]	6 (4.5%)

Legend: IQR interquartile range; LOS length of stay; IVH intraventricular hemorrhage (grade 3 and 4); BPD bronchopulmonary dysplasia; ROP retinopathy of prematurity; PDA persistent arterial duct; NEC necrotizing enterocolitis.

3.2. Blood Transfusion

The rate of patients receiving at least one packed red cell transfusion during their hospital stay was 31.8%. The cumulative blood transfusion volume during the entire hospital stay was 33.5 mL on average (IQR 20–53.75 mL) in patients who received at least one transfusion. Patients with and without a blood transfusion were demographically different (Table 2) with a higher birth weight and gestational age and a shorter duration of stay in non-transfused patients.

Table 2. Demographic differences between transfused and non-transfused patients.

Demographic Factor	Transfused Patients (n = 42)	Non-Transfused Patients (n = 90)	p (t-Test)
Birth weight [g, median, IQR]	755 (643–943)	1275 (1074–1415)	<0.001
Gestational age [weeks, median, IQR]	26 + 2 (25 + 3 − 29 + 5)	30 + 2 (28 + 5 − 31 + 5)	<0.001
LOS [days, median, IQR]	93 (70–103)	44 (33–59)	<0.001

Legend: IQR interquartile range; LOS length of stay.

3.3. Blood Sampling

The absolute amount of blood sampling is shown in Table 3. The median absolute amount of blood sampling [mL] during the initial four weeks of life was 16.5 mL (IQR 12.3–21.1 mL). Median sampling volume and median gestational age were different with 14.00 mL (IQR 12.05–16.20 mL)/gestational age 30 + 2 weeks (IQR 28 + 5 − 31 + 5 weeks) for non-transfused infants and 21.60 mL (IQR 17.51–29.40 mL)/26 + 2 weeks (IQR 25 + 3 − 29 + 5 weeks) for transfused infants.

Table 3. Absolute cumulative blood sampling volume [n = 132 VLBW infants].

Postnatal Age [Completed Weeks]	Non-Transfused Patients [mL; Median (IQR)]	Transfused Patients [mL; Median (IQR)]
0	6.18 (4.73–7.35)	8.20 (6.60–9.95)
1	8.65 (7.23–10.53)	11.50 (9.35–14.75)
2	10.33 (8.43–12.69)	14.98 (11.86–18.95)
3	12.45 (10.39–14.01)	17.15 (13.90–26.50)
4	14.00 (12.05–16.20)	21.60 (17.51–29.40)
5	15.50 (13.49–17.71)	22.10 (17.88–32.89)
6	17.68 (15.93–20.64)	23.20 (19.10–35.95)
7	19.45 (17.30–21.25)	25.50 (21.03–35.86)
8	20.90 (18.74–24.84)	30.83 (23.25–41.79)
9	26.45 (21.45–29.45)	34.63 (25.40–44.35)
10	31.45 (29.10–33.25	37.28 (25.11–47.11)
11	33.60 (32.08–35.13)	39.45 (29.50–49.00)
12	36.80 (35.25–37.60)	41.45 (31.38–53.75)
13	36.23 (35.01–37.44)	44.70 (34.70–55.10)
14		49.75 (43.99–60.01)
15		59.90 (45.70–70.05)
16		65.60 (62.65–87.35)
17		89.90 (77.13–123.05)
18		90.10 (78.80–124.13)
19		92.15 (80.75–126.50)
20		126.60 (109.43–143.78)

Legend: IQR interquartile range.

The amount of blood sampling during the total length of stay in relation to birth weight [mL/kg birth weight, median (IQR)] was 16.42 mL (IQR 9.86–32.65 mL) for the whole group; 12.78 mL (IQR 8.15–17.35 mL) for non-transfused infants and 39.42 mL (IQR 29.33–73.95 mL) for transfused infants (Figure 1).

The mean initial hematocrit in non-transfused neonates with 52.6% was significantly higher compared to 47.0% in neonates requiring transfusion during hospital stay ($p < 0.001$), whereas the hematocrit at discharge was not statistically different between the two groups (31.3% vs. 30.4%, $p = 0.34$) (Figure 1).

The time course of cumulative iatrogenic losses by blood sampling is presented in Table 4 and Figure 2A,B. The cumulative blood sampling volume was significantly different between patients requiring a transfusion and non-transfused patients. The time course of hematocrit is shown in Figure 2C.

There was a significant correlation between cumulative blood sampling volume and cumulative blood transfusion volume (Figure 3).

An analysis of the relative contribution of iatrogenic blood losses in the study sample of neonates treated in our unit is given in Figure 4.

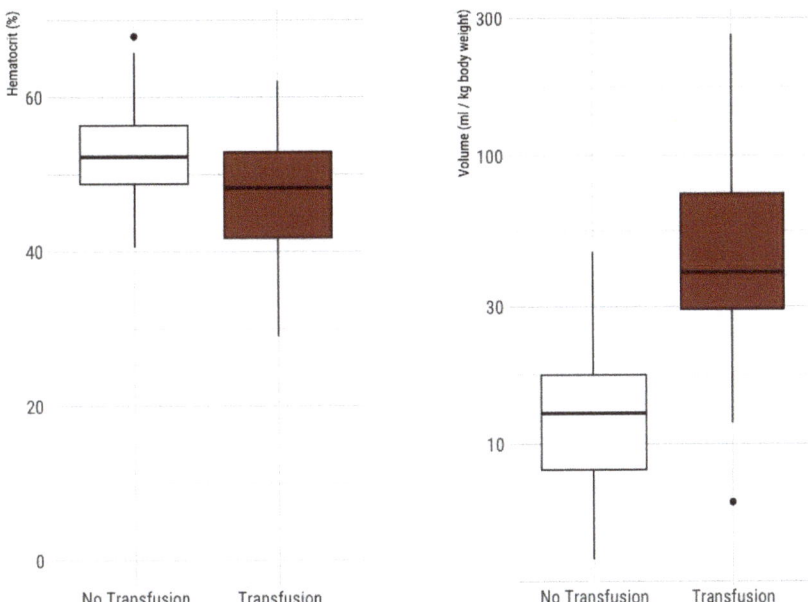

Figure 1. (**Left**) Comparison of hematocrit on admission between non-transfused and transfused VLBW infants. Boxplots show median, IQR, 95% confidence intervals, and outliers. The mean initial hematocrit in non-transfused neonates with 52.6% was significantly higher compared to 47.0% in neonates requiring at least one transfusion during hospital stay ($p < 0.001$). (**Right**) Comparison of cumulative blood sampling volume in VLBW infants during their hospital stay [mL/kg body weight at birth] between non-transfused and transfused VLBW neonates. Boxplots show median, IQR, 95% confidence intervals and outliers, y-axis logarithmic scale. Non-transfused neonates ($n = 90$) had significantly less median blood sampling volume 12.78 mL (IQR 8.15–17.35 mL) compared to neonates with one or more red blood cell transfusions during their hospital stay ($n = 42$) with a median cumulative sampling volume of 39.42 mL (IQR 29.33–73.95 mL).

Table 4. Chi-Square Test statistics for demographic and outcome factors associated with transfusions, factors ordered in ascending likelihood ratio for the necessity of red blood cell transfusion.

Factor	Likelihood Ratio (Fisher's Exact Test)	p
Sex	0.127	0.852 (n.s.)
Multiple gestation	0.127	0.852 (n.s.)
Delivery mode	0.140	0.740 (n.s.)
IVH	3.216	0.081 (n.s.)
BPD	7.165	0.012 *
Mortality	7.165	0.012 *
ROP	7.165	0.012 *
PDA treated operatively	9.432	0.009 *
NEC	9.432	0.009 *
PDA treated medically	12.892	0.000 *
Sepsis/Infection	30.087	0.000 *
Gestational age	92.743	0.001 *
Length of stay	131.353	0.000 *
Birth weight	136.013	0.000 *

Legend: n.s. no significance; * $p < 0.05$. LOS length of stay; IVH intraventricular hemorrhage (grade 3 and 4); BPD bronchopulmonary dysplasia; ROP retinopathy of prematurity; PDA persistent arterial duct; NEC necrotizing enterocolitis.

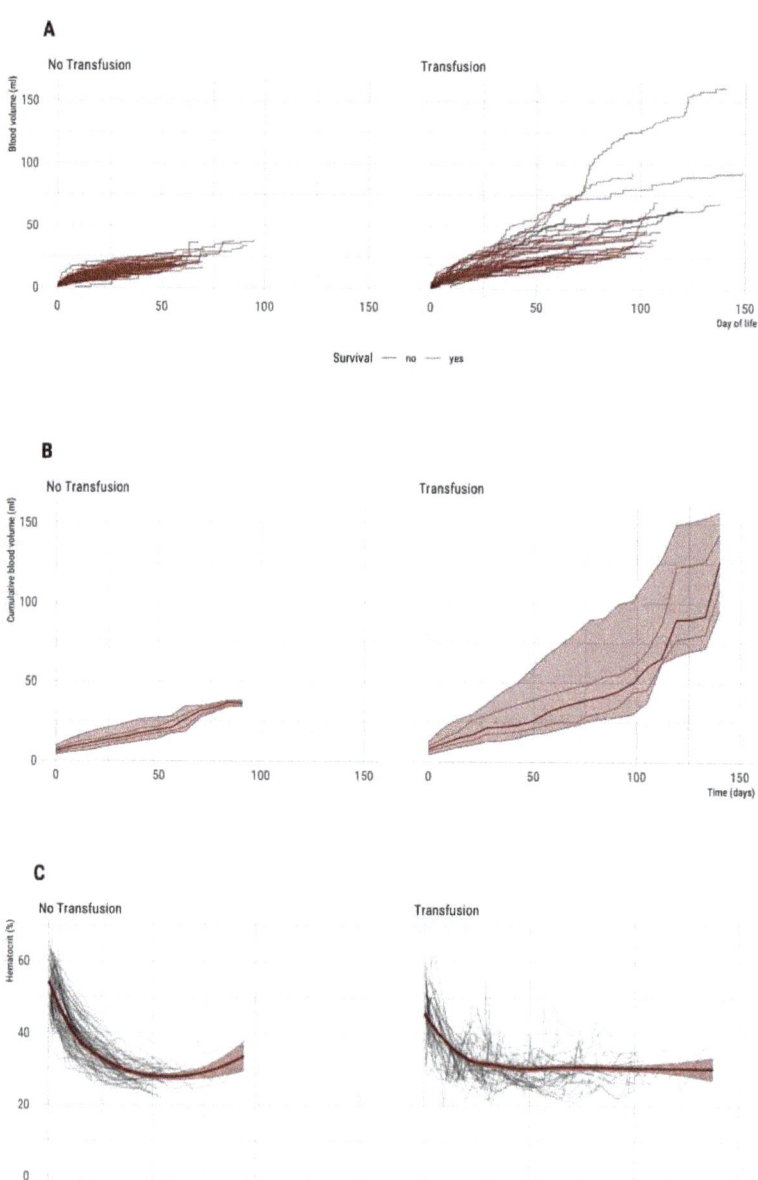

Figure 2. (**A–C**) Time course of cumulative blood sampling volume and hematocrit during entire hospital stay (*n* = 132 VLBW neonates included). Left: Non-transfused neonates (*n* = 90). Right: Neonates with one or more red cell transfusions (*n* = 42). (**A**) Absolute cumulative blood sampling volume [mL] over time. Each line represents an individual patient. (**B**) Median and percentiles (percentiles 5, 25, 50 75, 95) are given for a minimum of 3 patients per week, therefore plot truncated at 20 weeks. (**C**) Time course of hematocrit. Each grey line represents an individual patient. The dark red lines show smoothed average hematocrit, the dark red transparent ribbon the 95% CI of mean over time.

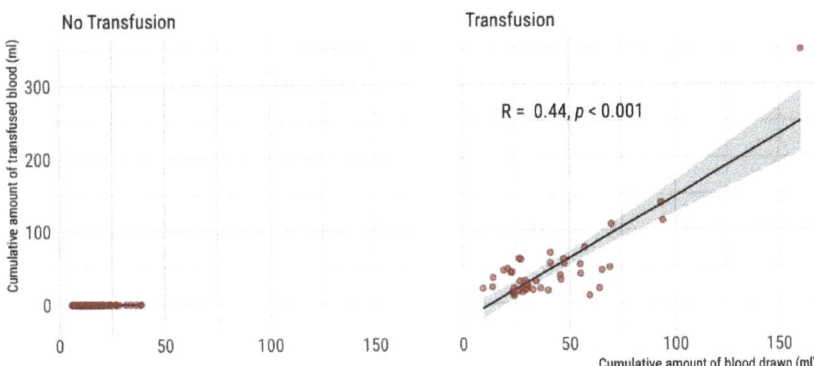

Figure 3. Correlation of cumulative blood sampling volume and cumulative amount of transfused blood during entire hospital stay (*n* = 132 VLBW neonates included). (**Left**) Non-transfused neonates (*n* = 90). (**Right**) Neonates with one or more red cell transfusions (*n* = 42). Two-sided Spearman's rank correlation coefficient rho and 95% CI is given.

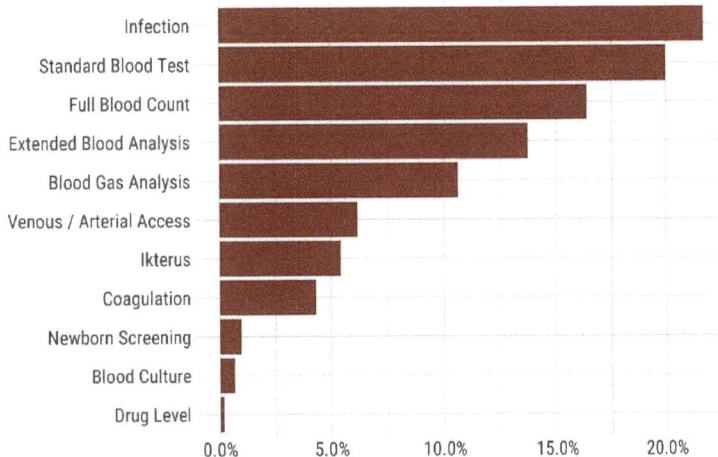

Figure 4. Relative amount [%] of iatrogenic blood loss during the hospital stay (*n* = 132 VLBW included neonates into the analysis). The bars represent the cumulative relative amount of blood loss associated with different laboratory investigations: Infection (sample including IL6), standard blood test (sample with C-reactive protein), full blood count, extended blood analysis (liver and renal function tests), blood gas analysis, losses during vascular access, icterus (bilirubin and liver function test), coagulation (clotting studies), newborn screening (neonatal newborn screening), blood culture, drug level.

3.4. Risk Factors for Necessity of Transfusion

Demographic parameters associated with the necessity for erythrocyte transfusion were birth weight, gestational age, and length of stay, whereas sex, delivery mode, and multiple gestations were not associated with an increased risk of a transfusion requirement. Outcome parameters significantly associated with the necessity for erythrocyte transfusion were sepsis/infection, PDA, NEC, ROP, fatal outcome. In contrast, IVH was not significantly associated with transfusions (Table 4).

A generalized logistic model, including time on invasive ventilation, the total amount of blood sampling, first hematocrit, and gestational age was calculated in order to identify independent risk factors for red blood cell transfusion during the hospital stay. The model identified the total amount of blood sampling and first hematocrit as independent predictors for a blood transfusion (Figure 5).

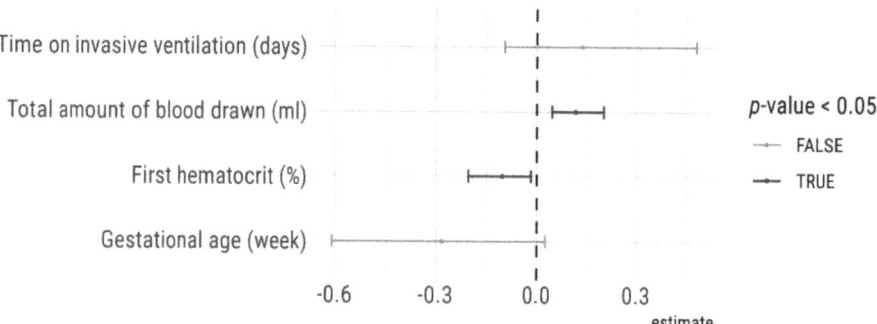

Figure 5. Predictors of transfusion deduced from a generalized logistic model. Cumulative blood sampling volume and hematocrit on admission were significant independent predictors of red blood cell transfusion during the hospital stay in the 132 VLBW included neonates into the analysis.

4. Discussion

This single-center retrospective study analyzed the amount of iatrogenic blood sampling and subsequent blood loss and requirements for packed red cell transfusions in VLBW infants during their entire hospital stay. The sample cohort comprised a non-selected cross-sectional and consecutive longitudinal group of VLBW neonates.

The median absolute amount of blood sampling during the initial four weeks of life was 16.5 mL (IQR 12.3–21.1 mL). The cumulative blood sampling volume was comparable to a recent publication on neonatal blood sampling in VLBW infants with a median blood loss of 19.6 mL during the first 28 days [8] and lower than in historical data [6,7]. Our unit strives to keep usage of umbilical vascular catheters restrictive and as short as possible. This may also contribute to a relatively low iatrogenic blood loss [9].

Demographic factors such as lower birth weight, lower gestational age, and longer length of stay were significantly associated with the necessity for erythrocyte transfusion, as well as several adverse neonatal outcome parameters (sepsis/infection, PDA, NEC, ROP, death). Thus, smaller VLBW patients with higher morbidity had a higher risk of receiving a transfusion.

In addition, a generalized logistic model identified both the cumulative amount of blood sampling (in mL/kg body weight) and the initial hematocrit as significant independent predictors of transfusion in the VLBW infants of our sample cohort.

The study finding of a higher hematocrit at birth in the group of non-transfused neonates supports the recommendations regarding delayed cord clamping at birth [3,4]. In a meta-analysis, delayed cord clamping increased the hematocrit at birth by 2.73%, resulting in a 10% reduction of red cell transfusions [4]. In our study, the initial hematocrit of non-transfused children was 11.9% higher than in transfused children (52.6% vs. 47.0%). Neonatal data showed an inverse correlation between hemoglobin at birth and the necessity for red blood cell transfusions during the hospital stay in VLBW neonates [14].

The study finding of a positive correlation between the amount of cumulative blood sampling and cumulative blood transfusion requirement implies, that all measures to spare blood, which is a valuable and limited resource for the patient, should be implemented [6–15,19]. Depending on local neonatal and laboratory practice the relative amount of iatrogenic blood losses may be distributed differently compared to our study sample (Figure 4) [10]. Neonatal patient blood management may include the use of umbilical cord or placental blood for admission laboratory values [13]. In addition, storage of maternal blood for ordering and crossmatching of blood products may minimize the amount of blood required for laboratory analyses. Setting point of care devices to minimal blood volumes, use of non-invasive monitoring methods, avoidance of "routine" blood sampling, strict indication, and supervision of blood tests by experienced personnel may help to avoid iatrogenic blood losses [9,12]. Cumulative documentation of blood draw volumes, possibly based on an automated calculation derived from a PDMS system, might also help raise neonatal team awareness in avoiding iatrogenic blood loss.

Perinatal medicine is well aware of the issue of placental transfusion at birth and the possible benefits of delayed cord clamping—providing additional blood volume to neonates [1–5,20,21] as part of initial neonatal management. The intention of this study is to emphasize the importance of the opposite side of the balance, i.e., avoidance of iatrogenic blood loss, especially in VLBW preterm infants as a part of good neonatal blood management [6–15,19].

Strengths and limitations: This analysis includes the entire hospital stay of a–compared to previously published data [6–9]—larger sample cohort of VLBW neonates over a longer time course. Blood sampling volumes were retrospectively deduced from the PDMS based on the locally minimally required amount of blood for standard laboratory investigations. This implies a complete cumulative capture of all blood samples, but potentially under-estimating blood sampling volumes in case of overfilled blood tubes. The unit policy adheres to restrictive transfusion triggers [16–18], but each transfusion was indicated at the physician's discretion in charge, implying a potential bias in the transfusion trigger. Statistical statements in association with neonatal morbidity are only possible to a limited extent, as the absolute number of patients with complications was low. Nevertheless, we identified the initial hematocrit and the total blood sampling volume as independent predictors for red blood cell transfusion in our patient sample.

5. Conclusions

In a patient sample of 132 VLBW neonates, cumulative iatrogenic blood losses during the entire hospital stay and the initial hematocrit were significant independent predictors for the necessity of packed red cell transfusions. Therefore, iatrogenic blood loss should be limited to a minimum in the interest of good patient blood management.

Author Contributions: Conceptualization, A.A., D.S. and M.E.B.; methodology, A.A., P.D. and M.E.B.; software, P.D. and M.E.B.; validation, A.A., P.D. and M.E.B.; formal analysis, A.A., P.D., C.U.E. and M.E.B.; investigation, A.A., P.D. and M.E.B.; resources, D.S.; data curation, A.A. and P.D.; writing—original draft preparation, M.E.B.; writing—review, editing, visualization, A.A., P.D., C.U.E., D.S. and M.E.B.; supervision, not applicable; project administration, M.E.B. Funding acquisition, no external funding. All authors have read and agreed to the published version of the manuscript.

Funding: This research received no external funding.

Institutional Review Board Statement: The study was conducted according to the guidelines of the Declaration of Helsinki. Ethical review and approval were waived for this study by the local Ethics Committee (Ethik-Kommission der Ärztekammer Hamburg) in concordance with the local Hamburg Chamber Act for the Medical Professions and Professional Code of Conduct for Hamburg Physicians (WF-075/21, 29 March 2021), as the retrospective study handled and presented totally anonymized data.

Informed Consent Statement: Patient consent was waived (Ethik-Kommission der Ärztekammer Hamburg, WF-075/21, 29 March 2021, see above IRB statement).

Data Availability Statement: The data are not publicly available due to patient privacy reasons.

Conflicts of Interest: The authors declare no conflict of interest.

References

1. Hooper, S.B.; Pas, A.T.; Lang, J.; van Vonderen, J.; Roehr, C.C.; Kluckow, M.; Gill, A.; Wallace, E.; Polglase, G. Cardiovascular transition at birth: A physiological sequence. *Pediatr. Res.* **2015**, *77*, 608–614. [CrossRef]
2. Yao, A. Distribution of blood between infant and placenta after birth. *Lancet* **1969**, *294*, 871–873. [CrossRef]

3. Madar, J.; Roehr, C.C.; Ainsworth, S.; Ersdal, H.; Morley, C.; Rüdiger, M.; Skåre, C.; Szczapa, T.; Pas, A.T.; Trevisanuto, D.; et al. European Resuscitation Council Guidelines 2021: Newborn resuscitation and support of transition of infants at birth. *Resuscitation* **2021**, *161*, 291–326. [CrossRef]
4. Fogarty, M.; Osborn, D.A.; Askie, L.; Seidler, A.L.; Hunter, K.; Lui, K.; Simes, J.; Tarnow-Mordi, W. Delayed vs early umbilical cord clamping for preterm infants: A systematic review and meta-analysis. *Am. J. Obstet. Gynecol.* **2018**, *218*, 1–18. [CrossRef] [PubMed]
5. Katheria, A.; Reister, F.; Essers, J.; Mendler, M.; Hummler, H.; Subramaniam, A.; Carlo, W.; Tita, A.; Truong, G.; Davis-Nelson, S.; et al. Association of Umbilical Cord Milking vs Delayed Umbilical Cord Clamping With Death or Severe Intraventricular Hemorrhage Among Preterm Infants. *JAMA* **2019**, *322*, 1877–1886. [CrossRef] [PubMed]
6. Nexø, E.; Christensen, N.C.; Olesen, H. Volume of blood removed for analytical purposes during hospitalization of low-birthweight infants. *Clin. Chem.* **1981**, *27*, 759–761. [CrossRef]
7. Obladen, M.; Sachsenweger, M.; Stahnke, M. Blood sampling in very low birth weight infants receiving different levels of intensive care. *Eur. J. Nucl. Med. Mol. Imaging* **1988**, *147*, 399–404. [CrossRef]
8. Counsilman, C.E.; Heeger, L.E.; Tan, R.; Bekker, V.; Zwaginga, J.J.; Pas, A.T.; Lopriore, E. Iatrogenic blood loss in extreme preterm infants due to frequent laboratory tests and procedures. *J. Matern. Neonatal Med.* **2021**, *34*, 2660–2665. [CrossRef] [PubMed]
9. Carroll, P.D.; Zimmerman, M.B.; Nalbant, D.; Gingerich, E.L.; An, G.; Cress, G.A.; Veng-Pedersen, P.; Widness, J.A. Neonatal Umbilical Arterial Catheter Removal Is Accompanied by a Marked Decline in Phlebotomy Blood Loss. *Neonatology* **2020**, *117*, 294–299. [CrossRef] [PubMed]
10. Madsen, L.P.; Rasmussen, M.K.; Bjerregaard, L.L.; Nøhr, S.B.; Ebbesen, F. Impact of blood sampling in very preterm infants. *Scand. J. Clin. Lab. Investig.* **2000**, *60*, 125–132. [CrossRef] [PubMed]
11. Puia-Dumitrescu, M.; Tanaka, D.T.; Spears, T.G.; Daniel, C.J.; Kumar, K.R.; Athavale, K.; Juul, S.E.; Smith, P.B. Patterns of phlebotomy blood loss and transfusions in extremely low birth weight infants. *J. Perinatol.* **2019**, *39*, 1670–1675. [CrossRef]
12. Jakacka, N.; Snarski, E.; Mekuria, S. Prevention of Iatrogenic Anemia in Critical and Neonatal Care. *Adv. Clin. Exp. Med.* **2016**, *25*, 191–197. [CrossRef] [PubMed]
13. Carroll, P.D.; Christensen, R.D. New and underutilized uses of umbilical cord blood in neonatal care. *Matern. Health Neonatol. Perinatol.* **2015**, *1*, 16. [CrossRef] [PubMed]
14. Ekhaguere, O.A.; Jr, F.H.M.; Bell, E.; Prakash, N.; Widness, J.A. Predictive factors and practice trends in red blood cell transfusions for very-low-birth-weight infants. *Pediatr. Res.* **2016**, *79*, 736–741. [CrossRef] [PubMed]
15. Crighton, G.L.; New, H.V.; Liley, H.G.; Stanworth, S.J. Patient blood management, what does this actually mean for neonates and infants? *Transfus. Med.* **2018**, *28*, 117–131. [CrossRef] [PubMed]
16. Whyte, R.; Kirpalani, H. Low versus high haemoglobin concentration threshold for blood transfusion for preventing morbidity and mortality in very low birth weight infants. *Cochrane Database Syst. Rev.* **2011**, *11*. [CrossRef]
17. Howarth, C.; Banerjee, J.; Aladangady, N. Red Blood Cell Transfusion in Preterm Infants: Current Evidence and Controversies. *Neonatology* **2018**, *114*, 7–16. [CrossRef] [PubMed]
18. Franz, A.R.; Engel, C.; Bassler, D.; Rüdiger, M.; Thome, U.H.; Maier, R.F.; Krägeloh-Mann, I.; Kron, M.; Essers, J.; Bührer, C.; et al. Effects of Liberal vs Restrictive Transfusion Thresholds on Survival and Neurocognitive Outcomes in Extremely Low-Birth-Weight Infants. *JAMA* **2020**, *324*, 560–570. [CrossRef]
19. Whitehead, N.S.; Williams, L.O.; Meleth, S.; Kennedy, S.M.; Ubaka-Blackmoore, N.; Geaghan, S.M.; Nichols, J.H.; Carroll, P.; McEvoy, M.T.; Gayken, J.; et al. Interventions to prevent iatrogenic anemia: A Laboratory Medicine Best Practices systematic review. *Crit. Care* **2019**, *23*, 1–11. [CrossRef]
20. Katheria, A.C.; Lakshminrusimha, S.; Rabe, H.; McAdams, R.; Mercer, J.S. Placental transfusion: A review. *J. Perinatol.* **2017**, *37*, 105–111. [CrossRef] [PubMed]
21. Rabe, H.; Gyte, G.M.; Díaz-Rossello, J.L.; Duley, L. Effect of timing of umbilical cord clamping and other strategies to influence placental transfusion at preterm birth on maternal and infant outcomes. *Cochrane Database Syst. Rev.* **2019**, *2019*, CD003248. [CrossRef] [PubMed]

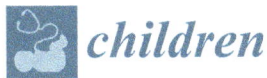

Case Report

Successful Postnatal Cardiopulmonary Resuscitation Due to Defibrillation

Lukas Peter Mileder [1,*], Nicholas Mark Morris [1], Stefan Kurath-Koller [2], Jasmin Pansy [1], Gerhard Pichler [1], Mirjam Pocivalnik [3], Bernhard Schwaberger [1], Ante Burmas [2] and Berndt Urlesberger [1]

[1] Division of Neonatology, Department of Pediatrics and Adolescent Medicine, Medical University of Graz, 8036 Graz, Austria; nicholas.morris@medunigraz.at (N.M.M.); jasmin.pansy@medunigraz.at (J.P.); gerhard.pichler@medunigraz.at (G.P.); bernhard.schwaberger@medunigraz.at (B.S.); berndt.urlesberger@medunigraz.at (B.U.)
[2] Division of Pediatric Cardiology, Department of Pediatrics and Adolescent Medicine, Medical University of Graz, 8036 Graz, Austria; stefan.kurath@medunigraz.at (S.K.-K.); ante.burmas@medunigraz.at (A.B.)
[3] Pediatric Intensive Care Unit, Department of Pediatrics and Adolescent Medicine, Medical University of Graz, 8036 Graz, Austria; mirjam.pocivalnik@medunigraz.at
* Correspondence: lukas.mileder@medunigraz.at; Tel.: +43-316-385-81052; Fax: +43-316-385-13953

Abstract: An asphyxiated term neonate required postnatal resuscitation. After six minutes of cardio-pulmonary resuscitation (CPR) and two doses of epinephrine, spontaneous circulation returned, but was shortly followed by ventricular fibrillation. CPR and administration of magnesium, calcium gluconate, and sodium bicarbonate did not improve the neonate's condition. A counter shock of five Joule was delivered and the cardiac rhythm immediately converted to sinus rhythm. The neonate was transferred to the neonatal intensive care unit and received post-resuscitation care. Due to prolonged QTc and subsequently suspected long-QT syndrome propranolol treatment was initiated. The neonate was discharged home on day 14 without neurological sequelae.

Keywords: neonate; resuscitation; ventricular fibrillation; defibrillation

1. Introduction

Postnatal cardiac arrest is most commonly a consequence of failure in transition from placental to pulmonary gas exchange and hence secondary to a disturbance in establishing sufficient aeration of the lungs. Cardiac arrest is defined as the cessation of blood circulation resulting from absent or ineffective cardiac mechanical activity, which in neonates is primarily due to asystole, severe bradycardia (<60 beats per minute (bpm)) or pulseless electrical activity [1]. In the case of postnatal cardiac arrest despite effective ventilation, resuscitation guidelines recommend cardio-pulmonary resuscitation (CPR) with a ratio of three chest compressions to one ventilation [2]. Although intravenous epinephrine is rarely required during resuscitation in the delivery room [3], resuscitation guidelines recommend its use "if the heart rate has not increased to 60/min or greater after optimizing ventilation and chest compressions ..." [2].

While defibrillation is one of the most effective interventions in the case of sudden cardiac arrest due to ventricular fibrillation (VF) or pulseless ventricular tachycardia in the adolescent and adult population, defibrillation is not mentioned in the neonatal resuscitation guidelines [2], and to our knowledge is yet to be reported in postnatal resuscitation.

2. Case Presentation

A male neonate was delivered at term ($40^{6/7}$ weeks of gestation, birth weight 3400 g) by emergency caesarean section due to persistent bradycardia after premature rupture of membranes with clear amniotic fluid. He initially presented with reduced muscle tone, cyanosis, and a heart rate between 60 and 100 bpm. The neonate did not respond to

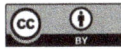

drying and tactile stimulation, and had only insufficient breathing efforts. Electrocardiogram (ECG) and pulse oximetry monitoring were initiated and continuous positive airway pressure via face mask was applied, rapidly followed by non-invasive positive pressure ventilation (PPV) due to persistent bradycardia. Non-invasive PPV did not result in visible thoracic excursions and the peak inspiratory pressure was slowly increased from 25 cm H_2O to 40 cm H_2O during the second minute of life, but not leading to the expected improvement in the neonate's condition. The attending neonatologist intubated the neonate, but no chest wall movement could be observed under invasive PPV und the neonate remained bradycardic around 40 bpm. CPR was commenced, but after doubting correct tube placement and failure to detect exhaled carbon dioxide (CO_2) with a colorimetric CO_2 detector the endotracheal tube was removed and CPR was continued under non-invasive PPV. The concentration of inspired oxygen was set to 1.0 and non-invasive PPV was delivered with a peak inspiratory pressure of 40 cm H_2O, which now resulted in adequate thoracic excursions. In minute 9 after birth, intraosseous vascular access had been established and 30 µg epinephrine (~9 µg/kg) and 5 mL isotonic fluid were administered due to persistent bradycardia. However, incorrect needle placement was suspected leading to a second intraosseous puncture on the contralateral tibia. This time correct needle placement could be confirmed and a second dose of epinephrine (100 µg, ~29 µg/kg), followed by 5 mL of isotonic fluid, were successfully administered. This led to a rapid increase in heart rate to above 100 bpm and chest compressions were stopped after a total of six minutes of CPR. The airway was cleared of viscous secretions, the neonate was rapidly re-intubated under vision and the correct tube position was verified clinically and by detection of CO_2 exhalation.

At 12 minutes after birth, approximately two minutes after the second dose of epinephrine and 90 s after return of spontaneous circulation, the ECG suddenly converted to VF with a heart rate of 280–340 bpm. During this episode the neonate deteriorated rapidly with clinical signs of shock, leading to a restart of CPR and the administration of 5 mL magnesium gluconate, 5 mL calcium gluconate 10%, and 5 mL sodium bicarbonate via the intraosseous access. After two minutes of CPR a defibrillator was available and self-adhesive pediatric defibrillation pads were placed in anterior-posterior position. A non-synchronized counter shock of five Joule was delivered causing an immediate conversion to sinus rhythm at a rate of 150–160 bpm with sufficient cardiac output. The neonate was transferred to the neonatal intensive care unit where standardized therapeutic hypothermia (72 h) was initiated because of hypoxic ischemic encephalopathy after perinatal asphyxia (Apgar 2/1/0). Postnatal resuscitation is summarized in Figure 1.

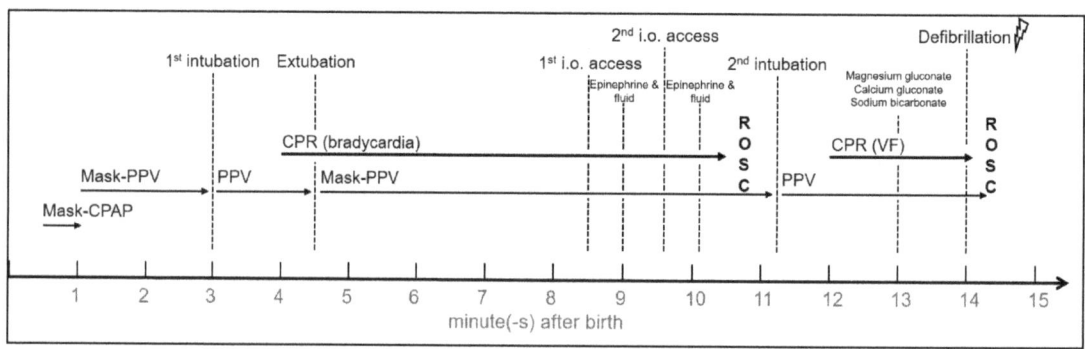

Figure 1. Time course of medical interventions (CPAP: continuous positive airway pressure; CPR: cardio-pulmonary resuscitation; i.o.: intraosseous; PPV: positive pressure ventilation; ROSC: return of spontaneous circulation; VF: ventricular fibrillation).

Before and during whole body cooling, we observed a prolonged QT interval corrected for heart rate (QTc) using Bazett's formula of 0.6 s without any further ECG abnormalities.

In response to the prolonged QTc, we initiated beta-blocker therapy with propranolol (2 mg/kg/day), and over the following days QTc decreased to stable values of 0.41 s. Complete echocardiographic evaluation was performed and did not show any structural abnormalities or congenital heart disease. Electrolytes were checked regularly during and after therapeutic hypothermia, and were all within normal ranges.

In the following, neither clinical signs nor laboratory findings made suggestion of any infection related issue. The neonate was extubated on day seven and in the comprehensive work-up including neurological examination, cranial sonography, electroencephalography, and magnetic resonance imaging no abnormalities were detected. After a further week of uneventful cardiac monitoring, the neonate was discharged home on day 14 of life with cardio-respiratory home monitoring and under continued propranolol treatment.

Genetic analysis revealed a mutation in the SCN5A gene (c.3911C>T, p.Thr1304Met). Extended genetic analyses found the identical gene mutation in the neonate's brother and mother, both of whom were asymptomatic with normal QTc. There were no cases of sudden cardiac death reported in the extended family.

At the age of 18 months, neurodevelopmental testing was unremarkable and showed normal development. At the latest cardiology follow-up at the age of 3.5 years, the boy was asymptomatic with normal QTc without anti-arrhythmic medication.

3. Discussion

Several aspects of this unusual case are worth discussing and have the potential to improve both knowledge and management of hemodynamically compromised neonates during postnatal resuscitation.

To our knowledge, this is the first reported case of a neonate who required defibrillation after birth. During infancy, VF is generally a rare event, with an incidence of only 0.52 per 100,000 person-years during the first year of life [4]. During the neonatal period VF may be caused either by long-QT syndrome (LQTS) [5] or an anomalous left coronary artery descending from the pulmonary artery [6], first of which is a known cause of sudden infant death syndrome [7].

In our case the neonate developed VF shortly after the administration of epinephrine. This appears to have triggered VF on the basis of preexisting QTc prolongation, which is known to increase susceptibility to arrhythmogenic factors. Epinephrine shortens the effective refractory time of the atria, atrioventricular (AV) node and ventricular myocardium, improves conduction via the AV node, and, therefore, may induce sustained ventricular arrhythmia [8]. The electrophysiological effects of epinephrine mainly result from stimulation of beta-receptors and while it also stimulates alpha-receptors, this seems not to affect the AV node. However, alpha-receptor stimulation increases the effective refractory time of the atria and ventricles, partially offsetting the shortening of refractory time mediated by beta-receptor stimulation [8]. Epinephrine administration itself has been associated with prolongation of QTc and induction of Torsades de Pointes [9]. Byrum et al. [10] also described VF in a neonate with Wolff-Parkinson-White syndrome associated with the use of digitalis, which exhibits positive bathmotropic properties similar to epinephrine. In addition, ischemia and reperfusion during postnatal cardiac arrest may have contributed to cardiac arrhythmia [11]. High inspiratory oxygen supplementation may have resulted in hyperoxemia, which then may have increased the susceptibility for VF [12]. Finally, therapeutic hypothermia may have induced or further aggravated QTc prolongation [13], as Vega et al. [14] showed (reversible) prolonged QTc in neonates undergoing therapeutic hypothermia due to hypoxic ischemic encephalopathy.

Due to initially prolonged QTc, empirical propranolol treatment was established. In addition, we found a mutation in the SCN5A gene, which is present in 5–10% of patients with LQTS [15]. The SCN5A gene encodes the α-subunit of the cardiac sodium channel Nav1.5, which initiates and transmits action potentials within the myocardium, and gain-of-function mutations in SCN5A may cause LQTS [16]. In untreated patients with LQTS, cardiac arrest or sudden cardiac death is the sentinel event in 13% of cases [17]. However, in our patient the SCN5A mutation discovered is not associated with LQTS. The fact that our patient's QTc normalized over time and that two family members carrying the same mutation were asymptomatic without QTc prolongation led us to exclude LQTS as an underlying condition, allowing us to discontinue beta-blocker treatment during follow-up. Furthermore, we had calculated QTc using Bazett's formula, which is known to overestimate QTc at high heart rates [18]. Applying different formulas for QT correction (e.g., Fridericia, Framingham, Hodges) may yield more accurate QTc in newborns especially with heart rates above 100 bpm [18].

Case reports on defibrillation in neonates include an incidence of fire ignited by a defibrillation attempt in a 10-day-old neonate with VF following heart surgery [19] and the need for electrical cardioversion during the first day of life in one preterm and one term neonate with narrow complex tachycardia [20]. Sauer et al. [5] described defibrillation in a 19-day-old neonate due to VF, which was associated with susceptibility to LQTS type 6. Hirakubo et al. [21] reported on a term neonate suffering from tuberous sclerosis with multiple cardiac tumors and (supra-)ventricular tachycardia, who developed VF requiring electrical cardioversion on day 12 after birth. However, postnatal resuscitation requiring defibrillation due to VF has not been reported yet. It has to be noted that the energy dose used in our patient (five Joule, i.e., ~1.5 Joule per kg) was lower than the recommended initial dose of two to four Joule per kg for infants or children suffering from VF [22]. Despite reports about the potential inadequacy of initial shock doses of two Joule per kg for termination of VF or pulseless ventricular tachycardia in infants and children [23], defibrillation was successful on the first attempt in our patient. We speculate that due to the short plasma half-life of epinephrine electrophysiological effects on the myocardium may have already been wearing off and that in this vulnerable state of arrhythmia a relatively low energy dose was sufficient. Nevertheless, we still regard the recommended energy dose of two to four Joule per kg for defibrillation of VF advisable [22].

From a clinical viewpoint, the severely compromised neonate was resuscitated according to published guidelines [1]. Immediate application of ECG leads allowed for rapid and continuous assessment of heart rate as well as early recognition of VF. This underlines the recommendation to use ECG monitoring during neonatal resuscitation [1,2]. Non-invasive PPV was initially not effective despite an increased peak inspiratory pressure, which at least in apneic preterm neonates is a common finding due to temporary airway obstruction [24]. The lack of exhaled CO_2 following the first intubation attempt we consider most likely due to a displaced endotracheal tube causing esophageal intubation, but must alternatively also consider the following reasons: (a) persistently high pulmonary vascular resistance due to initially insufficient lung aeration, (b) low cardiac output due to ineffective chest compressions, or (c) undetected tube occlusion. The approaching team suspected esophageal intubation and removed the endotracheal tube immediately. Colorimetric CO_2 detectors are useful to indicate correct endotracheal tube placement after lung aeration and consecutive increase in lung perfusion. They have also been used to identify patent airways during non-invasive PPV [25], whereas continuous measurement of end-tidal CO_2 may be used to guide and optimize chest compressions during CPR [26]. Current resuscitation guidelines recommend "umbilical venous catheterization as the primary method of vascular access during newborn infant resuscitation in the delivery room", but define intraosseous vascular access as "reasonable alternative" [2]. At our institution the choice of emergency vascular access (umbilical venous catheter or intraosseous access) during neonatal resuscitation is at the treating neonatologist's individual discretion; in the described case intraosseous access was chosen primarily and could be established on the second attempt, providing us with an effective route for administration of emergency drugs. In a previous study we found that although infrequently required, intraosseous access was successfully used during resuscitation of preterm and term neonates with a moderate overall success rate of 75% [27]. No study so far has directly compared drug administration between the umbilical venous and the intraosseous route; however, Schwindt et al. [28] compared umbilical venous catheterization versus intraosseous access in the simulated environment and found significantly reduced time to successfully establish intraosseous access. Scrivens et al. [29] included 41 neonates in their systematic literature review of intraosseous access, and concluded that it "should be available on neonatal units and considered for early use in neonates where other access routes have failed".

When considering the crisis resource management, one very fortunate aspect of this unusual resuscitation scenario was the time of day, which happened to be on a weekday at the time of handover. This meant that several neonatologists and one pediatric intensive care specialist were readily available and rapidly involved. These personnel resources allowed for prompt and efficient delivery of resuscitative measures, and likely contributed to the overall excellent outcome of the patient.

4. Conclusions

We describe the rare clinical presentation of a neonate with perinatal asphyxia, who required postnatal resuscitation and defibrillation due to VF following epinephrine administration. Based on this case we suggest that medical professionals managing neonatal resuscitation be aware of the possible need for defibrillation, even though it may be very rare. Institutional simulation-based training of neonatal resuscitation should therefore include scenarios involving cardiac arrest due to shockable heart rhythms (i.e., VF and pulseless ventricular tachycardia) to prepare neonatal resuscitation teams to manage such infrequent events adequately. In neonates with evident QTc prolongation epinephrine should be used with caution due to its arrhythmogenic properties, especially the higher recommended dosage of 30 μg/kg [2]. Finally, we consider it appropriate to have a defibrillator, allowing for weight-adapted, gradual titration of the energy level, and appropriately sized pediatric defibrillation pads available in every delivery room.

Author Contributions: L.P.M. conceptualized the manuscript, collected clinical data, drafted the initial manuscript, and reviewed and revised the manuscript. N.M.M. and S.K.-K. assisted with data collection and interpretation, and critically reviewed the manuscript for important intellectual content. J.P., G.P., M.P., B.S., A.B., and B.U. supervised data collection and assisted with data interpretation, and critically reviewed the manuscript for important intellectual content. All authors approved the final manuscript as submitted and agree to be personally accountable for each author's own contributions and for ensuring that questions related to the accuracy or integrity of any part of the work, even ones in which the author was not personally involved, are appropriately investigated, resolved, and documented in the literature. All authors have read and agreed to the published version of the manuscript.

Funding: This research received no external funding.

Institutional Review Board Statement: Ethics committee approval was not required for this case description, as we did not conduct original research in humans and described the patient's case retrospectively and without identifying information, i.e., in pseudo-anonymized manner.

Informed Consent Statement: Written informed consent was obtained from the patient's parents prior to publication.

Conflicts of Interest: The authors declare no conflict of interest.

References

1. Wyllie, J.; Bruinenberg, J.; Roehr, C.C.; Rüdiger, M.; Trevisanuto, D.; Urlesberger, B. European Resuscitation Council Guidelines for Resuscitation 2015: Section 7. Resuscitation and support of transition of babies at birth. *Resuscitation* **2015**, *95*, 249–263. [CrossRef]
2. Wyckoff, M.H.; Wyllie, J.; Aziz, K.; de Almeida, M.F.; Fabres, J.; Fawke, J.; Guinsburg, R.; Hosono, S.; Isayama, T.; Kapadia, V.S.; et al. Neonatal Life Support: 2020 International Consensus on Cardiopulmonary Resuscitation and Emergency Cardiovascular Care Science with Treatment Recommendations. *Circulation* **2020**, *142*, 185–221. [CrossRef]
3. Perlman, J.M.; Risser, R. Cardiopulmonary Resuscitation in the Delivery Room. *Arch. Pediatr. Adolesc. Med.* **1995**, *149*, 20–25. [CrossRef]
4. Tseng, W.-C.; Wu, M.-H.; Chen, H.-C.; Kao, F.-Y.; Huang, S.-K. Ventricular Fibrillation in a General Population—A National Database Study. *Circ. J.* **2016**, *80*, 2310–2316. [CrossRef] [PubMed]

5. Sauer, C.W.; Marc-Aurele, K.L. A Neonate with Susceptibility to Long QT Syndrome Type 6 who Presented with Ventricular Fibrillation and Sudden Unexpected Infant Death. *Am. J. Case Rep.* **2016**, *17*, 544–548. [CrossRef] [PubMed]
6. Walker, T.C.; Renno, M.S.; Parra, D.A.; Guthrie, S.O. Neonatal ventricular fibrillation and an elusive ALCAPA: Things are not al-ways as they seem. *BMJ Case Rep.* **2016**. [CrossRef]
7. Schwartz, P.J.; Priori, S.G.; Dumaine, R.; Napolitano, C.; Antzelevitch, C.; Stramba-Badiale, M.; Richard, T.A.; Berti, M.R.; Bloise, R. A Molecular Link between the Sudden Infant Death Syndrome and the Long-QT Syndrome. *N. Engl. J. Med.* **2000**, *343*, 262–267. [CrossRef] [PubMed]
8. Morady, F.; Nelson, S.D.; Kou, W.H.; Pratley, R.; Schmaltz, S.; De Buitleir, M.; Halter, J.B. Electrophysiologic effects of epinephrine in humans. *J. Am. Coll. Cardiol.* **1988**, *11*, 1235–1244. [CrossRef]
9. Woosley, R.L.; Romero, K.; Heise, C.W.; Gallo, T.; Tate, J. Summary of Torsades de Pointes (TdP) Reports Associated with Intravenous Drug Formulations Containing the Preservative Chlorobutanol. *Drug Saf.* **2019**, *42*, 907–913. [CrossRef] [PubMed]
10. Byrum, C.J.; Wahl, R.A.; Behrendt, D.M.; Dick, M. Ventricular fibrillation associated with use of digitalis in a newborn infant with Wolff-Parkinson-White syndrome. *J. Pediatr.* **1982**, *101*, 400–403. [CrossRef]
11. Chenliu, C.; Sheng, X.; Dan, P.; Qu, Y.; Claydon, V.E.; Lin, E.; Hove-Madsen, L.; Sanatani, S.; Tibbits, G.F. Ischemia–reperfusion destabilizes rhythmicity in immature atrioventricular pacemakers: A predisposing factor for postoperative arrhythmias in neonate rabbits. *Heart Rhythm* **2016**, *13*, 2348–2355. [CrossRef] [PubMed]
12. Wittnich, C.; Torrance, S.M.; Carlyle, C.E. Effects of hyperoxia on neonatal myocardial energy status and response to global is-chemia. *Ann. Thorac. Surg.* **2000**, *70*, 2125–2131. [CrossRef]
13. Khan, J.N.; Prasad, N.; Glancy, J.M. QTc prolongation during therapeutic hypothermia: Are we giving it the attention it de-serves? *Europace* **2010**, *12*, 266–270. [CrossRef]
14. Vega, L.; Boix, H.; Albert, D.; Delgado, I.; Castillo, F. Corrected QT interval during therapeutic hypothermia in hypoxic is-chaemic encephalopathy. *An. Pediatr. (Barc.)* **2016**, *85*, 312–317. [CrossRef] [PubMed]
15. Mizusawa, Y.; Horie, M.; Wilde, A.A. Genetic and Clinical Advances in Congenital Long QT Syndrome. *Circ. J.* **2014**, *78*, 2827–2833. [CrossRef] [PubMed]
16. Wilde, A.A.N.; Amin, A.S. Clinical Spectrum of SCN5A Mutations: Long QT Syndrome, Brugada Syndrome, and Cardiomyopa-thy. *JACC Clin. Electrophysiol.* **2018**, *4*, 569–579. [CrossRef]
17. Priori, S.G.; Schwartz, P.J.; Napolitano, C.; Bloise, R.; Ronchetti, E.; Grillo, M.; Vicentini, A.; Spazzolini, C.; Nastoli, J.; Bottelli, G.; et al. Risk Stratification in the Long-QT Syndrome. *N. Engl. J. Med.* **2003**, *348*, 1866–1874. [CrossRef] [PubMed]
18. Luo, S.; Michler, K.; Johnston, P.; Macfarlane, P.W. A comparison of commonly used QT correction formulae: The effect of heart rate on the QTc of normal ECGs. *J. Electrocardiol.* **2004**, *37*, 81–90. [CrossRef]
19. Theodorou, A.A.; Gutierrez, J.A.; Berg, R.A. Fire Attributable to a Defibrillation Attempt in a Neonate. *Pediatrics* **2003**, *112*, 677–679. [CrossRef]
20. Cornwell, L.; Mukherjee, R.; Kelsall, A. Problems with the use of self-adhesive electrode pads in neonates. *Resuscitation* **2006**, *68*, 425–428. [CrossRef]
21. Hirakubo, Y.; Ichihashi, K.; Shiraishi, H.; Momoi, M.Y. Ventricular Tachycardia in a Neonate with Prenatally Diagnosed Cardiac Tumors: A Case with Tuberous Sclerosis. *Pediatr. Cardiol.* **2005**, *26*, 655–657. [CrossRef] [PubMed]
22. Maconochie, I.K.; Aickin, R.; Hazinski, M.F.; Atkins, D.L.; Bingham, R.; Couto, T.B.; Guerguerian, A.M.; Nadkarni, V.M.; Ng, K.C.; Nuthall, G.A.; et al. Pediatric Life Support: 2020 International Consensus on Cardiopulmonary Resuscitation and Emergency Cardiovascular Care Science with Treatment Recommendations. *Circulation* **2020**, *142*, 140–184. [CrossRef] [PubMed]
23. Tibballs, J.; Carter, B.; Kiraly, N.J.; Ragg, P.; Clifford, M. External and internal biphasic direct current shock doses for pediatric ventricular fibrillation and pulseless ventricular tachycardia*. *Pediatr. Crit. Care Med.* **2011**, *12*, 14–20. [CrossRef] [PubMed]
24. Finer, N.N.; Rich, W.; Wang, C.; Leone, T. Airway Obstruction during Mask Ventilation of Very Low Birth Weight Infants during Neonatal Resuscitation. *Pediatrics* **2009**, *123*, 865–869. [CrossRef]
25. Leone, T.A.; Lange, A.; Rich, W.; Finer, N.N. Disposable Colorimetric Carbon Dioxide Detector Use as an Indicator of a Patent Airway during Noninvasive Mask Ventilation. *Pediatrics* **2006**, *118*, e202–e204. [CrossRef]
26. Hamrick, J.T.; Hamrick, J.L.; Bhalala, U.; Armstrong, J.S.; Lee, J.-H.; Kulikowicz, E.; Lee, J.K.; Kudchadkar, S.R.; Koehler, R.C.; Hunt, E.A.; et al. End-Tidal CO2-Guided Chest Compression Delivery Improves Survival in a Neo-natal Asphyxial Cardiac Arrest Model. *Pediatr. Crit. Care Med.* **2017**, *18*, e575–e584. [CrossRef] [PubMed]
27. Mileder, L.P.; Urlesberger, B.; Schwaberger, B. Use of Intraosseous Vascular Access during Neonatal Resuscitation at a Tertiary Center. *Front. Pediatr.* **2020**, *8*, 571285. [CrossRef] [PubMed]
28. Schwindt, E.M.; Hoffmann, F.; Deindl, P.; Waldhoer, T.J.; Schwindt, J.C. Duration to Establish an Emergency Vascular Access and How to Accelerate It: A Simulation-Based Study Performed in Real-Life Neonatal Resuscitation Rooms. *Pediatr. Crit. Care Med.* **2018**, *19*, 468–476. [CrossRef]
29. Scrivens, A.; Reynolds, P.R.; Emery, F.E.; Roberts, C.; Polglase, G.R.; Hooper, S.B.; Roehr, C.C. Use of Intraosseous Needles in Neonates: A Systematic Review. *Neonatology* **2019**, *116*, 305–314. [CrossRef]

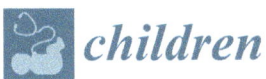

Review

Accuracy of Pulse Oximetry in the Presence of Fetal Hemoglobin—A Systematic Review

Ena Pritišanac [1,2], Berndt Urlesberger [1,2], Bernhard Schwaberger [1,2] and Gerhard Pichler [1,2,*]

1. Research Unit for Neonatal Micro- and Macrocirculation, Medical University of Graz, Auenbruggerplatz 34/II, 8036 Graz, Austria; ena.pritisanac@medunigraz.at (E.P.); berndt.urlesberger@medunigraz.at (B.U.); bernhard.schwaberger@medunigraz.at (B.S.)
2. Division of Neonatology, Department of Pediatrics, University Hospital Graz, Auenbruggerplatz 30, 8036 Graz, Austria
* Correspondence: gerhard.pichler@medunigraz.at; Tel.: +43-316-385-80520

Abstract: Continuous monitoring of arterial oxygen saturation by pulse oximetry (SpO2) is the main method to guide respiratory and oxygen support in neonates during postnatal stabilization and after admission to neonatal intensive care unit. The accuracy of these devices is therefore crucial. The presence of fetal hemoglobin (HbF) in neonatal blood might affect SpO2 readings. We performed a systematic qualitative review to investigate the impact of HbF on SpO2 accuracy in neonates. PubMed/Medline, Embase, Cumulative Index to Nursing & Allied Health database (CINAHL) and Cochrane library databases were searched from inception to January 2021 for human studies in the English language, which compared arterial oxygen saturations (SaO2) from neonatal blood with SpO2 readings and included HbF measurements in their reports. Ten observational studies were included. Eight studies reported SpO2-SaO2 bias that ranged from −3.6%, standard deviation (SD) 2.3%, to +4.2% (SD 2.4). However, it remains unclear to what extent this depends on HbF. Five studies showed that an increase in HbF changes the relation of partial oxygen pressure (paO2) to SpO2, which is physiologically explained by the leftward shift in oxygen dissociation curve. It is important to be aware of this shift when treating a neonate, especially for the lower SpO2 limits in preterm neonates to avoid undetected hypoxia.

Keywords: neonate; fetal hemoglobin; oxygen saturation monitoring; pulse oximetry

1. Introduction

Continuous arterial oxygen saturation measured by pulse oximetry (SpO2) is the primary monitoring to guide respiratory and oxygen support in neonates during postnatal stabilization and after admission to a neonatal intensive care unit (NICU) [1,2]. The recent resuscitation guidelines recommend specific pre-ductal SpO2 targets during postnatal transition based on the 25th percentile of SpO2 values in healthy term neonates that required no medical interventions at birth (2 min 65%, 5 min 85%, 10 min 90%) [1,3].

Before the 1980s, transcutaneous oxygen tension measurement (tc-pO2) was a common monitoring method in the NICU. Because of the practical aspects (regular calibration and repositioning of the electrodes, skin irritations, underestimation of partial oxygen pressure (paO2) in older neonatal patients) pulse oximetry was introduced into neonatal care as a better and more convenient monitoring method [4–7].

Pulse oximetry measures SpO2 by illuminating the tissue and detecting changes in the absorption of oxygenated and deoxygenated blood hemoglobin at two wavelengths: 660 nm (red) and 940 nm (infrared). In order to establish the pulse oximeter's measure of SpO2, the ratio of absorbance at these wavelengths is calculated and calibrated against direct measurements of arterial oxygen saturation from blood samples (SaO2). For this purpose, blood samples are taken from healthy adult volunteers under room air (normoxia) and in artificially acquired hypoxic environments to achieve hypoxemia [8,9].

The difference (bias) between SpO2 and SaO2 reported in adults is 3–4%, with a tendency for overestimation of SpO2 in critically ill mechanically ventilated patients [10–12]. However, studies conducted in mechanically ventilated neonates and children reported an even greater bias, particularly at lower SpO2 values. For instance, in the largest conducted study in children, the median bias of SpO2 versus SaO2 was as high as 6% for a SpO2 range of 81% to 85% [13]. Moreover, within the saturation target range for preterm infants (89–95%), pulse oximetry exceeded the 4% error quality margin in the latest published study, which included 1908 neonates. SpO2 values were overestimated by an average of 2.9% with a standard deviation (SD) of 5.8% in this study [14].

The oxygen carrying capacity of blood depends primarily on the hemoglobin molecule. Fetal hemoglobin (HbF) is the main oxygen carrier during pregnancy. From the 20th week of gestation, HbF is gradually replaced by adult hemoglobin (HbA) and declines to its adult levels by approximately six months after birth [15,16]. HbF exhibits a significantly higher affinity for oxygen, which enables oxygen extraction from the blood of the mother to the fetus via the placenta at lower partial oxygen pressures and leads to the shift of the oxyhemoglobin dissociation curve (ODC) to the left (shown in Figure 1) [17,18].

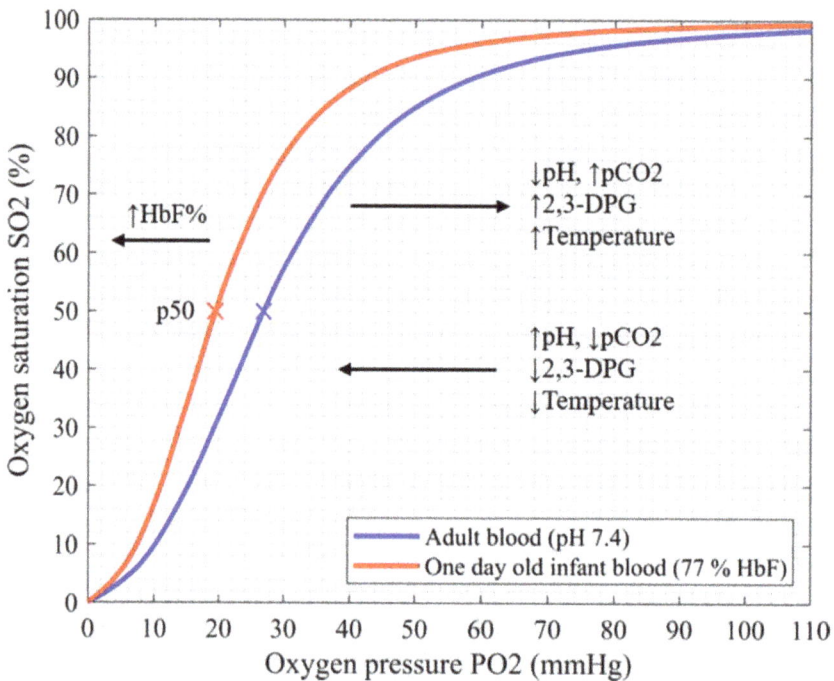

Figure 1. Oxyhemoglobin dissociation curve of fetal and adult hemoglobin shows the relationship between pO2 and SO2. For the saturation of 50%, the corresponding pO2 values (p50) are indicated (×). The factors that change the hemoglobin affinity for oxygen are indicated. HbF (red), fetal hemoglobin; pCO2, partial pressure of carbon dioxide; 2,3-DPG, diphosphoglycerate.

The prenatal HbF expression and conversion to HbA is regulated by a set of evolutionarily conserved genes and is not affected by the birth event itself. HbF values at birth are therefore particularly high in very low birth-weight neonates (HbF > 90%) [19]. However, in term neonates, these values can vary considerably among individuals, as reported in the largest conducted study in more than 150,000 newborns (mean HbF 82%, range 5–100%) [20]. Higher HbF values were observed in newborns exposed to risk factors for maternal or fetal hypoxia and for sudden infant death syndrome (SIDS) [21]. Furthermore, higher HbF values were reported to reduce the incidence of retinopathy of prematurity (ROP) in at-risk preterms, suggesting that HbF could be a protective factor for oxygen-related tissue injury in preterm neonates [22].

HbF content in the blood is often expressed as a percentage of total hemoglobin or fraction of fetal hemoglobin (FHbF) and can be measured by several methods. These include the alkali denaturation method, electrophoresis, spectroscopy, and high-performance liquid chromatography, which is the most accurate method and the gold standard. The differentiation between fetal and adult hemoglobin in a sample is based on the existence of gamma-chain peaks, which are characteristic of HbF. The level of HbF can be determined by measuring the total chromatogram gamma-globin chain areas expressed as a percentage of total Hb [23].

However, because of its wide availability, visible absorption spectroscopy performed by a hemoximeter or a blood-gas analyzer is the most commonly used method in clinical studies [24,25]. The optical system of a hemoximeter is designed to measure the concentration of total hemoglobin, oxygen saturation, and fractions of oxyhemoglobin, carboxyhemoglobin, deoxyhemoglobin, methemoglobin, and HbF. HbF does not have the same visible absorption spectrum as HbA due to a slight variation in molecular structure [26]. If not taken into account, the presence of HbF in a sample will interfere with the results of oxygen saturation and the carboxyhemoglobin. Newer models of the hemoximeter (since 1992) use a linear relationship to adjust the SaO2 and oxyhemoglobin readings by the measured level of HbF [27].

Since the calibration curves of pulse oximeters use SaO2 measurements from the blood samples of healthy adults (with almost no HbF), the accuracy of SpO2 values in the presence of HbF is questionable. The aim of this review was, therefore, to summarize the studies which examined the effect of HbF on pulse oximetry monitoring in human neonates.

2. Materials and Methods

Articles were identified using the stepwise approach specified in the Preferred Reporting Items for Systematic Reviews and Meta-Analyses (PRISMA) statement [28].

2.1. Search Strategy

A systematic search of Pubmed/Medline, Embase, Cumulative Index to Nursing & Allied Health (CINAHL) and Cochrane library was performed from the date of inception of the databases to January 2021 to identify articles that concerned HbF and oxygen saturation monitoring by pulse oximetry in term and preterm neonates. Only human studies written in the English language were selected. Search terms included: newborn, neonate, preterm, term, infant, HbF, hemoglobin F, fetal hemoglobin, after birth, postnatal, oxygenation, arterial oxygen saturation, pulse oximetry, SaO2 and SpO2 (Supplementary Figure S1, Tables S1 and S2). Studies on fetal hemoglobin addressing sickle cell anemia and thalassemia were excluded. Additional published reports were identified through a manual search of references in retrieved articles and in review articles. The search was last updated on 24 January 2021.

2.2. Study Selection

Identified articles were independently evaluated by two authors (E.P., G.P.) by reviewing the titles and abstracts. If an uncertainty remained regarding the eligibility for inclusion, the full text was reviewed. The two reviewers independently selected relevant abstracts, critically appraised the full texts of the selected articles, and assessed the methodological quality of the studies. Data were analyzed qualitatively. Extracted data included the characterization of study type, patient characteristics, methods, and results.

3. Results

Our initial search identified 2024 articles. After the removal of duplicates, 1822 articles were screened for inclusion. Exclusion criteria included absence of reliable HbF measurements or non-invasive oxygenation monitoring in term or preterm neonates (shown in Figure 2). Ten observational studies fulfilled the inclusion criteria [4–7,29–34]. No randomized controlled trial was identified. All studies performed measurements of HbF and non-invasive oxygen saturation monitoring by pulse oximetry at the upper and/or lower extremity in neonates in the first days and weeks after birth and determined blood oxygenation parameters. The study populations included preterm and term neonates with a range of gestational ages from 24 to 42 weeks of gestation. Studies are presented in Tables 1 and 2 according to the HbF measurement method.

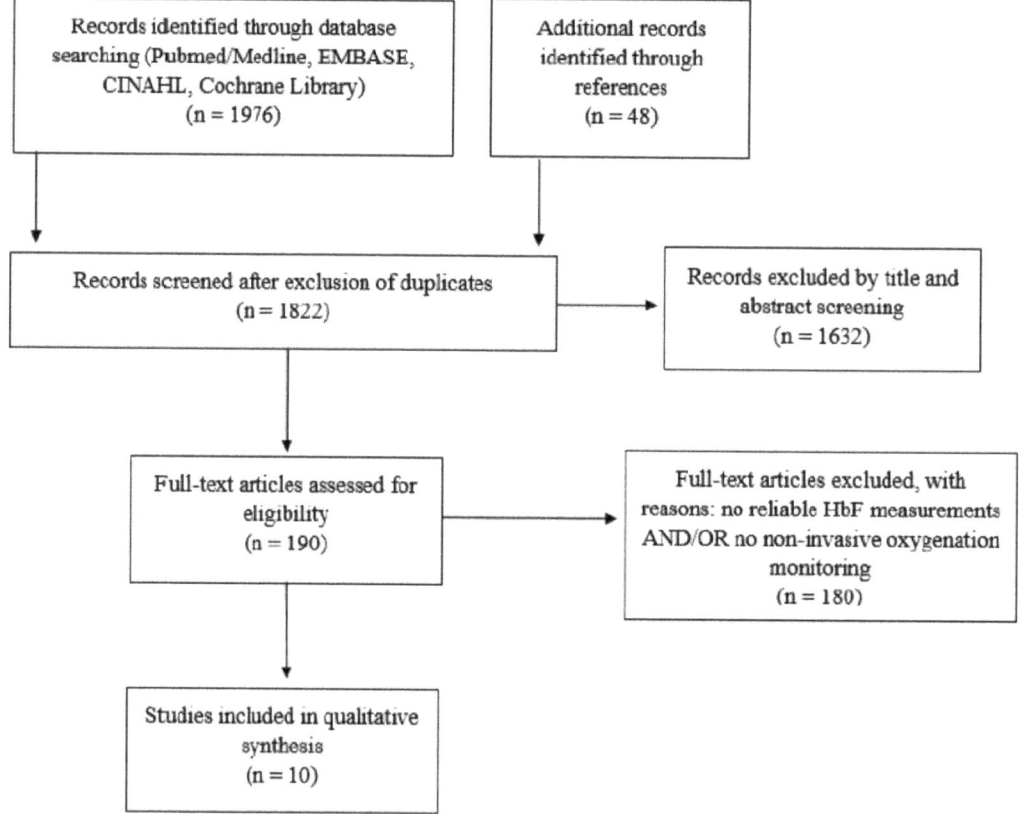

Figure 2. Study selection flow diagram.

Table 1. Studies before 1992 comparing SpO2 monitoring to invasively measured blood oxygenation parameters.

Ref	1st Author, Year	Number of Patients/ HbF Blood Samples	Blood Sample Type	HbF Measurement Method	Gestation Distribution (Weeks)	Time of Sample Collection and Non-Invasive Monitoring	Blood Oxygenation Parameters	Blood Gas Analyzer /Hemoximeter	Pulse Oximeter (Company Name)	Additional Bedside Oxygenation Monitoring Device (Company Name)	Relevant Results
[32].	Durand, 1986	75/140	Arterial	Alkali denaturation method	24–42	1–14 days + 30–153 days after birth	paO2, SaO2	Radiometer BMS3 Mark II / Co-oximeter IL 282	Nellcor N-100 (Hayward, CA, USA)	tc-pO2 Oxygen electrode (Novametrix, Wallingford, CT, USA)	HbF values of 4.3% to 95% did not influence the accuracy of pulse oximeter readings.
[7].	Ramanathan, 1987	68/132	Arterial	Alkali denaturation method	25–31	1–6 days + 20–80 days after birth	paO2, SaO2	Radiometer BMS3 Mark II / Co-oximeter IL 282	Nellcor N-100 (Hayward, CA, USA)	tc-pO2 Oxygen electrode (Novametrix, Wallingford, CT, USA)	HbF values of 4.3% to 92.2% did not influence the accuracy of pulse oximeter readings.
[33].	Wimberley, 1987	18/18	Arterial	Alkali denaturation method	25–34	Within 5 days after birth	paO2, SaO2	ABL300/ Hemoximeter OSM3	Ohmeda Biox 3700	tc-pO2 Radiometer TCM3	FHbF ranged from 44–97%. The variations in the levels of HbF, pH, pCO2 and 2,3-DPG resulted in a variable paO2-SaO2 relation.
[4].	Jennis, 1987	26/49	Arterial	Electrophoresis	24–40	1–49 days after birth	SaO2	Co-oximeter IL 282	Nellcor N-100 (Hayward, CA, USA)	NA	FHbF > 50% generated a 2.8% to 3.6% error (underestimation) in SpO2 reading.
[5].	Praud, 1989	71/52	Arterial	Electrophoresis and alkali denaturation method	25–40	1–14 days after birth + 4.5–38 weeks after birth	SaO2	Hemoximeter OSM2	Nellcor N-100 (Hayward, CA, USA)	NA	For FHbF < 50% and SaO2 ≤ 95%, SpO2 was overestimated.

FHbF = fraction of fetal hemoglobin, HbF = fetal hemoglobin, NA = not applicable, paO2 = partial arterial oxygen pressure, SaO2 = arterial blood oxygen saturation, SpO2 = peripheral arterial oxygen saturation measured by pulse-oximetry, tc-pO2 = transcutaneous oxygen tension, 2,3-DPG = 2,3- diphosphoglycerate.

Table 2. Hemoximetry studies (after 1992) comparing SpO2 monitoring to invasively measured blood oxygenation parameters.

Ref	1st Author, Year	Number of Patients/ HbF Blood Samples	Blood Sample Type	HbF Measurement Method	Gestation Distribution (Weeks)	Time of Sample Collection and Non-Invasive Monitoring	Blood Oxygenation Parameters	Blood Gas Analyzer/Hemoximeter	Pulse Oximeter (Company Name)	Additional Bedside Oxygenation Monitoring Device (Company Name)	Relevant Results
[6]	Rajadurai, 1992	22/64	Arterial	Visible absorption spectroscopy (hemoximeter)	25–36	1 h–73 days after birth	Functional SaO2 *	ABL30 Analyzer/ Hemoximeter OSM3	Nellcor N-100 (Hayward, CA, USA)	NA	Pulse oximeter saturations were unaffected by FHbF values which ranged from 0 to 100%.
[29]	Shiao, 2005	20/210	Arterial and venous	Visible absorption spectroscopy (hemoximeter)	24–34	First 5 days after birth	paO2, SaO2, SvO2, HbO2	Hemoximeter OSM3	Nellcor NPB 290 (Pleasanton, CA, USA)	NA	Bias of SpO2 vs HbO2 was +1.6% (2SD 5.6) and SpO2 vs SaO2 −0.6% (2SD 5.9). There was no statistical analysis of HbF contribution to the bias.
[30]	Shiao, 2006	39/188	Arterial and venous	Visible absorption spectroscopy (hemoximeter) + HPLC	25–38	First 5 days after birth	paO2, SaO2, SvO2, HbO2	Hemoximeter OSM3	Nellcor NPB 290 (Tyco Healthcare, Mansfield, MA, USA)	NA	Lower HbF levels after the transfusion resulted in lower SpO2 for the same paO2 range of 50–75 mmHg. There was no statistical analysis of HbF contribution to the SpO2-SaO2 bias.
[31]	Shiao, 2007	78/771	Arterial and venous	Visible absorption spectroscopy (hemoximeter)	25–38	First 5 days after birth (every 6–8 h)	paO2, SaO2, HbO2	Hemoximeter OSM3	Nellcor (NPB 290, Pleasanton, CA, USA)	SaO2m, SvO2m *** Oximetric 3-wavelength monitors (Abbott, Chicago, IL, USA)	Bias of SpO2 vs HbO2 in arterial blood samples was 2.5% (SD 3.1). There was no statistical analysis of HbF contribution to the SpO2-SaO2 bias.
[34]	Nitzan, 2018	14/28	Arterial	Visible absorption spectroscopy (hemoximeter)	24–33	Within 12 h before and after the blood transfusion (first 5 days after birth)	paO2, SaO2	ABL 90 FLEX	Nellcor (Covidien-Medtronic, Mansfield, MA, USA)	NA	HbF declined significantly after transfusion and FiO2 increased by >12% to keep SpO2 within the same range.

FHbF = fraction of fetal hemoglobin, HbF = fetal hemoglobin, HbO2 = oxyhemoglobin, HPLC = high performance liquid chromatography, NA = not applicable, paO2 = partial arterial oxygen pressure, SaO2 = arterial blood oxygen saturation, SvO2 = venous blood oxygen saturation, SpO2 = peripheral arterial oxygen saturation measured by pulse-oximetry, SD = standard deviation. *Functional SaO2 = (HbO2/100 − HbCO- HbMet) × 100, **SO2 = SaO2 and SvO2, *** SaO2m = arterial blood oxygen saturation monitoring, SvO2m = venous blood oxygen saturation monitoring (measured through umbilical catheters by using Oximetric 3 monitors of 3-wavelength technology).

Five studies conducted before 1992 used alkali denaturation or electrophoresis (Table 1), whereas five studies initiated after 1992 used a hemoximeter for the HbF measurement. (Table 2) All studies compared the non-invasive SpO2 readings to invasively measured blood oxygenation parameters, most commonly SaO2, and included HbF in the analyses.

One out of the five studies conducted before 1992 found a 2.8–3.6% underestimation in SpO2 readings in relation to higher HbF levels [4], two found no bias in SpO2 readings in relation to HbF [7,32], and two reported inconclusive results [5,33]. Out of the five studies conducted after 1992, one reported no SpO2-SaO2 bias in relation to HbF [6], three studies reported an overestimation of SpO2 with higher HbF but did not provide statistical evidence to support this statement [29–31], and one study reported a decrease in SaO2-SpO2 bias following transfusion of adult blood to the neonates and consequential HbF decline. It remains unclear whether this decrease can be attributed to HbF alone [34].

4. Discussion

To our knowledge, this is the first systematic review on the influence of HbF on SpO2 monitoring in human neonates. Based on the results of the majority of the included studies, a SpO2-SaO2 difference (bias) can be detected when the SpO2 (%) readings are compared to the direct measurements of SaO2 (%) or HbO2 (%) in neonatal blood. Reported mean SpO2-SaO2 bias ranged from -3.6% (SD 2.3) to $+4.2$% (SD 2.4) (Table S2). Although there have been indications that the bias could be influenced by HbF, none of the included studies provided an adequate statistical analysis to prove this statement.

We included ten studies in our analysis and divided them in two groups according to the technical characteristics and HbF measurement methods (Tables 1 and 2).

The five studies listed in Table 1 were conducted before the automatic correction of SaO2 for the presence of HbF by the hemoximeter (before 1992) [4,5,7,32,33]. Therefore, the corrections were performed retrospectively using a formula suggested by Cornellison et al. [35]. SpO2-SaO2 bias, which could be attributed to HbF, was detected in two studies [4,5]. The first study found a SpO2 underestimation of 2.8% to 3.6% for higher HbF values (FHbF > 50%) [4]. The second study reported a SpO2 overestimation for the lower HbF values (FHbF < 50%, SpO2-SaO2 bias +4.2% (SD 2.4)) and a decrease in SpO2-SaO2 bias for the higher HbF (for FHbF > 50%, SpO2-SaO2 bias +0.9% (SD 1.8)) [5]. Two of the five studies reported no significant effect of HbF on SpO2 accuracy [7,32]. Nevertheless, these two studies included patients with wide variations in HbF levels (FHbF 4–95%) and reported only the mean difference between SpO2 and SaO2 for all patients. The fifth study of the period before 1992 observed the effects of multiple factors (HbF, pH, pCO2, 2,3-DPG) on ODC in neonates and found that all of the parameters influenced ODC and therefore affected the corresponding SpO2 [33] (Figure 1). As the SpO2-SaO2 bias was not tested for HbF alone, the reported results are difficult to interpret.

Five studies conducted after 1992 used a hemoximeter for HbF measurements and adopted the automatic correction for SaO2 that accounts for the presence of HbF [6,29–31,34]. Out of these, one study found pulse oximeter saturations to be unaffected by HbF. It is important to mention that the 22 preterm neonates included in this study received multiple transfusions of adult blood which led to a rapid postnatal decline in HbF levels in the study population (FHbF 0–16% after 2 weeks). Moreover, the study reported an average SpO2-SaO2 bias from all of the acquired measurements irrespective of the HbF level at the time of the blood sampling [6].

The three larger studies by Shiao et al. reported primarily an HbF effect on SaO2 and HbO2 measurements from neonatal blood samples [29–31]. Although the authors mentioned the SpO2-SaO2 and SpO2-HbO2 bias, there was no statistical evidence that these could be attributed to HbF alone.

In their first study on 210 neonatal blood samples, the authors compared different measurement modes of the hemoximeter: the HbA-mode (adult mode) and the HbF-mode (fetal mode). They found that the blood saturation values were 4% to 7% higher using the HbA-mode as compared to the HbF mode (which assumed FHbF of 80%). The analyses with the HbA-mode overestimated both arterial and venous saturation from neonatal blood samples. Regarding the SpO2-SaO2 comparisons, a SpO2-SaO2 bias of −0.59% (2SD 5.93) for the HbF mode vs. −5.69% (2SD 5.96) for the HbA mode was reported. However, the bias was tested only for the arterial saturation range of 97.5% (SD 3.16) and there was no statistical analysis of HbF contribution to the SpO2-SaO2 bias. Based on these results, it is difficult to assess pulse oximeters' accuracy for the different saturation ranges as well as the HbF contribution to the biases [29].

In their largest study, Shiao and Ou reported that the bias between SpO2 and HbO2 in arterial blood samples was as high as 2.5% (SD 3.1) for the arterial saturation range of 96.9% (SD 3.18). However, any influence of HbF is only reported on blood-derived oxygen saturation parameters and was not tested for SpO2-SaO2 bias. Nevertheless, the authors presented several ODC based on the paO2 and SaO2 of their samples and showed that the ODC in neonates was not only left-shifted but also steeper when compared to adults. For paO2 values between 50 and 75 mmHg (normoxemia), SpO2 ranged from 95% to 97% in neonates as compared to 85% to 94% in adults [31].

This narrow SpO2 range is based on the physiological characteristics of HbF. The study conducted on blood samples of extremely low birth weight neonates with very high HbF levels showed that a paO2 of 41 mmHg should be adequate to saturate 90% of HbF at a physiological pH. Therefore, the paO2 range of 45 to 60 mmHg could be defined as safe and preferable for this group of patients [36]. However, at paO2 of 50 mmHg, HbF is already 95% saturated. Consequently, further increase in paO2 leads to a minimal increase in saturation. (Figure 1) These observations further stress the importance of accurate SpO2 measurements and correct SpO2 targets to avoid undetected hypoxic or hyperoxic episodes.

Finally, the last included study, which investigated the effect of transfusion of adult blood and the consequential HbF decline on oxygenation parameters in neonates, found that there was a significant increase in paO2 after the transfusion (51 ± 8 mmHg vs 57 ± 7 mmHg, $p < 0.001$) with almost no changes in SpO2 ($94 \pm 2\%$ vs $93 \pm 1\%$, $p = 0.4$). This was achieved by an increase in FiO2 (>12%) applied to the infants to keep the SpO2 within the set goal [34]. However, it is not clear from this study whether the results reflect only the decrease in HbF or whether the changes in other parameters, such as pH or methemoglobin after the transfusion, might have influenced the described changes as well.

Based on the ten included studies, a SpO2-SaO2 bias can be detected by direct comparison of SpO2 readings to SaO2 in neonatal blood after the correction for HbF, but it is unclear to what extent this can be attributed to the HbF alone. An increase in HbF changes the relation of SpO2 to paO2, which is physiologically explained by the leftward shift in the ODC. It is important to be aware of this shift when treating a neonate, especially for the lower SpO2 limits in preterm neonates. Because of the fetal ODC form (Figure 1), a potential undetected hypoxia is particularly pronounced in the lower saturation ranges, i.e. for SpO2 < 90% where the curve is steep and becomes less detectable at its flat part (SpO2 > 95%). From this point of view, it can be assumed that there is only a low risk of undetected hyperoxemia when using an upper alarm limit of 95%. This was already shown in a study on three different pulse oximeters (Agilent Viridia, Masimo SET, Nellcor Oxismart), which detected hyperoxemia with 93–95% sensitivity for the upper alarm limit of 95% [37].

The question of optimal oxygen-saturation targeting for preterm neonates in order to avoid hypoxic and/or hyperoxic organ damage has been a subject of numerous, large, randomized controlled clinical trials [38–44]. Lower SpO2 target ranges (85–89%) have led to a decreased risk of retinopathy of prematurity but an increased risk of mortality [45]. If we took the ODC characteristics of HbF into account, the lower target ranges may have resulted in lower SaO2 values, as one would expect, and could have potentially resulted in more significant undetected hypoxemia in preterm infants. This may also have contributed to the reported increased rate of mortality and necrotizing enterocolitis in these patients. In addition, red blood cell transfusions, which are often required in preterm infants, lead to an increase in HbA relative to HbF, thus resulting in an ODC shift to the right. If the

SpO2 target ranges are set higher, the ODC shift to the right after a transfusion may lead to hyperoxemia and increase the incidence of retinopathy of prematurity.

Finally, there are additional limitations of the included studies. The changes in the ODC positions (and consequently of SaO2) based on the differences in pH, temperature, and pCO2 (Figure 1) were not investigated in most of the studies. The studies also did not report the influence of oxygen supplementation on the SpO2-SaO2 bias. The largest study in neonates, which compared more than twenty-seven thousand SpO2 readings to SaO2 and paO2, however, reported a three-fold higher likelihood of SpO2 overestimation in infants treated with supplemental oxygen [14]. An additional explanation for the SpO2 differences in neonates and adults is that the sensors used in the calibration process of pulse oximeters have a different optical-path length in an adult compared to an infant, which may affect the accuracy of pulse oximeters in neonates [9,46]. As different measurement methods for HbF were used within the studies, this fact is a further limitation for the interpretation of the HbF levels and for the comparison of the studies. HPLC as a gold standard was only used in one study and when compared to the HbF measurements by a hemoximeter, a bias of 23% (SD 9) was detected [30].

5. Conclusions

In studies that compared non-invasive SpO2 monitoring by pulse oximetry to oxygen saturation measurements from blood samples in preterm and term infants and included HbF measurements in their reports, the majority found a SpO2-SaO2 bias, but it remains unclear whether this can be explained by the high fractions of HbF in neonatal blood alone. As hemoximeters today usually correct for the presence of HbF, SaO2 values of those devices likely reflect the paO2 of neonatal blood correctly. Based on the physiological characteristics of fetal ODC, there might be an influence of HbF on SpO2 readings, resulting mostly in an overestimation of SpO2 for the lower saturation ranges. Further prospective studies on a larger sample size are needed to support this statement.

Supplementary Materials: The following are available online at https://www.mdpi.com/article/10.3390/children8050361/s1; Figure S1: table, Table S1: PRISMA Checklist. Table S2: Summary of the most important numerical data from the included studies.

Author Contributions: Conceptualized and designed the review, conducted systematic search of literature, drafted the initial manuscript, and reviewed and edited the manuscript, E.P. and G.P.; designed the tables and reviewed and edited the manuscript, E.P. and B.S.; critically reviewed the manuscript for important intellectual content, E.P., G.P., B.S. and B.U. All authors approved the final manuscript as submitted and agree to be accountable for all aspects of the work. All authors have read and agreed to the published version of the manuscript.

Funding: This research received no external funding.

Acknowledgments: The authors would like to thank Thomas Reid Alderson and Iva Pritišanac for critically reading the manuscript and Thomas Suppan for his help with the figures.

Conflicts of Interest: The authors declare no conflict of interest.

References

1. Madar, J.; Roehr, C.C.; Ainsworth, S.; Ersdal, H.; Morley, C.; Rüdiger, M.; Skåre, C.; Szczapa, T.; Te Pas, A.; Trevisanuto, D.; et al. European Resuscitation Council Guidelines 2021: Newborn resuscitation and support of transition of infants at birth. *Resuscitation* **2021**, *161*, 291–326. [CrossRef]
2. Aziz, K.; Lee, H.C.; Escobedo, M.B.; Hoover, A.V.; Kamath-Rayne, B.D.; Kapadia, V.S.; Magid, D.J.; Niermeyer, S.; Schmölzer, G.M.; Szyld, E.; et al. Part 5: Neonatal Resuscitation 2020 American Heart Association Guidelines for Cardiopulmonary Resuscitation and Emergency Cardiovascular Care. *Pediatrics* **2021**, *147* (Suppl. 1), e2020038505E. [CrossRef] [PubMed]
3. Dawson, J.A.; Kamlin, C.O.F.; Vento, M.; Wong, C.; Cole, T.J.; Donath, S.M.; Davis, P.G.; Morley, C.J. Defining the reference range for oxygen saturation for infants after birth. *Pediatrics* **2010**, *125*, e1340–e1347. [CrossRef] [PubMed]
4. Jennis, M.S.; Peabody, J.L. Pulse oximetry: An alternative method for the assessment of oxygenation in newborn infants. *J. Pediatr.* **1987**, *79*, 524–528.

5. Praud, J.P.; Gaultier, C.L.; Carofilis, A.; Lacaille, F.; Dehan, M.; Bridey, F. Accuracy of two wavelength pulse oximetry in neonates and infants. *Pediatr. Pulmonol.* **1989**, *6*, 180–182. [CrossRef]
6. Rajadurai, V.S.; Walker, A.M.; Yu, V.Y.H.; Oates, A. Effect of fetal hemoglobin on the accuracy of pulse oximetry in preterm infants. *J. Paediatr. Child Health* **1992**, *28*, 43–46. [CrossRef]
7. Ramanathan, R.; Durand, M.; Larrazabal, C. Pulse oximetry in very low birth weight infants with acute and chronic lung injury. *Pediatrics* **1987**, *79*, 612–617.
8. Wukitsch, M.W.; Petterson, M.T.; Tobler, D.R.; Pologe, J.A. Pulse oximetry: Analysis of theory, technology, and practice. *J. Clin. Monit.* **1988**, *4*, 290–301. [CrossRef] [PubMed]
9. Nitzan, M.; Romem, A.; Koppel, R. Pulse oximetry: Fundamentals and technology update. *Med. Devices* **2014**, *7*, 231–239. [CrossRef]
10. Louw, A.; Cracco, C.; Cerf, C.; Harf, A.; Duvaldestin, P.; Lemaire, F.; Brochard, L. Accuracy of pulse oximetry in the intensive care unit. *Intensive Care Med.* **2001**, *27*, 1606–1613. [CrossRef]
11. Perkins, G.D.; McAuley, D.F.; Giles, S.; Routledge, H.; Gao, F. Do changes in pulse oximeter oxygen saturation predict equivalent changes in arterial oxygen saturation? *Crit. Care* **2003**, *7*, R67. [CrossRef] [PubMed]
12. Jubran, A.; Tobin, M.J. Reliability of pulse oximetry in titrating supplemental oxygen therapy in ventilator-dependent patients. *Chest* **1990**, *97*, 1420–1425. [CrossRef] [PubMed]
13. Ross, P.; Newth, C.; Khemani, R. Accuracy of pulse oximetry in children. *Pediatrics* **2014**, *133*, 22–29. [CrossRef] [PubMed]
14. Wackernagel, D.; Blennow, M.; Hellström, A. Accuracy of pulse oximetry in preterm and term infants is insufficient to de-termine arterial oxygen saturation and tension. *Acta Paediatr.* **2020**, *109*, 2251–2257. [CrossRef] [PubMed]
15. Oski, F.A.; Delivoria-Papadopoulos, M. The shift to the left. *Pediatrics* **1971**, *48*, 853–856. [PubMed]
16. Sankaran, V.G.; Orkin, S.H. The Switch From Fetal to Adult Hemoglobin. *Cold Spring Harb. Perspect. Med.* **2013**, *3*, a011643. [CrossRef]
17. Bunn, H.F.; Briehl, R.W. The interaction of 2,3-diphosphoglycerate with various human hemoglobins. *J. Clin. Investig.* **1970**, *49*, 1088–1095. [CrossRef]
18. Orzalesi, M.M.; Hay, W.W. The regulation of oxygen affinity of fetal blood. I. In vitro experiments and results in normal infants. *Pediatrics* **1971**, *48*, 857–864.
19. Bard, H. Postnatal fetal and adult hemoglobin synthesis in early preterm newborn infants. *J. Clin. Investig.* **1973**, *52*, 1789–1795. [CrossRef]
20. Wilson, K.; Hawken, S.; Murphy, M.S.; Atkinson, K.M.; Potter, B.K.; Sprague, A.; Walker, M.; Chakraborty, P.; Little, J. Postnatal prediction of gestational age using newborn fetal hemoglobin levels. *EBioMedicine* **2017**. [CrossRef]
21. Cochran-Black, D.L.; Cowan, L.D.; Neas, B.R. The relation between newborn hemoglobin F fractions and risk factors for sudden infant death syndrome. *Arch. Pathol. Lab. Med.* **2001**, *125*, 211–217. [CrossRef] [PubMed]
22. Stutchfield, C.J.; Jain, A.; Odd, D.; Wiliams, C.; Markham, R. Foetal haemoglobin, blood transfusion, and retinopathy of prematurity in very preterm infants: A pilot prospective cohort study. *Eye* **2017**, *31*, 1451–1455. [CrossRef] [PubMed]
23. Inoue, H.; Takabe, F.; Maeno, Y.; Iwasa, M. Identification of fetal hemoglobin in blood stains by high performance liquid chro-matography. *Z. Rechtsmed.* **1989**, *102*, 437–444. [CrossRef] [PubMed]
24. Davis, M.D.; Walsh, B.K.; Sittig, S.E.; Restrepo, R.D. AARC Clinical practice guideline: Blood gas analysis and hemoximetry: 2013. *Respir. Care* **2013**, *58*, 1694–1703. [CrossRef]
25. *ABL800 FLEX Reference Manual from Software Version 6.00*; Code number: 989-963; Radiometer: Copenhagen, Denmark, 2008.
26. Zijlstra, W.G.; Buursma, A.; Meeuwsen-van der Roest, W.P. Absorption spectra of human fetal and adult oxyhemoglobin, de-oxyhemoglobin, carboxyhemoglobin, and methemoglobin. *Clin. Chem.* **1991**, *37*, 1633–1638. [CrossRef]
27. Krzeminski, A. *How Is Fetal Hemoglobin Determined and Corrected for in the OSM3, the ABL 510, and the ABL 520?* Radiometer: Copenhagen, Denmark, 1992; pp. 1–4.
28. Moher, D.; Shamseer, L.; Clarke, M.; Ghersi, D.; Liberati, A.; Petticrew, M.; Shekelle, P.; Stewart, L.A. Preferred reporting items for systematic review and meta-analysis-protocols (Prisma P) 2015 statement. *Syst. Rev.* **2015**, *4*, 1. [CrossRef]
29. Shiao, S.Y.P.K. Effects of fetal hemoglobin on accurate measurements of oxygen saturation in neonates. *J. Perinat. Neonatal Nurs.* **2005**, *19*, 348–361. [CrossRef]
30. Shiao, S.Y.P.K.; Ou, C.N.; Pierantoni, H. The measurement of accurate fetal hemoglobin and related oxygen saturation by the hemoximeter. *Clin. Chim. Acta* **2006**, *374*, 75–80. [CrossRef]
31. Shiao, S.Y.; Ou, C.N. Validation of oxygen saturation monitoring in neonates. *Am. J. Crit. Care* **2007**, *16*, 168–178. [CrossRef]
32. Durand, M.; Ramanathan, R. Pulse oximetry for continuous oxygen monitoring in sick newborn infants. *J. Pediatr.* **1986**, *109*, 1052–1056. [CrossRef]
33. Wimberley, P.D.; Helledie, N.R.; Friis-Hansen, B.; Fogh-Andersen, N.; Olesen, H. Pulse oximetry versus transcutaneous pO2 in sick newborn infants. *Scand. J. Clin. Lab. Investig.* **1987**, *188*, 19–25. [CrossRef]
34. Nitzan, I.; Hammerman, C.; Mimouni, F.B.; Bin-Nun, A. Packed red blood cells transfusions in neonates: Effect on FiO2 and PaO2/SaO2 ratio and implications for neonatal saturation targeting. *J. Perinatol.* **2018**, *38*, 693–695. [CrossRef]
35. Cornelissen, P.J.H.; van Woensel, C.L.M.; van Oel, W.C.; de Jong, P.A. Correction factors for hemoglobin derivatives in fetal blood, as measured with the IL 282 Co-oximeter. *Clin. Chem.* **1983**, *29*, 1555–1556. [CrossRef]

36. Émond, D.; Lachance, C.; Gagnon, J.; Bard, H. Arterial partial pressure of oxygen required to achieve 90% saturation of hae-moglobin in very low birth weight newborns. *Pediatrics* **1993**, *91*, 602–604.
37. Bohnhorst, B.; Peter, C.S.; Poets, C.F. Detection of hyperoxaemia in neonates: Data from three new pulse oximeters. *Arch. Dis. Child. Fetal Neonatal Ed.* **2002**, *87*, F217–F219. [CrossRef] [PubMed]
38. Support Study Group of the Eunice Kennedy Shriver NICHD Neonatal Research Network; Carlo, W.A.; Finer, N.N.; Walsh, M.C.; Rich, W.; Gantz, M.G.; Laptook, A.R.; Yoder, B.A.; Faix, R.G.; Das, A.; et al. Target ranges of oxygen saturation in extremely pre-term infants. *N. Engl. J. Med.* **2010**, *362*, 1959–1969.
39. Vaucher, Y.E.; Peralta-Carcelen, M.; Finer, N.N.; Carlo, W.A.; Gantz, M.G.; Walsh, M.C.; Laptook, A.R.; Yoder, B.A.; Faix, R.G.; Das, A.; et al. Neurodevelopmental outcomes in the early CPAP and pulse oximetry trial. *N. Engl. J. Med.* **2012**, *367*, 2495–2504. [CrossRef] [PubMed]
40. Schmidt, B.; Whyte, R.K.; Asztalos, E.V.; Moddemann, D.; Poets, C.; Rabi, Y.; Solimano, A.; Roberts, R.S.; the Canadian Oxygen Trial (COT) Group. Effects of targeting higher vs lower arterial oxygen saturations on death or disability in extremely preterm infants: A randomized clinical trial. *JAMA* **2013**, *309*, 2111–2120. [CrossRef]
41. Group BIUKC; Group BIAC; Group BINZC; Stenson, B.J.; Tarnow-Mordi, W.O.; Darlow, B.A.; Simes, J.; Juszczak, E.; Askie, L.; Battin, M.; et al. Oxygen saturation and outcomes in preterm infants. *N. Engl. J. Med.* **2013**, *368*, 2094–2104.
42. Darlow, B.A.; Marschner, S.L.; Donoghoe, M.; Battin, M.R.; Broadbent, R.S.; Elder, M.J.; Hewson, M.P.; Meyer, M.P.; Ghadge, A.; Graham, P.; et al. Randomized controlled trial of oxygen saturation targets in very pre-term infants: Two year outcomes. *J. Pediatr.* **2014**, *165*, 30–35. [CrossRef] [PubMed]
43. The BOOST-II Australia and United Kingdom Collaborative Groups; Tarnow-Mordi, W.O.; Stenson, B.J.; Kirby, A.; Juszczak, E.; Donoghoe, M.; Deshpande, S.; Morley, C.; King, A.; Doyle, L.W.; et al. Outcomes of two trials of oxygen-saturation targets in preterm infants. *N. Engl. J. Med.* **2016**, *374*, 749–760. [PubMed]
44. Khadawardi, E.; Al Hazzani, F. Oxygen saturation and outcomes in preterm infants: The BOOST II United Kingdom, Australia, and New Zealand Collaborative Groups. *J. Clin. Neonatol.* **2013**, *2*, 73–75. [CrossRef]
45. Lakshminrusimha, S.; Manja, V.; Mathew, B.; Suresh, G.K. Oxygen targeting in preterm infants: A physiologic interpretation. *J. Perinatol.* **2015**, *35*, 8–15. [CrossRef] [PubMed]
46. Poets, C.F. Noninvasive monitoring and assessment of oxygenation in infants. *Clin. Perinatol.* **2019**, *46*, 417–433. [CrossRef] [PubMed]

Article

Cardiac Output and Cerebral Oxygenation in Term Neonates during Neonatal Transition

Nariae Baik-Schneditz [1,2,3], Bernhard Schwaberger [1,2,3], Lukas Mileder [1,2,3], Nina Höller [1,2,3], Alexander Avian [4], Berndt Urlesberger [1,2,3] and Gerhard Pichler [1,2,3,*]

1. Division of Neonatology, Department of Paediatrics and Adolescent Medicine, Medical University of Graz, 8036 Graz, Austria; nariae.baik@medunigraz.at (N.B.-S.); bernhard.schwaberger@medunigraz.at (B.S.); lukas.mileder@medunigraz.at (L.M.); nina.hoeller@medunigraz.at (N.H.); berndt.urlesberger@medunigraz.at (B.U.)
2. Research Unit for Neonatal Micro- and Macrocirculation, Division of Neonatology, Medical University of Graz, 8036 Graz, Austria
3. Research Unit for Cerebral Development and Oximetry, Division of Neonatology, Medical University of Graz, 8036 Graz, Austria
4. Institute for Medical Informatics, Statistics and Documentation, Medical University of Graz, 8036 Graz, Austria; alexander.avian@medunigraz.at
* Correspondence: gerhard.pichler@medunigraz.at; Tel.: +43-316-385-80520

Abstract: The immediate transition from foetus to neonate includes substantial changes, especially concerning the cardiovascular system. Furthermore, the brain is one of the most vulnerable organs to hypoxia during this period. According to current guidelines for postnatal stabilization, the recommended parameters for monitoring are heart rate (HR) and arterial oxygen saturation (SpO_2). Recently, there is a growing interest in advanced monitoring of the cardio-circulatory system and the brain to get further objective information about the neonate's condition during the immediate postnatal transition after birth. The aim of the present study was to combine cardiac output (CO) and brain oxygenation monitoring in term neonates after caesarean section in order to analyse the potential influence of CO on cerebral oxygenation during neonatal transition. This was a monocentric, prospective, observational study. For non-invasive cardiac output measurements, the electrical velocimetry (EV) method (Aesculon Monitor, Osypka Medical, CA, USA) was used. The pulse oximeter probe for SpO_2 and HR measurements was placed on the right hand or wrist. The cerebral tissue oxygen index (cTOI) was measured using a NIRO-200NX monitor with the near-infrared spectroscopy (NIRS) transducer on the right frontoparietal head. Monitoring started at minute 1 and was continued until minute 15 after birth. At minutes 5, 10, and 15 after birth, mean CO was calculated from six 10 s periods (with beat-to-beat analysis). During the study period, 99 term neonates were enrolled. Data from neonates with uncomplicated transitions were analysed. CO showed a tendency to decrease until minute 10. During the complete observational period, there was no significant correlation between CO and cTOI. The present study was the first to investigate a possible correlation between CO and cerebral oxygenation in term infants during the immediate neonatal transition. In term infants with uncomplicated neonatal transition after caesarean section, CO did not correlate with cerebral oxygenation.

Keywords: cardiac output; cerebral oxygenation; term neonates; neonatal transition

1. Introduction

To standardize the assessment of the condition of newborns during the immediate transition period after birth, Virginia Apgar developed a scoring system [1] that is nowadays widely used all over the world. However, there is significant inter- and intra-observer variability when the Apgar score is used [2,3]. In order to improve postnatal assessment, the latest guidelines recommend, besides clinical evaluation, monitoring of heart rate (HR) and arterial oxygen saturation (SpO$_2$) with pulse oximetry and optionally with electrocardiography (ECG) in the delivery room [4]. However, these monitoring methods do not provide comprehensive information about potentially compromised cardio-circulatory status resulting in compromised oxygen delivery to various organs. One of the most vital organs certainly is the brain [5]. Oxygen delivery to the brain depends on the oxygen content of the blood (haemoglobin concentration and oxygen saturation) and cerebral perfusion. Cerebral perfusion depends on cardiac output (CO) and vascular resistance, whereby the evaluation of these cardio-circulatory parameters in the first minutes after birth remains challenging. Concerning cardio-circulation, centiles of HR during the first minutes after birth have already been published [6]. Our study group recently published reference ranges for blood pressure in the first minutes after birth [7]. Furthermore, we proved the feasibility of non-invasive CO measurements in term neonates during neonatal transition in the delivery room using the electrical velocimetry (EV) method [8]. The aim of the present study was to investigate whether there is a significant correlation between non-invasively monitored CO and cerebral oxygenation in term neonates during the neonatal transition period. We hypothesized that higher CO might be correlated with higher cerebral oxygenation.

2. Materials and Methods

This was a monocentric, prospective, observational study conducted from September 2013 to March 2017 at the Division of Neonatology, Department of Paediatrics and Adolescent Medicine, Medical University of Graz. The study was approved by the Regional Committee on Biomedical Research Ethics (EC number: 25-342 ex 12/13). Informed parental consent was obtained antenatally before neonates were included in the study.

Neonates born by caesarean section were included. After the neonates were fully delivered, a stopwatch was started. After cord clamping, which was routinely performed within 30 s, neonates were brought to the resuscitation table and placed under an overhead heater in the supine position. Measurements were performed during the first 15 min after birth. For non-invasive CO measurements, the Aesculon monitor (Osypka Medical, La Jolla, CA, USA) was used. Before starting the measurement, the skin was cleaned from vernix and the four surface electrodes were placed on the left forehead, left side of the neck, left hemithorax, and left thigh.

CO was calculated as an average out of six 10 s periods (with beat-to-beat analysis). The data from these 10 s periods were only accepted if the signal quality index (SQI) was $\geq$80%. The pulse oximeter probe for SpO$_2$ and HR measurements (IntelliVue MP 30 Monitor, Philips, Amsterdam, The Netherlands) was placed on the right hand or wrist. The cerebral tissue oxygenation index (cTOI) was measured using a NIRO-200NX monitor (Hamamatsu Photonics, Hamamatsu, Japan). The near-infrared spectroscopy (NIRS) sensor was positioned on the right frontoparietal head and secured with a cohesive conforming bandage (Peha-haft, Harmann, Heidenheim, Germany).

Resuscitation was performed according to latest guideline recommendations [4,9]. We only analysed data from neonates who had uncomplicated neonatal transition periods (without any need for respiratory and/or medical support). All variables were stored using the multichannel system alpha-trace digital MM (BEST Medical Systems, Vienna, Austria) for subsequent analyses. Values of SpO$_2$ and HR were stored every second, and the sampling rate of cTOI was 2 Hz.

Baseline characteristics are presented as mean $\pm$ standard deviation (SD) for normally distributed continuous variables and medians with interquartile range (IQR) when the distribution was skewed. Categorical variables are given with numbers and percentages. Changes in CO (mL/kg/min), cTOI (%), SpO$_2$ (%) and HR (beats per minute) were analysed using a linear mixed-effects model with a fixed effect for time and a first-order autoregressive covariance structure. Estimated mean scores with 95% confidence intervals (CI) are given for the analysed variables for 5, 10, and 15 min. To analyse possible associations between CO and cerebral oxygenation, correlation analyses (Spearman's rank correlation coefficient) were performed separately at minutes 5, 10, and 15 after birth. A *p*-value < 0.05 was considered statistically significant. Statistical analyses were performed using IBM SPSS Statistics 26.0.0 (IBM Corporation, Armonk, NY, USA).

3. Results

During the study period, 99 term neonates were enrolled. The demographic and clinical characteristics of the study population are presented in Table 1.

Table 1. Demographic and clinical characteristics of the study population.

	Study Population (*n* = 99)
Gestational age (weeks)—median (IQR)	38.8 (38.3–39.3)
Birth weight (g)—mean (SD)	3296 ± 492
Body length (cm)—median (IQR)	51 (49–52)
Head circumference (cm)—median (IQR)	35 (34–36)
Female sex—*n* (%)	54 (54.5)
Apgar score at 5 min—median (IQR)	10 (10–10)
Apgar score at 10 min—median (IQR)	10 (10–10)
Umbilical artery pH—median (IQR)	7.29 (7.27–7.31)
Maternal spinal anaesthesia—*n* (%)	99 (100%)

3.1. Course of CO, cTOI, SpO$_2$, and HR at Minutes 5, 10, and 15 after Birth

The courses of vital parameters at the time points 5, 10, and 15 min after birth are presented in Table 2. CO decreased from minute 5 to 10 and significantly increased afterwards. cTOI and SpO$_2$ showed a statistically significant increase from minute 5 to 10 after birth. Additionally, SpO$_2$ rose significantly from minute 10 to minute 15, but after considering the number of values, this increase is not relevant for clinical praxis. HR did not change from minute 5 to 10 or 15.

Table 2. Courses of vital parameters at 5, 10, and 15 min after birth.

	Minute 5 after Birth	Minute 10 after Birth	Minute 15 after Birth	*p*-Value Minute 5 to 10/Minute 10 to 15
cTOI (%) mean (95% CI)	63.8 (61.9–65.8)	73.2 (71.3–75.0)	73.1 (71.2–75.0)	<0.001/0.935
SpO$_2$ (%) mean (95% CI)	81.2 (79.6–82.8)	93.4 (91.9–95.0)	95.2 (93.6–96.8)	<0.001/0.024
HR (beats per minute) Mean (95% CI)	152 (148–156)	151 (147–155)	153 (149–157)	0.618/0.308
CO (mL/kg/min) Mean (95% CI)	199.8 (188.3–211.4)	187.5 (177.3–197.7)	198.0 (187.7–208.3)	0.019/0.019

3.2. Correlation between CO and cTOI at minutes 5, 10 and 15 after birth

There was no correlation between CO and cTOI during the first 15 min after birth (Table 3/Figures 1 and 2).

Table 3. Correlation analyses between CO and cTOI.

		cTOI
	Minute 5 after birth	
	ρ	0.170
	p-value	0.351
	Minute 10 after birth	
Cardiac output	ρ	0.074
	p-value	0.629
	Minute 15 after birth	
	ρ	0.265
	p-value	0.071

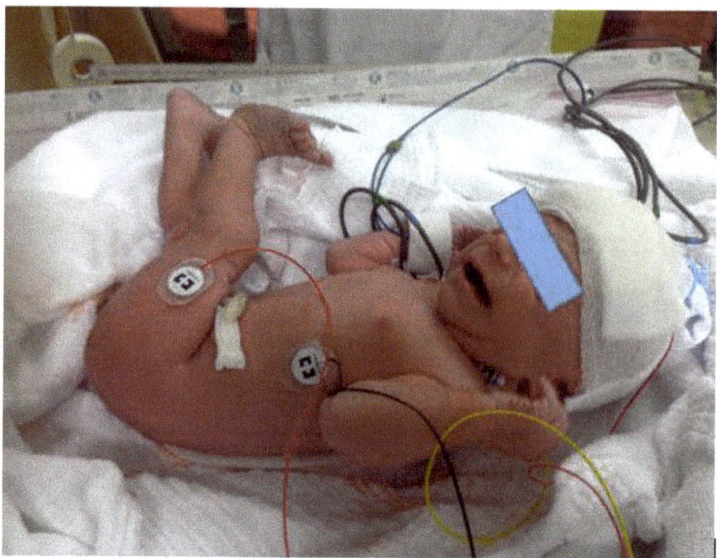

Figure 1. Neonate with four surface electrodes on the left forehead, left side of the neck, left hemithorax, and left thigh for non-invasive CO measurement.

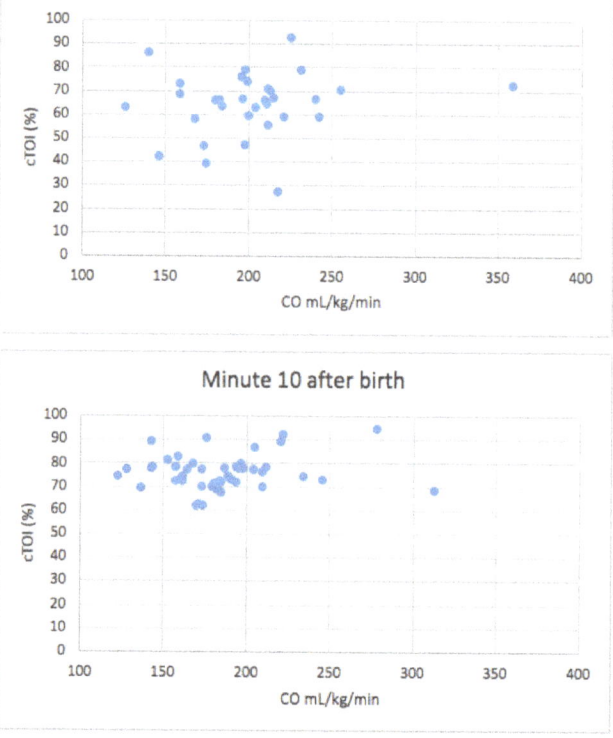

Figure 2. Cont.

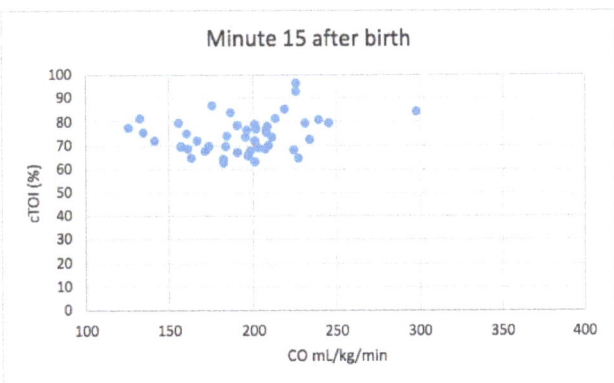

Figure 2. Correlation analyses between CO and cTOI at minute 5, 10, and 15 after birth.

4. Discussion

To our knowledge, this is the first study presenting correlation analyses between CO and cerebral oxygenation in term infants during the immediate neonatal transition. As the brain is a vulnerable organ, it is important to better understand oxygen delivery to the brain during this time. We hypothesized that higher CO would result in higher cerebral oxygenation, as oxygen delivery is dependent on CO and oxygen content. However, in our study population of 99 term infants delivered by caesarean section, we could not observe any significant correlation between CO and cerebral oxygenation.

Most published haemodynamic changes during the immediate neonatal transition described an increase in heart rate and a decrease in pulmonary vascular resistance after cord clamping and lung aeration [10–15]. Some research groups have published data showing changes in cardiac output in recent studies, mostly using echocardiography [13,14]. In the present study, we observed a significant decrease in cardiac output from minute 5 (199 mL/kg/min) until minute 10 (187 mL/kg/min). Afterwards, CO rose again until minute 15 (198 mL/kg/min) after birth. In a study using echocardiography, Van Vonderen et al. [15] described an increase in cardiac output from minute 2 (151 mL/kg/min) to minute 5 (203 mL/kg/min), and afterwards a stable tendency until minute 10 (201 mL/kg/min). A further study described an increasing tendency of cardiac output in the first 20 min after birth, which did not reach significance. CO was 168 mL/kg/min at p1, 186 mL/kg/min at p2, and 189 mL/kg/min at p3 [10]. These findings are comparable with the results in the present study.

Compared with echocardiography, EV provides the opportunity to monitor CO continuously and objectively. Additionally, the feasibility of this method has already been proven in the delivery room in term infants after caesarean section [8], and in vaginally born neonates receiving delayed cord clamping [9].

Noori et al. [10] compared EV measurements with echocardiography in 20 healthy neonates during the first two days after birth. They performed left ventricular output measurements with EV and echocardiography. There was no significant difference between these two methods, confirming that EV measurements have comparable accuracy and precision to echocardiography for CO measurements when the EV SQI was $\geq$80% [10].

Several studies have described lower cerebral oxygenation values in preterm neonates immediately after birth, resulting in cerebral injury in the following days [11,12]. As a recent study described a possible association between lower left ventricular output measured by echocardiography and the development of intraventricular haemorrhage during the first day of life in extremely preterm infants [13], the authors raised the question of whether CO immediately after birth has an impact on cerebral oxygenation. As a first step, we wanted to investigate whether there is an impact of CO on cerebral oxygenation in term infants during neonatal transition. However, in contrast to our hypothesis, we did not find such a correlation in healthy term neonates. Nonetheless, this finding is in accordance with a recent observation in term neonates that mean arterial blood pressure had no significant impact on cerebral oxygenation [16]. In contrast, there was a significant association between blood pressure and cerebral oxygenation in preterm neonates during neonatal transition [16]. These contradictory results may be a sign of intact vascular autoregulation in term neonates and potentially impaired autoregulation in preterm neonates. In the present study of term infants during uncomplicated transition without any need for respiratory and/or medical support, our results further emphasize the intact cerebral autoregulation in neonates born at term. With this knowledge, the next step should be CO monitoring in compromised term and preterm neonates to better understand the underlying (patho)physiological processes in those infants.

We recognize several limitations in this study. First, we only included neonates born by caesarean section. Due to technical reasons, not all of the measurements were able to be performed in the delivery room next to the mother. Since all neonates after caesarean section were brought to the resuscitation table and observed by a neonatologist for 10 to 15 min, we only performed measurements on those neonates. We did not include vaginally born neonates to avoid delaying immediate bonding with the mother. Therefore, we do not have any information about cardiac output measurements in vaginally born neonates. Recent studies showed that the mode of delivery might influence haemodynamic parameters and cerebral oxygenation during neonatal transition [6,17,18]. We may have observed some differences in vaginally born neonates. Additionally, in these neonates, cord clamping time was within 30 s, as this was the routine procedure during the observational period. Delayed cord clamping might have resulted in better oxygenation in these neonates. Second, our study population contains exclusively term neonates. In our study population, we observed stable values concerning cardiac output during the immediate neonatal transition. The next interesting question would be whether there are observable differences in very low birth weight preterm neonates needing extended respiratory and/or medical support. Third, since we only accepted and analysed cardiac output measurements, if the signal quality index was >80%, to guarantee the reproducibility with the other already approved methods, we had to exclude 76% of NICOM measurements. In many cases, the activity and movements of the neonates influenced the NICOM measurements. Further studies are needed before introducing this method into routine clinical practice.

5. Conclusions

The present work is the first study to investigate a possible correlation between CO and cerebral oxygenation in term infants during immediate neonatal transition. In term infants with uncomplicated neonatal transition after caesarean section, there was no significant correlation between CO and cerebral oxygenation at 5, 10, or 15 min after birth.

Author Contributions: Conceptualization, N.B.-S., B.U. and G.P.; methodology, N.B.-S., B.S., G.P., L.M. and A.A.; software, A.A.; validation, N.H., A.A. and N.B.-S.; formal analysis, N.B.-S., B.S. and B.U.; investigation, N.B.-S., L.M., N.H.; resources, G.P.; data curation, B.U.; writing—original draft preparation, N.B.-S., G.P.; writing—review and editing, N.B.-S., B.S., L.M., B.U., N.H., G.P. and A.A.; supervision, G.P. project administration, N.B.-S. All authors have read and agreed to the published version of the manuscript.

Funding: This research received no external funding.

Institutional Review Board Statement: The study was conducted according to the guidelines of the Declaration of Helsinki and approved by the Regional Committee on Biomedical Research Ethics (EC number: 25-342 ex 12/13), Medical University of Graz.

Informed Consent Statement: Informed parental consent was obtained antenatally before neonates were included in the study.

Acknowledgments: We would like to thank the parents for allowing us to study their infants, as well as all the midwives, nurses, and physicians involved in the treatment of these neonates.

Conflicts of Interest: The authors declare no conflict of interest.

References

1. Apgar, V. A proposal for a new method of evaluation of the newborn infant. *Curr. Res. Anesth. Analg.* **1953**, *32*, 260–267. [CrossRef] [PubMed]
2. O'Donnell, C.P.; Kamlin, C.O.; Davis, P.G.; Carlin, J.B.; Morley, C.J. Clinical assessment of infant colour at delivery. *Arch. Dis. Child. Fetal Neonatal. Ed.* **2007**, *92*, F465–F467. [CrossRef] [PubMed]
3. O'Donnell, C.P.; Kamlin, C.O.; Davis, P.G.; Carlin, J.B.; Morley, C.J. Interobserver variability of the 5-minute Apgar score. *J. Pediatr.* **2006**, *149*, 486–489. [CrossRef] [PubMed]
4. Wyllie, J.; Bruinenberg, J.; Roehr, C.C.; Rüdiger, M.; Trevisanuto, D.; Urlesberger, B. European Resuscitation Council Guidelines for Resuscitation 2015: Section 7. Resuscitation and support of transition of babies at birth. *Resuscitation* **2015**, *95*, 249–263. [CrossRef] [PubMed]
5. Baik, N.; Urlesberger, B.; Schwaberger, B.; Freidl, T.; Schmölzer, G.M.; Pichler, G. Cardiocirculatory monitoring during immediate fetal-to-neonatal transition: A systematic qualitative review of the literature. *Neonatology* **2015**, *107*, 100–107. [CrossRef]
6. Dawson, J.A.; Kamlin, C.O.F.; Wong, C.; Pas, A.B.T.; Vento, M.; Cole, T.J.; Donath, S.M.; Hooper, S.B.; Davis, P.G.; Morley, C.J. Changes in heart rate in the first minutes after birth. *Arch. Dis. Child. Fetal Neonatal. Ed.* **2010**, *95*, F177–F181. [CrossRef]
7. Pichler, G.; Cheung, P.Y.; Binder, C.; O'Reilly, M.; Schwaberger, B.; Aziz, K.; Urlesberger, B.; Schmölzer, G.M. Blood Pressure in Term and Preterm Infants Immediately after Birth. *PLoS ONE* **2014**, *9*, e114504. [CrossRef]
8. Freidl, T.; Baik, N.; Pichler, G.; Pichler, G.; Schwaberger, B.; Zingerle, B.; Avian, A.; Urlesberger, B. Haemodynamic Transition after Birth: A New Tool for Non-Invasive Cardiac Output Monitoring. *Neonatology* **2016**, *111*, 55–60. [CrossRef] [PubMed]
9. Katheria, A.C.; Wozniak, M.; Harari, D.; Arnell, K.; Petruzzelli, D.; Finer, N.N. Measuring cardiac changes using electrical impedance during delayed cord clamping: A feasibility trial. *Matern. Health Neonatal. Perinatol.* **2015**, *1*, 15. [CrossRef] [PubMed]
10. Noori, S.; Wlodaver, A.; Gottipati, V.; McCoy, M.; Schultz, D.; Escobedo, M. Transitional changes in cardiac and cerebral hemodynamics in term neonates at birth. *J. Pediatr.* **2012**, *160*, 943–948. [CrossRef] [PubMed]
11. Fuchs, H.; Lindner, W.; Buschko, A.; Almazam, M.; Hummler, H.D.; Schmid, M.B. Brain oxygenation monitoring during neonatal resuscitation of very low birth weight infants. *J. Perinatol.* **2012**, *32*, 356–362. [CrossRef] [PubMed]
12. Baik, N.; Urlesberger, B.; Schwaberger, B.; Schmölzer, G.M.; Avian, A.; Pichler, G. Cerebral haemorrhage in preterm neonates: Does cerebral regional oxygen saturation during the immediate transition matter? *Arch. Dis. Child. Fetal Neonatal. Ed.* **2015**, *100*, F422–F427. [CrossRef] [PubMed]
13. Noori, S.; McCoy, M.; Anderson, M.P.; Ramji, F.; Seri, I. Changes in cardiac function and cerebral blood flow in relation to peri/intraventricular hemorrhage in extremely preterm infants. *J. Pediatr.* **2014**, *164*, 264–270.e1–e3. [CrossRef] [PubMed]
14. Van Vonderen, J.J.; Roest, A.A.; Siew, M.L.; Walther, F.J.; Hooper, S.B.; Pas, A.B.T. Measuring physiological changes during the transition to life after birth. *Neonatology* **2014**, *105*, 230–242. [CrossRef] [PubMed]
15. Van Vonderen, J.J.; Roest, A.A.; Siew, M.L.; Blom, N.A.; Van Lith, J.M.; Walther, F.J.; Hooper, S.B.; Pas, A.B.T. Noninvasive measurements of hemodynamic transition directly after birth. *Pediatr. Res.* **2014**, *75*, 448–452. [CrossRef] [PubMed]
16. Baik, N.; Urlesberger, B.; Schwaberger, B.; Avian, A.; Mileder, L.; Schmölzer, G.M.; Pichler, G. Blood Pressure during the Immediate Neonatal Transition: Is the Mean Arterial Blood Pressure Relevant for the Cerebral Regional Oxygenation? *Neonatology* **2017**, *112*, 97–102. [CrossRef] [PubMed]
17. Gonzales, G.F.; Salirrosas, A. Pulse oxygen saturation and neurologic assessment in human neonates after vaginal and cesarean delivery. *Int. J. Gynaecol. Obstet.* **1998**, *63*, 63–66. [CrossRef]
18. Urlesberger, B.; Kratky, E.; Rehak, T.; Pocivalnik, M.; Avian, A.; Czihak, J.; Müller, W.; Pichler, G. Regional oxygen saturation of the brain during birth transition of term infants: Comparison between elective cesarean and vaginal deliveries. *J. Pediatr.* **2011**, *159*, 404–408. [CrossRef] [PubMed]

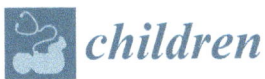

Brief Report

In-Silico Evaluation of Anthropomorphic Measurement Variations on Electrical Cardiometry in Neonates

David B. Healy [1,2], Eugene M. Dempsey [1,2,3], John M. O'Toole [1,2] and Christoph E. Schwarz [1,2,3,4,*]

1 Department of Neonatology, Cork University Maternity Hospital, Wilton, T12 K8AF Cork, Ireland; david.healy@ucc.ie (D.B.H.); g.dempsey@ucc.ie (E.M.D.); jotoole@ucc.ie (J.M.O.)
2 Department of Paediatrics & Child Health, University College Cork, T12 K8AF Cork, Ireland
3 INFANT Research Centre, Wilton, T12 K8AF Cork, Ireland
4 Department of Neonatology, University Children's Hospital, 72076 Tübingen, Germany
* Correspondence: C.Schwarz@med.uni-tuebingen.de; Tel.: +49-7071-29-82811

Abstract: Non-invasive cardiac output methods such as Electrical Cardiometry (EC) are relatively novel assessment tools for neonates and they enable continuous monitoring of stroke volume (SV). An in-silico comparison of differences in EC-derived SV in relation to preset length and weight was performed. EC (ICON, Osypka Medical) was simulated using the "demo" mode for various combinations of length and weight representative of term and preterm infants. One-centimetre length error resulted in a SV-change of 1.8–3.6% (preterm) or 1.6–2.0% (term) throughout the tested weight ranges. One-hundred gram error in weight measurement resulted in a SV-change of 5.0–7.1% (preterm) or 1.5–1.8% (term) throughout the tested length ranges. Algorithms to calculate EC-derived SV incorporate anthropomorphic measurements. Therefore, inaccuracy in physical measurement can impact absolute EC measurements. This should be considered in the interpretation of previous findings and the design of future clinical studies of EC-derived cardiac parameters in neonates, particularly in the preterm cohorts where a proportional change was noted to be greatest.

Keywords: infant; premature; term; bio-impedance; non-invasive cardiac output monitoring

Citation: Healy, D.B.; Dempsey, E.M.; O'Toole, J.M.; Schwarz, C.E. In-Silico Evaluation of Anthropomorphic Measurement Variations on Electrical Cardiometry in Neonates. *Children* **2021**, *8*, 936. https://doi.org/10.3390/children8100936

Academic Editor: Bernhard Schwaberger

Received: 20 September 2021
Accepted: 14 October 2021
Published: 18 October 2021

Publisher's Note: MDPI stays neutral with regard to jurisdictional claims in published maps and institutional affiliations.

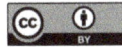

Copyright: © 2021 by the authors. Licensee MDPI, Basel, Switzerland. This article is an open access article distributed under the terms and conditions of the Creative Commons Attribution (CC BY) license (https://creativecommons.org/licenses/by/4.0/).

1. Introduction

Neonatal non-invasive evaluation of cardiac output (CO) is typically performed with echocardiography. Electrical cardiometry (EC) enables a continuous assessment of CO in newborns. Parameters, including stroke volume (SV) and, multiplied by heart rate (HR), cardiac output (CO), are recorded as absolute values or indexed for body weight. While EC is now increasingly used in clinical research in neonates [1], including the delivery room and neonatal intensive care unit [1–5], further research and development of the technology is required before it can be appropriately utilized in clinical practice to potentially guide management.

In EC, the distance between electrodes influences the recorded parameters and, as such, an initial calibration using weight and length is required. Therefore, inaccurate anthropomorphic measurements might affect EC-derived parameters. Measurement is particularly challenging in the delivery room, and in previous studies, predetermined standardized measurements were employed [2–5]. Inaccuracy may become significant where absolute values are used to delineate 'normative ranges'. Thus, our aim was to evaluate the effect size of differences in length and weight on EC-derived SV estimates for preterm and term infants in a simulation study.

2. Materials and Methods

The ICON monitor (Osypka Medical, Berlin, Germany) was used in "demonstration mode", which provides an identical set of electrical impedance changes for each repetition representative for an adult patient. As sex does not have an effect on the measurements calculated by the ICON monitor (unpublished data and confirmed by the manufacturer), all measurements were performed as for a male on day 1 postnatally. Weight can be set to increments of 25 g (<1 kg) or 50 g (>1 kg) and length can be input in increments of 0.1 cm on the monitor. We used a representative range of weights and lengths (term: weight 3.0–4.2 kg, length 48–56 cm/preterm: weight 0.5–1.5 kg, length 28–40 cm). SV for each combination of weight and length was documented after a 2-min cycling period. A linear regression model was fitted to the data to find an analytical expression for the dependency of SV on weight and length. Models were developed separately for the term and preterm data using an ordinary least squares fit (Python 3.9 with statsmodel 0.12). The dependent variable was SV. Potential independent variables were weight [kg], length [cm], and the weight-by-length interaction. Models with all combinations of the independent variables were compared using the Akaike information criterion.

3. Results

Figure S1 (Online Supplementary) illustrates the dependence of SV on weight and length. For a term infant with a length of 51 cm, every 100-g difference from the median weight of 3.5 kg led to a change in SV of 1.7%. For preterm infants, this effect was found to be more influential on the resultant SV measurement; e.g., for a 34-cm infant, each 100-g increase or decrease from 1 kg led to a relative change in measured SV of 6.1%. In contrast every 1-cm change in length resulted in a 1.8% relative change in SV for median weight term infants and 2.7% for median weight preterm infants.

The SV regression models for the preterm and term data both included length and weight-by-length as independent variables (see Table 1). Relative SVs, normalized to the median of the variable, are presented in Table S1 (term) and Table S2 (preterm) (Online Supplementary).

Table 1. Coefficients of linear regression model of stroke volume.

	Preterm Model Coefficient (95% CI)	Term Model Coefficient (95% CI)
intercept [mL]	0.1503 (0.079 to 0.221)	0.4801 (0.423 to 0.537)
length [cm]	0.0141 (0.012 to 0.016)	0.0298 (0.029 to 0.031)
weight × length [kg × cm]	0.0285 (0.028 to 0.029)	0.0160 (0.016 to 0.016)

4. Discussion

We quantified the effect of weight and length on EC-derived SV estimates. Differences in anthropometric measures, and thereby, differences in intrathoracic intravascular volumes, lead to differences in SV measurements. The effects were more pronounced in preterm infants compared to term infants. Therefore, inaccurate estimates or measurements of these anthropometric values can lead to clinically relevant changes in SV.

While, in adults, such a small proportional error makes a clinically irrelevant difference, in infants, errors in anthropomorphic measurement could lead to significant discrepancies in SV. Furthermore, as CO equals SV times HR, the effect of the naturally higher newborn HR on CO estimation leads to amplification of the initial weight or length error. For example, from our simulation data, overestimation of a preterm infant's weight by 250 g and their length by 2 cm would subsequently result in a 0.33-mL error in SV. Based on a HR of 160 bpm in a 1-kg neonate, this would result in an error of almost 53 mL/s/kg/min in CO. In term infants, however, the relative error in SV is lower, and the amplification of the error is less pronounced due to slightly lower HR. Therefore, for a 200-g weight and a 2-cm length overestimation, the calculated error in CO would be 12.4 mL/s/kg/min for a 3.4-kg neonate.

Even the error in a single measurement (i.e., weight or length) can still lead to relevant change. For example, a 2-cm measurement inaccuracy would lead to almost 15 mL/s/kg/min in CO error for a 1-kg baby. The effect of length as a component in the algorithm calculation is important and raises important clinical concerns, as accurate measurement in neonates is not always straightforward [6]. Due to the expected inaccuracy in length, it is common in neonatology to index output by weight and not by body surface area. However, as EC parameters depend on the distance between outer and inner electrodes, calibration with length is necessary to adjust for differences in distance caused by body length. The ability to input weight only to the closest 25 g should also be considered as a factor when evaluating cardiac indices in extremely preterm infants, where seemingly small weight differences may also lead to clinically relevant distinctions in CO. This is particularly the case for the smallest preterm infants, in whom 25 g can represent up to 5% of a weight difference.

Accounting for this, researchers should be aware of the potential for algorithmic reproduction of weight and length estimation errors resulting in "abnormal" EC-derived parameters. Noori et al. mentioned calibration within the EC algorithm in 2012 [7]. However, few studies since then have reported how calibration for weight or length was addressed. This is pertinent in the delivery room. Previous studies used pre-set or standardized weight and length for term infants in the delivery setting [2–5]. In one study, EC measurements were performed during intact cord management, therefore relying solely on estimates [2]. As this will result in miscalibration, EC-derived parameters should only be used to provide trends, until weight and length are verified. Of note, only flow related measurements are affected (i.e., SV or CO), whereas other EC parameters are not (e.g., thoracic fluid content). While we would not currently recommend the use of EC for the determination of absolute CO values to guide clinical management decisions yet, it may be possible to improve accuracy in the delivery room research setting. Use of resuscitaires with in-built weighing scales could rapidly provide more accurate estimates of weight, or, where these are not available, the equipment could be pre-set based on the average weight for the gestational age or by using the estimated fetal weight derived from antenatal ultrasound scans. Length could be quickly estimated by employing a fixed ruler attached to the resuscitaire, without significant interference to clinical management of the baby.

When used in the research setting, it is feasible that correct measurements could be used in conjunction with raw data during analysis to produce more accurate estimates. However, without in-depth knowledge of the algorithm, this could have unreliable results. To enable the accurate investigation of cardiac parameters in the early transitional period and improve technological development, manufacturers could integrate an option for post-hoc correction of data based on reliable anthropomorphic measurements.

5. Limitations

This study is an *in-silico* study and does not reflect the complexity and variability of delivery room situations or other real-life scenarios. However, this enables high comparability as the parameters obtained by EC always use the same data sets of electrical impedance changes and HR; therefore, only the pre-set parameters affected changes in SV values. As the simulation is based on adult data, the absolute values of CO should not be interpreted and only the changes incurred by the alteration of weight and length are meaningful. The algorithm itself, including the method of calibration is kept confidential by the manufacturer. Inclusion of the weight–length interaction term in the linear-regression modelling indicates a nonlinear relation between weight, length, and SV. Plots of raw data in Figure S1, however, do suggest that the dominant relation is linear. Therefore, this *in-silico* study provides information to users on the effect size and, by this, the relevance of accurate weight and length measurement for EC.

Supplementary Materials: The following are available online at https://www.mdpi.com/article/10.3390/children8100936/s1, Figure S1: 3D-Visualisation of raw data, Table S1: Relative stroke volume estimates for term infants, Table S2: Relative stroke volume estimates for preterm infants.

Author Contributions: D.B.H. participated in study design, simulations, data analysis, and participated in writing the initial manuscript. E.M.D. participated in study design and critically reviewed the analysis and the manuscript. J.M.O. participated in data processing, performed analysis, and critically reviewed the manuscript. C.E.S. participated in study design, simulations, data processing and analysis, and participated in writing the initial manuscript. All authors read and approved the final manuscript.

Funding: Supported by Deutsche Forschungsgemeinschaft (DFG, German Research Foundation) Project number 420536451.

Institutional Review Board Statement: Not applicable.

Informed Consent Statement: Not applicable.

Data Availability Statement: All relevant data generated or analyzed during this study are included in this article or its supplementary material. Further enquiries can be directed to the corresponding author.

Acknowledgments: Thanks to Osypka Medical for providing an ICON device and technical advice and by this, supporting this study. We want to acknowledge the supported by Deutsche Forschungsgemeinschaft (DFG German Research Foundation) Project number 420536451. JOT was supported by Science Foundation Ireland (15/SIRG/3580).

Conflicts of Interest: Osypka Medical provided an ICON device to perform this study as well as technical support. Beside this, the authors have no conflict of interest to declare.

References

1. O'Neill, R.; Dempsey, E.M.; Garvey, A.A.; Schwarz, C.E. Non-invasive Cardiac Output Monitoring in Neonates. *Front. Pediatr.* **2020**, *8*, 614585. [CrossRef] [PubMed]
2. Katheria, A.C.; Wozniak, M.; Harari, D.; Arnell, K.; Petruzzelli, D.; Finer, N.N. Measuring cardiac changes using electrical impedance during delayed cord clamping: A feasibility trial. *Matern. Health Neonatol. Perinatol.* **2015**, *1*, 15. [CrossRef] [PubMed]
3. Freidl, T.; Baik, N.; Pichler, G.; Schwaberger, B.; Zingerle, B.; Avian, A.; Urlesberger, B. Haemodynamic Transition after Birth: A New Tool for Non-Invasive Cardiac Output Monitoring. *Neonatology* **2017**, *111*, 55–60. [CrossRef] [PubMed]
4. Baik-Schneditz, N.; Schwaberger, B.; Mileder, L.; Holler, N.; Avian, A.; Koestenberger, M.; Urlesberger, B.; Martensen, J.; Pichler, G. Sex related difference in cardiac output during neonatal transition in term neonates. *Cardiovasc. Diagn. Ther.* **2021**, *11*, 342–347. [CrossRef] [PubMed]
5. Baik-Schneditz, N.; Schwaberger, B.; Mileder, L.; Holler, N.; Avian, A.; Urlesberger, B.; Pichler, G. Cardiac Output and Cerebral Oxygenation in Term Neonates during Neonatal Transition. *Children* **2021**, *8*, 439. [CrossRef] [PubMed]
6. Wood, A.J.; Raynes-Greenow, C.H.; Carberry, A.E.; Jeffery, H.E. Neonatal length inaccuracies in clinical practice and related percentile discrepancies detected by a simple length-board. *J. Paediatr. Child Health* **2013**, *49*, 199–203. [CrossRef]
7. Noori, S.; Drabu, B.; Soleymani, S.; Seri, I. Continuous non-invasive cardiac output measurements in the neonate by electrical velocimetry: A comparison with echocardiography. *Arch. Dis. Child. Fetal Neonatal Ed.* **2012**, *97*, F340–F343. [CrossRef] [PubMed]

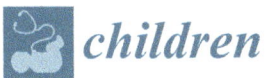

Article

Neonatal Multisystem Inflammatory Syndrome (MIS-N) Associated with Prenatal Maternal SARS-CoV-2: A Case Series

Ravindra Pawar [1,*], Vijay Gavade [2], Nivedita Patil [1], Vijay Mali [1,3], Amol Girwalkar [4,5], Vyankatesh Tarkasband [5], Sanjog Loya [2], Amit Chavan [2], Narendra Nanivadekar [6], Rahul Shinde [7], Uday Patil [2] and Satyan Lakshminrusimha [8]

1. Department of Pediatrics, Dr. D Y Patil Medical College Hospital and Research Institute, Kolhapur 416003, MH, India; patilnivedita8@gmail.com (N.P.); dr.vijaymali@gmail.com (V.M.)
2. Masai Children's Hospital, Kolhapur 416002, MH, India; vijaygavade@gmail.com (V.G.); sanjog877@gmail.com (S.L.); dramit.chavan15@gmail.com (A.C.); drudayspatil@gmail.com (U.P.)
3. NICE Advanced Neonatal Care Centre and Children's Clinic, Kolhapur 416008, MH, India
4. Ratna NICU, Kolhapur 416003, MH, India; amolgirwalkar@gmail.com
5. Department of Pediatrics, Apple Saraswati Multispeciality Hospital, Kolhapur 416003, MH, India; drt_vyankatesh@yahoo.co.in
6. Niramay Pediatric Nursing Home and Eye Care Centre, Kolhapur 416001, MH, India; narendrananivadekar@gmail.com
7. Samarth Nursing Home, Kolhapur 416002, MH, India; drrahulshinde@gmail.com
8. UC Davis Children's Hospital, Sacramento, CA 95817, USA; slakshmi@ucdavis.edu
* Correspondence: drravipawar@gmail.com

Citation: Pawar, R.; Gavade, V.; Patil, N.; Mali, V.; Girwalkar, A.; Tarkasband, V.; Loya, S.; Chavan, A.; Nanivadekar, N.; Shinde, R.; et al. Neonatal Multisystem Inflammatory Syndrome (MIS-N) Associated with Prenatal Maternal SARS-CoV-2: A Case Series. *Children* **2021**, *8*, 572. https://doi.org/10.3390/children8070572

Academic Editor: Bernhard Schwaberger

Received: 4 June 2021
Accepted: 30 June 2021
Published: 2 July 2021

Publisher's Note: MDPI stays neutral with regard to jurisdictional claims in published maps and institutional affiliations.

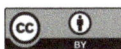

Copyright: © 2021 by the authors. Licensee MDPI, Basel, Switzerland. This article is an open access article distributed under the terms and conditions of the Creative Commons Attribution (CC BY) license (https://creativecommons.org/licenses/by/4.0/).

Abstract: Multisystem inflammatory syndrome in children (MIS-C) is a post-infectious immune-mediated condition, seen 3–5 weeks after COVID-19. Maternal SARS-CoV-2 may potentially cause a similar hyperinflammatory syndrome in neonates due to transplacental transfer of antibodies. We reviewed the perinatal history, clinical features, and outcomes of 20 neonates with features consistent with MIS-C related to maternal SARS-CoV-2 in Kolhapur, India, from 1 September 2020 to 30 April 2021. Anti-SARS-CoV-2 IgG and IgM antibodies were tested in all neonates. Fifteen singletons and five twins born to eighteen mothers with a history of COVID-19 disease or exposure during pregnancy presented with features consistent with MIS-C during the first 5 days after birth. Nineteen were positive for anti-SARS-CoV-2 IgG and all were negative for IgM antibodies. All mothers were asymptomatic and therefore not tested by RTPCR-SARS-CoV-2 at delivery. Eighteen neonates (90%) had cardiac involvement with prolonged QTc, 2:1 AV block, cardiogenic shock, or coronary dilatation. Other findings included respiratory failure (40%), fever (10%), feeding intolerance (30%), melena (10%), and renal failure (5%). All infants had elevated inflammatory biomarkers and received steroids and IVIG. Two infants died. We speculate that maternal SARS-CoV-2 and transplacental antibodies cause multisystem inflammatory syndrome in neonates (MIS-N). Immunomodulation may be beneficial in some cases, but further studies are needed.

Keywords: neonate; multisystem inflammatory syndrome in children (MIS-C); anti SARS-CoV-2 antibodies; COVID-19

1. Introduction

COVID-19, caused by SARS-CoV-2, is a global public health crisis with a large recent surge in India. As of 24 June 2021, 179 million individuals were infected worldwide, with India contributing to half of all new daily cases in April–May 2021 [1]. Initial studies showed that children were spared of severe COVID-19 [2–4]. However, recently case reports of children experiencing a potentially life threatening pediatric inflammatory multisystem syndrome (PIMS)—also called multisystem inflammatory syndrome in children (MIS-C)—have been described [5–7].

MIS-C is a new disease in children, the exact mechanism of which is still unclear. It is thought to be due to immune dysregulation following exposure to SARS CoV-2 [8]. It usually presents as fever and multiorgan involvement, with blood investigations showing increased inflammatory markers weeks after exposure to SARS-CoV-2 [5,6,8]. MIS-C has clinical and serological similarities with Kawasaki disease and the severe COVID-19 cytokine storm seen in adults [9]. However, its pathophysiology and immunological response is different, and may be mediated by autoantibodies [10]. More than 80% of children with MIS-C have specific IgM and IgG antibodies against SARS-CoV-2, but only about one-third are positive for SARS-CoV-2 by RTPCR [5,11,12].

Unlike MIS-C, where SARS-CoV-2 infection and multisystem inflammation occur in the same subject, a few case reports suggest neonatal multisystem inflammation [13] occurs secondary to maternal SARS-CoV-2 infection [14–17]. A few weeks after the first wave of COVID-19 in Kolhapur, India, we found an increase in the number of neonates with structurally normal hearts who presented with conduction abnormalities and were born to mothers with a past history of COVID-19. Specifically, these neonates presented with prolonged QTc with 2:1 Atrioventricular (AV) block or thrombosis similar to older children with MIS-C within the first week after birth [18]. We present a case series of 20 neonates with multisystem involvement, hyperinflammatory syndrome and positive anti SARS-CoV-2 IgG antibodies, temporally related to maternal antenatal SARs-CoV-2 exposure. To our knowledge, this is the largest series of MIS-C presenting in the early neonatal period.

2. Materials and Methods

Access to chart reviews and publication was approved by the Institutional Ethics Committee (IEC) of the Dr D Y Patil Medical College Hospital and Research Institute, at Dr D Y Patil University, Kolhapur, India. Informed consent was obtained from parents/guardians for using clinical data and photographs. Neonates who met the criteria in Table 1 (with four exceptions, as explained below) and that were admitted to seven NICUs in Kolhapur between 1 September 2020 and 30 April 2021 were included. These criteria were modified from CDC criteria for MIS-C and interim guidance from AAP to accommodate lack of fever in neonates and source of primary infection (mother, instead of the child) [19,20]. Neonates with signs consistent with MIS-C, maternal history of COVID-19, and positive for anti-SARS CoV-2 antibodies were included. However, infants with these symptoms and culture positive sepsis, or proven infective pathology in other organ systems (e.g., meningitis, urinary tract infection, etc.) were excluded. Infants with low Apgar scores (≤ 3 at 5 min) and evidence of birth asphyxia were excluded. Preterm infants with findings attributable to early gestation (such as respiratory distress presenting immediately after birth and transient hypotension) were excluded. IgG and IgM against SARS CoV-2 were detected using VIDAS® SARS-COV-2 kits (BioMerieux SA, Marcy-I'Etiole, France), with MINIVIDAS using ELFA: enzyme linked fluorescent assay. Data are presented as median (range) or number (%).

We differentiated neonates presenting with multisystem inflammatory syndrome in the first week after birth secondary to possible maternal COVID-19 infection (labeled in this article as MIS-N), from neonates who had early onset neonatal COVID-19 or late-onset neonatal COVID-19 and subsequently present with multisystem inflammation during 2–4 weeks after birth (labeled in this article as MIS-C) (Figure 1). In patients with MIS-C, multisystem inflammation was secondary to prior COVID-19 in the same subject. However, in MIS-N, multisystem inflammation in the neonate was secondary to COVID-19 in the mother with passive transmission of antibodies.

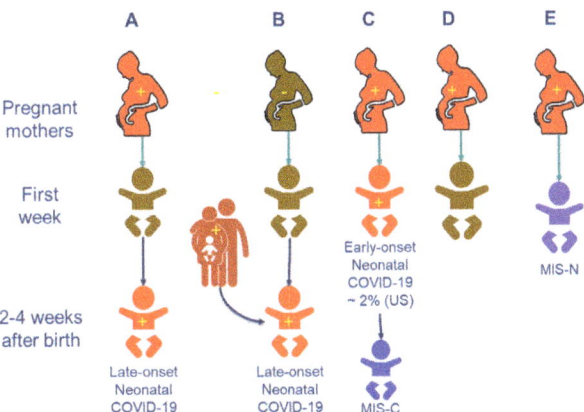

Figure 1. Various presentations of SARS-CoV-2 infection and its sequences in the neonatal period. Red colored subjects with a '+' sign indicate COVID-19 positive patients. Pregnant mother A has COVID-19 and her baby is negative at birth but contracts late-onset COVID-19 due to transmission from the mother. Pregnant mother B has no COVID-19 but her neonate develops late-onset neonatal infection due to exposure to a family member 2–4 weeks after birth. Pregnant mother C is COVID-19 positive during the perinatal period and transmits the virus to her offspring during birth leading to early-onset infection in the neonate. This baby can potentially develop MIS-C 2–4 weeks later (a rare occurrence) [16]. Pregnant mother D has COVID-19 during pregnancy but the neonate remains healthy. Pregnant mother E has COVID-19 disease or exposure to SARS-COV-2 during pregnancy and the baby develops multisystem inflammation secondary to passive transfer of antibodies leading to MIS-N (multisystem inflammatory syndrome in neonates) [14].

Table 1. Proposed inclusion criteria for neonatal multisystem inflammatory syndrome (MIS-N) secondary to maternal SARS CoV-2 exposure or infection.

(1) A neonate aged <28 days at the time of presentation
(2) Laboratory or epidemiologic evidence of SARS-CoV-2 infection in the mother
- Positive SARS-CoV-2 testing by RT-PCR, serology (IgG or IgM), or antigen during pregnancy
- Symptoms consistent with SARS CoV-2 infection during pregnancy
- COVID-19 exposure with confirmed SARS CoV-2 infection during pregnancy
- Serological evidence (positive IgG specific to SARS CoV-2 but not IgM) in the neonate

(3) Clinical criteria:
- Severe illness necessitating hospitalization AND
- Two or more organ systems affected [i.e., cardiac, renal, respiratory, hematologic, gastrointestinal, dermatologic, neurological, temperature instability (fever or hypothermia)] OR
- Cardiac AV conduction abnormalities OR coronary dilation or aneurysms (without involvement of a second organ system)

(4) Laboratory evidence of inflammation
- One or more of the following: an elevated CRP, ESR, fibrinogen, procalcitonin, D-dimer, ferritin, LDH, or IL-6; elevated neutrophils or reduced lymphocytes; low albumin

(5) No alternative diagnosis (such as birth asphyxia–cord pH $\leq$ 7.0 and Apgar score $\leq$ 3 at 5 min; viral or bacterial sepsis–confirmed blood culture; maternal lupus resulting in neonatal AV conduction abnormalities; presence of these findings indicating an alternate diagnosis excludes MIS-N).

3. Results

Clinical characteristics of 20 neonates are shown in Table 2. Individual patient characteristics are shown in Table 3. Three infants (# 17, 18 and 19 in Table 3) had IgG anti SARS-CoV-2 levels below the cut-off but were included because of maternal history and typical presentation (AV block or dilated coronaries). Case # 20 only had a cardiac thrombus without other organ involvement but was included due to maternal history, high IgG levels, elevated inflammatory markers, and lack of other explanation for the thrombus.

Table 2. Characteristics of patients with suspected MIS-N.

Characteristic	Median (Range) or Number (%)	Comments
Maternal age	26.5 years (20–34 years)	
Maternal symptoms (n = 18):		
Asymptomatic	11 (61.2%)	
Symptomatic	7 (38.8)	
Trimester when positive or had exposure	First–1 (5.5%), Second–2 (11.1%), Third–15 (83.3%)	
Mode of delivery–Cesarean	7 (38.8%)	
Gestational age at birth (n = 20)	34 weeks (27–38 weeks)	Term ($\geq$37 weeks)–3 (15%) Late preterm (34–36 weeks)–13 (65%) <33 weeks–4 (20%)
Birth weight (kg)	2.15 (1–4)	
Sex	Male (10), Female (10)	
Multiplicity	Singleton–15 Twins–5	
Neonate–age at presentation	Day 2 (day 1 to day 5)	Day 1 (<24 h of birth)–7 (35%)
Organ system involvement		
• Cardiac	18 (90%)	
• Hematologic/thrombosis	2 (10%)-thrombosis; 2 (10%)-GI bleed	
• Respiratory	11 (55%)-requiring ventilator/CPAP	
• Gastrointestinal	6 (30%)	
• Neurological	2 (10%)	
• Cutaneous	1 (5%)	
• Renal	1 (5%)	
• Fever/temperature instability	2 (10%)	
Investigations:		Normal values
• CRP	24 (9–62)	0-6 mg/L
• Procalcitonin	2.05 (1.3–51)	<0.5 ng/mL
• D-dimer	5932 (2820–12,000)	<2700 ng/mL
• LDH	1315 (793–6424)	290-775 U/L
• NT-Pro BNP	24,300 (7361–>30,000)	<11,987 pg/mL for 0-2 days, <5918 pg/mL for 3-11 days
• Blood culture	No growth in all infants	No growth
Cardiac findings		
• Arrhythmia	11 (44%)	
• Dilated coronaries	2 (12%)	
• Intracardiac thrombus	2 (8%)	One thrombus in LPA, one in RA
• Shock/ cardiac dysfunction	5 (20%)	
Infant's serology		
• IgM SARS CoV-2	0.0 (0–0) COI	Cut-off-Index (COI) $\geq$ 1 is positive, for both IgG and IgM
• IgG SARS CoV-2	3.49 (0.07–74.39) COI	
Therapy		
• Steroids	20 (100%)	IV Methylprednisolone 2 mg/kg/day
• IVIG	20 (100%)	1–2 g/kg
• LMWH	14 (70%)	1.5 mg/kg/dose, twice a day
• Inotropes	12 (60%)	IV Milrinone, Adrenaline, Dobutamine, Dopamine
Outcome		
• Mortality	2 (10%)	One due to necrotizing enterocolitis One due to Multiorgan dysfunction

3.1. Maternal Features

Of the 18 mothers (three with twin pregnancy), seven (38.8%) were symptomatic for COVID-19 during pregnancy, three (16.6%) were asymptomatic but RT-PCR positive for COVID-19, and eleven (61.1%) were asymptomatic but had history of close contact with COVID-19 cases (usually a confirmed case in the family). Fifteen mothers (83.3%) were symptomatic or had contact during the last trimester of pregnancy, (five (27.7%) within the last 4 weeks before delivery), two (11.1%) during second trimester and one (5.5%) in the first trimester of pregnancy. None of them had symptomatic COVID-19 or febrile illness during admission for delivery, and none were tested for COVID -19 RT-PCR during the admission for delivery. Five mothers (27.7%) had an antenatal ultrasound scan showing fetoplacental compromise (reduced flow in uterine artery or umbilical artery and/or diastolic notch, diastolic flow reversal, fetal ascites, pericardial and pleural effusion). Mothers whose infants presented with cardiac conduction abnormalities were tested for lupus antibodies and were negative.

3.2. Resuscitation at Birth and Post-Resuscitation Period

Two neonates did not cry immediately after birth and two had significant respiratory distress in the delivery room. These four (20%) neonates required positive pressure ventilation (PPV) and subsequently required conventional mechanical ventilation on the day of birth. Sixteen (80%) neonates did not require any PPV in the delivery room. However, three of these infants required respiratory support (invasive mechanical ventilation or CPAP) on the day of birth in the NICU.

3.3. Clinical Presentation

The most common presentation involved the cardiovascular system (Table 3). Eleven had rhythm disorders, of which nine presented with prolonged QTc interval with 2:1 AV block (Figure 2A,D,G,J,M). With immunomodulatory therapy with methylprednisolone and intravenous immunoglobulin (IVIG), 2:1 AV block disappeared first (Figure 2B,E,H,K,N), followed by normalization of QTc (C, F, I, L, O), in all of the nine neonates. One neonate had an episode of supraventricular tachycardia (SVT), requiring a short course of beta blockers, and one infant had bradycardia with tall, peaked T waves and broad QRS due to hyperkalemia secondary to acute renal failure. Shock with or without cardiac dysfunction on echocardiography was seen in five neonates. Two neonates had significant coronary dilatation on day one of life (Figure 3A–C). One neonate had a thrombus almost completely occluding the left pulmonary artery (LPA) (Figure 3D), requiring systemic thrombolysis with Alteplase (t-PA, 3 doses), and low molecular weight heparin (LMWH) for six weeks. One neonate had an intracardiac thrombus at the inferior vena cava–right atrial junction (Figure 3E), which partly resolved at discharge, after LMWH therapy.

Eleven neonates required either mechanical ventilation (n = 8) or CPAP (n = 3), for respiratory distress syndrome associated with prematurity, shock, or respiratory depression. Two neonates presented with fever on day one of life. Two neonates did not cry immediately after birth but had Apgar scores >3 by 5 min of age. One infant presented with convulsions on day 4 and was admitted on day 6 with multiorgan failure leading to death.

Feeding intolerance and gastric aspirates were seen in 6 neonates, of which two had brownish gastric aspirates. Two had lower gastrointestinal bleeding, of which one had tarry stools (melena) (Figure 3I) and one had blood in stools on day 8 of life (with a normal coagulation profile).

Anti-SARS-CoV-2 IgM antibodies were negative in all the neonates, and IgG antibodies (cut-off-index (COI) ≥1 considered reactive) were positive (COI value > 1) in 17 (85%) neonates. Two (10%) had levels below positive cut-off, and one (5%) had no detectable levels. RTPCR for SARS-CoV-2 was not done in any of the neonates as the Indian Academy of Pediatrics Guidelines recommend this test after birth if mothers are symptomatic, or tested positive within 14 days before birth, or if there is history of contact with COVID-19 positive persons in the postnatal period. [21]

Table 3. Clinical features, treatments, and outcomes of suspected patients with Neonatal Inflammatory Multisystem Syndrome (MIS-C) associated with SARS-CoV-2 infection.

Subject Number	Age at Presentation/ Sex/Weight/Gestation	Maternal COVID-19 Status	Neonatal Serology (All Were IgM-ve)	Lab Studies (Values)	Clinical Features	Treatment	Outcome
1 *	Day 1/F 4 kg 38 weeks	asymptomatic, RTPCR +ve 3 weeks before delivery	IgG +ve on day 1	Elevated CRP (14), PCT (1.3), Ferritin (1500), D Dimer (5088).	Fever on day 1, hypotension; echo-LV dysfunction	Inotropes Steroids IVIG	Discharged on day 13
2 *	Day 1/M 2.02 kg 35 weeks	asymptomatic, COVID-19 contact 8 weeks before delivery,	IgG +ve on day 2	Elevated CRP (9), D-Dimer (5100), Ferritin (393), LDH (1183), NT Pro BNP (>30,000)	Antenatal scan showing fetoplacental compromise; shock on day 1, Echo—mild LV dysfunction and bilateral pleural effusions	LMWH Steroids IVIG	Discharged on day 14
3 *	Day 4/F 2 kg 33 weeks	asymptomatic COVID-19 contact 6 weeks before delivery, IgG +ve	IgG +ve on day 6	Elevated CRP (10), d-dimer (3020), Ferritin (407)	RDS, severe bradycardia with prolonged QTc and 2:1 AVB from day 4 of life (Figure 2A,B)	Surfactant MV, Steroids IVIG	Sinus rhythm at discharge on day 16 (Figure 2C)
4 *	Day 1/M 2 kg 36 weeks	asymptomatic COVID-19 contact 6 weeks before delivery,	IgG +ve on day 1	Elevated CRP (12), D Dimer (6848), NT Pro BNP (>25,000), LDH (1158)	Antenatal scan showing dilated RA/RV, pericardial and pleural effusions and ascites; Respiratory distress, PPV at birth, shock; echo–dilated hypertrophied RV with dysfunction, moderate TR, large thrombus at LPA origin on day 3 (Figure 3D,E)	LMWH, Alteplase, Inotropes, MV, IVIG, Steroids	Discharged on day 19; LMWH and Aspirin x 6 weeks, complete resolution of thrombus at 8 weeks echo
5 *	Day 3/M 3.5 kg 38 weeks	Febrile illness at 7 months of gestation	IgG +ve on day 5	Elevated CRP (60.2), PCT (2.1), D Dimer (6483), Ferritin (878), LDH (793), leucocytosis (18,600).	Grunting, tachypnea, and lethargy, feeding intolerance, intermittent bradycardia, hypotension	Inotropes, MV, Steroids, IVIG	Discharged on day 13
6 *	Day 2/M 2.3 kg 34 weeks	Febrile illness 2 weeks before delivery	IgG +ve on day 12	Elevated CRP (24), d dimer (4200), thrombocytopenia (39 × 10^9/L)	feeding intolerance, decreased activity from day 2, brown gastric aspirates on day 4, treated like NEC, bleeding continued with rash, pedal edema, oral and skin lesions, skin peeling (Figure 3G,H)	CPAP, Inotropes, LMWH, Steroids, IVIG	Discharged on day 38

Table 3. Cont.

Subject Number	Age at Presentation/ Sex/Weight/Gestation	Maternal COVID-19 Status	Neonatal Serology (All Were IgM-ve)	Lab Studies (Values)	Clinical Features	Treatment	Outcome
7 *	Day 3/F 1.4 kg 34 weeks	Asymptomatic RTPCR +ve, 5th month of gestation	IgG +ve on day 5	Elevated CRP (50), D Dimer (5100), normal coagulation profile	Antenatal scan showing fetoplacental compromise; LBW. Brownish gastric aspirates from day 3, frank malena (Figure 3I) from day 6, episodes of SVT from day 8; Echo- bilateral pleural and pericardial effusion.	Beta- blockers, Steroids, IVIG	Discharged on day 20
8 * 2nd of twins †	Day 2/M 1.9 kg 32 weeks	Asymptomatic RTPCR positive at 3rd month of gestation	IgG +ve on day 1	Elevated CRP (43), IL-6 (116), D Dimer (6600)	distress at birth, bradycardia with prolonged QTc and 2:1 AVB on day 2 of life	MV and CPAP, inotropes, Steroids, IVIG	Sinus rhythm at discharge on day 23
9 * Twin 1	Day2/F 1.9 kg 33 weeks	Asymptomatic COVID-19 contact 8 weeks before delivery	IgG +ve on day 4	Elevated CRP (35), D Dimer (10,000)	Antenatal scan showing fetoplacental compromise, bradycardia with prolonged QTc and 2:1 AVB from day 2	IVIG, Steroids, LMWH,	Sinus rhythm at discharge on day 18
10 * Twin 2	Day 2/M 1.6 kg 33 weeks	Asymptomatic COVID-19 contact 8 weeks before delivery	IgG +ve on day 5	Elevated D Dimer (10,000), LDH (977)	Antenatal scan showing feto-maternal compromise, feeding intolerance, bradycardia with prolonged QTc and 2:1 AVB from day 2,	IVIG, steroids, LMWH	Sinus rhythm at discharge on day 18
11 * Twin 1	Day 4/F 2.05kg 34 weeks	Febrile illness 3 weeks before delivery–IgG level below cutoff	IgG +ve on day 4	Elevated PCT (1.8), D Dimer (4840), NT Pro BNP (> 25,000)	bradycardia with prolonged QTc and 2:1 AVB on day 4 (Figure 2D,E)	IVIG, steroids, LMWH, inotropes, CPAP	Sinus rhythm at discharge on day 11 (Figure 2F)
12 * Twin 2	Day 4/M 2.1 kg 34 weeks	Febrile illness 3 weeks before delivery–IgG level below cutoff	IgG +ve on day 4	Elevated PCT (1.4), D Dimer (5932)	bradycardia with prolonged QTc and 2:1 AVB on day 4 (Figure 2G,H)	IVIG, steroids, LMWH, inotropes, CPAP	Sinus rhythm at discharge on day 11 (Figure 2I)

Table 3. Cont.

Subject Number	Age at Presentation/ Sex/Weight/Gestation	Maternal COVID-19 Status	Neonatal Serology (All Were IgM-ve)	Lab Studies (Values)	Clinical Features	Treatment	Outcome
13 *	Day 3/F 1 kg 27 weeks	Asymptomatic COVID-19 contact 8 weeks before delivery	IgG +ve on day	Elevated PCT (51), D Dimer (10,000), LDH (6424), NT Pro BNP (25,000)	Extreme PT, Extreme LBW, bradycardia with prolonged QTc and 2:1 AVB with 2:1 AV block on day 4 (Figure 2J,K); sinus rhythm on day 7 (Figure 2L)	IVIG, Steroids, LMWH, MV	day 9 abdominal distension, NEC → death on day 11
14 *	Day 2/M 2.4 kg 36 weeks	Asymptomatic COVID-19 contact 10 weeks before delivery, IgG +ve	IgG +ve on day 6	Elevated CRP (11), D Dimer (4700), LDH (2143)	not accepting feeds on day2, Cardiomegaly on X-ray chest, cardiogenic shock on day 5, echo (Figure 3A)-dilated coronaries # (LMCA Z score = + 4.2, RCA Z score = +4.9) severe TR, mild MR, ASD, PDA, Severe PAH,	IVIG, steroids, LMWH, Inotropes, PPV, Aspirin	Discharged on day 14; Coronaries normalized at discharge, Tab Aspirin x 6 weeks
15 *	Day 4/M 2 kg 36 weeks	Asymptomatic COVID-19 contact 4 weeks before delivery	IgG +ve on day 6	Elevated CRP (18), BUN (99.2), serum Creatinine (1.9), NT Pro BNP (14,500), Potassium (6.9 mEq/L)	Admitted on day 6, Seizures, shock, bradycardia, acute renal failure, hyperkalemia, Echo-small ASD, dilated all four chambers, mild LV dysfunction	IVIG, Steroids, MV, Inotropes, Peritoneal dialysis,	Death on day 8-Multi-organ dysfunction
16 *	Day 1/F 2 kg 36 weeks	Asymptomatic COVID-19 contact 4 weeks before delivery, IgG +ve	IgG +ve on day 1	Elevated CRP (62), PCT (2.4), D Dimer (9734), NT Pro BNP (7361).	Fever on day 1, feeding intolerance, vomiting, tachypnea, desaturation on day 2	IVIG, Steroids	Discharged on day 10
17	Day 2/F 1.5 kg 32 weeks	Asymptomatic COVID-19 contact 10 weeks before delivery	IgG -ve	Elevated CRP (18), D Dimer (12,000)	RDS, bradycardia with prolonged QTc and 2:1 AVB on day 3	IVIG, steroids, inotropes, CPAP	Sinus rhythm at discharge on day 13
18	Day 2/F 1.5 kg 32 weeks	Febrile illness 8 weeks before delivery	IgG below cut-off level	Elevated CRP (25), D Dimer (10,000), NT Pro BNP (23,700)	bradycardia with prolonged QTc and 2:1 AVB on day 2 (Figure 2M,N)	IVIG, steroids	Sinus rhythm at discharge on day 14 (Figure 2O)

Table 3. Cont.

Subject Number	Age at Presentation/ Sex/Weight/Gestation	Maternal COVID-19 Status	Neonatal Serology (All Were IgM-ve)	Lab Studies (Values)	Clinical Features	Treatment	Outcome
19	Day 1/M 1.9 kg 34 weeks	Febrile illness 6 weeks before delivery; IgG below cutoff levels, IgM -ve	IgG below cutoff levels	Elevated D Dimer (2820), LDH (2661), NT Pro BNP (>25,000), thrombocytopenia (93 × 10^9/L)	Antenatal scan showing pleural, pericardial effusions, and ascites; not cried after birth; LBW, pitting edema over chest wall, hepatomegaly, tachypnea, crepitations; Echo (Figure 3C)—dilated coronaries # , (LMCA Z score = +2.7, LAD Z score = +2.7, RCA Z score = +2), large PDA, mild TR and MR, normal function (on inotropes), bilateral moderate pleural effusion;	IVIG, Steroids, LMWH, Inotropes, Lasix, MV, Aspirin	Discharged on day 15; Coronaries normal, Aspirin x 6 weeks.
20	Day 1/ F 2.7 kg 38 weeks	Febrile illness 6 weeks before delivery. IgG +ve	IgG +ve on day 2	Elevated CRP (53), D Dimer (3942), LDH (804), NT Pro BNP (17,018)	Not cried after birth, mottling and poor peripheral pulsations, hypotension; Echo (Figure 2F)-day 4-intracardiac thrombus in RA, normal LV function	PPV, surfactant, Inotropes, IVIG, Steroids, LMWH, MV	Discharged on day 24; LMWH x 6 weeks, thrombus decreased in size at 4 weeks echo

Normal ranges and units for lab values: CRP 0-6 mg/L; D-Dimer < 2740 ng/mL; NT Pro-BNP < 11,987 pg/mL for 0-2 days, <5918 pg/mL for 3–11 days; procalcitonin <0.5 ng/mL; LDH 290-775 U/L (for 0-4 days of life); IL-6 < 7 pg/mL; Ferritin = 25-200 ng/mL; BUN 2-19 mg/dL; serum creatinine 0.3-1 mg/dL; patients with (*) met the inclusion criteria mentioned in Table 1. Patients 17-19 did not have a positive IgG SARS CoV-2 level above the laboratory cut-off–however, patients had EKG consistent with AV block; patient 20 had delayed cry and might have had perinatal depression but had Apgar scores > 3 by 5 min but an unexplained intracardiac thrombus in the right atrium. † Twin A was positive for IgG SARS CoV-2 but other clinical features were consistent with prematurity. # Z scores for coronary diameter were calculated based on Kobayashi et al. [22]. Abbreviations: -ve = negative; +ve = positive; M = male, F = female; ASD = atrial septal defect; AVB = atrioventricular block; BUN = blood urea nitrogen; CKMB = creatinine kinase myocardial band; CNS = central nervous system; COVID-19 = corona virus disease 2019; CPAP = continuous positive airway pressure; CRP = C-reactive protein; IgG = immunoglobulin G, IgM = immunoglobulin M, IL-6 = interleukin-6; IVIG = intravenous immunoglobulin; LAD = left anterior descending coronary artery; LBW = low birth weight, LDH = lactate dehydrogenase; LMCA = left main coronary artery; LMWH = low molecular weight heparin; LPA = left pulmonary artery; LV = left ventricle; MR = mitral regurgitation; MV = mechanical ventilation; NEC = necrotizing enterocolitis; NT Pro BNP = N-terminal pro-B-type natriuretic peptide; PAH = p ulmonary artery hypertension; PCT = procalcitonin; PDA = patent ductus arteriosus; PPHN = persistent pulmonary hypertension of the newborn; PPV = positive pressure ventilation; PT = preterm; QTc = corrected QT interval; RA and RV = right atrium and ventricle; RCA = right coronary artery; RT-PCR = reverse transcription-polymerase chain reaction; SVT = supraventricular tachycardia; TR = tricuspid regurgitation.

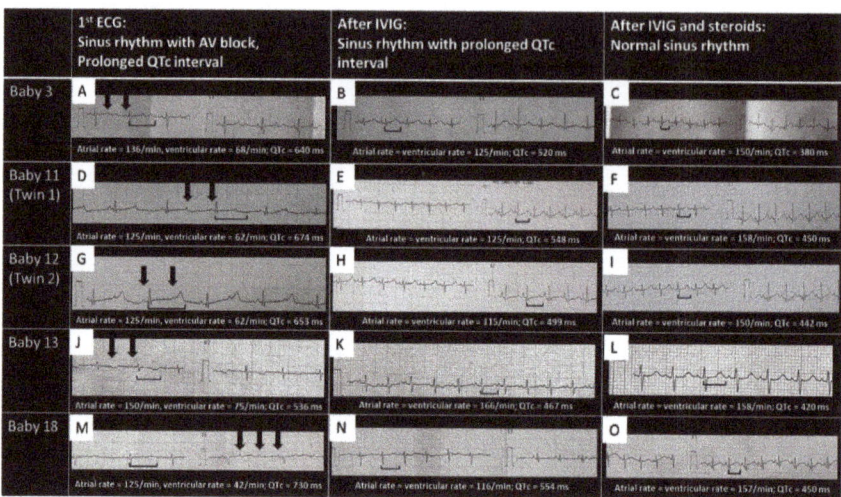

Figure 2. Representative EKGs of neonates presenting with bradycardia. Baby number sequence is the same as in Table 3. The first column showing EKGs at presentation (**A,D,G,J,M**), with sinus rhythm, prolonged QT interval and atrio-ventricular block. Middle column showing sinus rhythm and prolonged QT interval (**B,E,H,K,N**). The last column showing sinus rhythm with normal QT interval (**C,F,I,L,O**). Black arrows = atrial beats; horizontal square bracket = QT interval; QTc = corrected QT interval; ms = milliseconds. QTc values in the figure are derived by the formula QTc = QT/$\sqrt{RR}$.

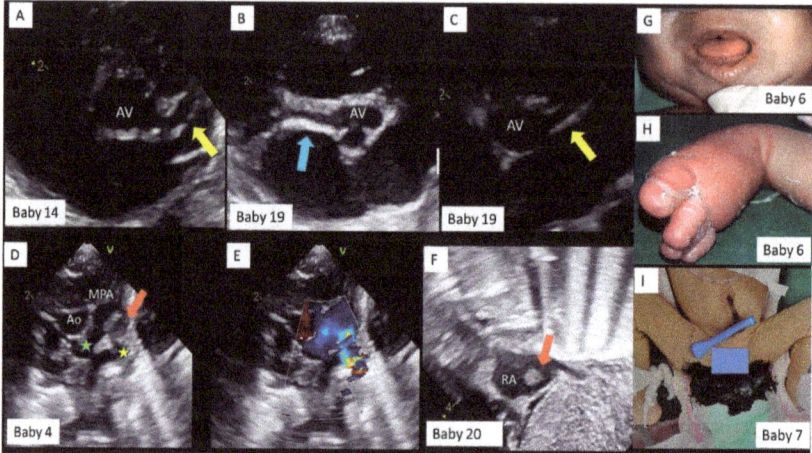

Figure 3. Echocardiography and clinical findings in neonates with MIS-C. Baby number sequence is the same as in Table 3. Transthoracic echocardiography, parasternal short axis view in Baby #14 (**A**) and Baby #19 (**B,C**). The left main and left anterior descending coronary artery (yellow arrow) and the right coronary artery (blue arrow) are significantly dilated. AV = aortic valve. Transthoracic echocardiography and color doppler, parasternal short axis view in Baby #4 (**D**), showing aorta (Ao) and main pulmonary artery (MPA) bifurcation, with a large thrombus (red arrow) obstructing the left pulmonary artery (yellow star) origin and causing flow turbulence on color doppler (**E**), but normal flows across right pulmonary artery (green star). Transthoracic echocardiography subcostal bi-caval view in Baby #20 (**F**), showing a thrombus (red arrow) in right atrium (RA). Baby #6, showing oral and muco-cutaneous lesions (**G**) and, pedal edema and skin peeling (**H**) and Baby #7 with black, tarry stools (melena, **I**).

To summarize, we present a case series of 20 neonates born to mothers with a history of SARS-CoV-2 infection or exposure to COVID-19 patients. The majority of infants were late preterm, with equal sex distribution and presented with cardiac (90%), respiratory (55%) or gastrointestinal (30%) signs with elevated inflammatory markers and positive IgG SARS-CoV-2 titers. These infants were managed with supportive therapy, methylprednisolone, IVIG and was associated with a 10% mortality. Our protocol for diagnosis and management of MIS-N is shown in Table 4.

Table 4. Protocol for laboratory investigations and management of MIS-N.

Laboratory investigations need to be titrated based on clinical presentation. [9]
1. Initial laboratory evaluation (suspected cases without cardiac involvement)
    a. Complete Blood Count (CBC) with differential
    b. Inflammatory markers: ESR, CRP, Procalcitonin
    c. Urinalysis
    d. Blood culture
    e. Imaging as clinically indicated (respiratory or gastrointestinal signs):
        i. Chest X-ray
        ii. Abdominal X-ray or ultrasound if concerning physical findings.
2. If initial labs concerning for MIS-C, or cases with cardiac involvement without alternate explanation (ESR > = 40 mm or CRP > =5mg/dL in addition to 1 of the following: lymphopenia with absolute lymphocyte count <1000/mm^3, platelets <150,000/mm^3, albumin < = 3g/dL, hyponatremia Na < 135 mEq/L), consider the following evaluation:
    a. Cardiac markers: troponin T/I and BNP or NT-Pro-BNP
    b. Twelve-lead electrocardiogram (EKG)
    c. Other markers of inflammation: ferritin, LDH, IL-6
    d. Coagulation panel: PT, PTT, D-dimer, fibrinogen
    e. Mother and baby's Serology for SARS-CoV-2
    f. Mother and baby's SARS-CoV-2 PCR from nasopharyngeal swab
    g. Echocardiogram (transthoracic)–may be done in the presence of hypotension/shock or suspicion for cardiac dysfunction; this may aid in the diagnosis of coronary aneurysms

Management of neonates with MIS-N is predominantly supportive.
1. Respiratory support to optimize gas exchange and maintain oxygen saturations in the 90–97% range and $PaCO_2$ in the 40–50 mmHg will minimize pulmonary vasoconstriction and reduce the risk of PPHN.
2. Fluid resuscitation along with the use of inotropes and vasopressors is often needed to optimize perfusion.
3. Empiric antibiotics as per discretion of the provider may be considered pending blood culture results.

Specific therapy for MIS-C includes the use of anticoagulants, steroids, IVIG and anti-inflammatory agents. As shown in the case reports in Tables 2 and 3, neonates have received treatment with immunomodulatory therapies (IVIG, methylprednisolone, anti-platelet agents (aspirin), and anticoagulants (unfractionated heparin or low molecular weight heparin). Further studies are required to evaluate the benefits and risks of these therapies in MIS-C in neonates. Pending further studies, we recommend the following approach to MIS-C in neonates.
1. Infants with moderate to severe MIS-N may benefit from systemic glucocorticoid therapy. Methylprednisolone or prednisolone are commonly used.
2. Intravenous immunoglobulin (IVIG) is indicated in severe MIS-N requiring ICU care with cardiovascular involvement plus at least 1 other system involvement (cardiovascular involvement defined by: shock, left ventricular dysfunction, coronary artery abnormality, severe conduction abnormality, significant troponin elevation, new valvular regurgitation). Presence of coronary or peripheral aneurysms is also an indication for IVIG. Infants who meet criteria for Kawasaki disease should also receive IVIG. [23] Caution should be exercised during IVIG among neonates due to the potential risk of necrotizing enterocolitis. [24]
3. Anticoagulants: Children with MIS-N can present with vasculitis and thrombosis. [25] The incidence of thrombosis is higher in MIS-C in older children than infants and young children. [25] While low-dose aspirin, unfractionated heparin or enoxaparin are recommended in children with MIS-C, its routine use is not recommended in neonates, especially preterm infants at risk for intraventricular hemorrhage (IVH). In term infants at risk of thrombosis, and those with central lines, low-dose aspirin should be considered. Critically ill infants, admitted to the ICU with MIS-N with signs of thrombosis may benefit from prophylactic enoxaparin or unfractionated heparin. Close monitoring of PT, PTT, fibrinogen and D-dimer is necessary during anticoagulation.
4. Tocilizumab (an anti-IL-6 receptor antibody) has been used in children with MIS-C. There is no experience with the use of this therapy in neonates.

Note: During the neonatal period, MIS-N is relatively rare. More common causes for cardiac dysfunction and elevated Troponin or BNP such as perinatal asphyxia should be considered. The use of glucocorticoids and IVIG should be limited to indications outlined above.

Abbreviations are same as in Table 3.

4. Discussion

We present a case series of neonates born to mothers with a history of SARS-CoV-2 infection or exposure to a COVID-19 patient during pregnancy and presenting with features that cannot be explained by other causes. Whether these findings are unrelated to maternal COVID-19 or due to an inflammatory process induced by the transplacental passage of antibodies directed against autoantigens is not clear. However, the unusually high frequency of findings such as atrioventricular conduction abnormalities, resembling cardiac findings in older children with MIS-C [18], and response to immunomodulatory therapy with intravenous immunoglobulin (IVIG) and steroids suggests that "multisystem inflammatory syndrome in the neonate (MIS-N)" deserves further study [26]. We present this case series to increase awareness of this possibility amongst all care providers, especially obstetricians, pediatricians, pediatric cardiologists, and neonatologists.

We speculate that maternal infection with SARS CoV-2 results in development of protective IgG antibodies against spike protein of the virus (similar to a response following vaccination) [27]. These antibodies cross the placenta (with IgA versions in breastmilk) to provide passive immunity to the newborn [27]. In some genetically susceptible children, autoantibodies triggered by SARS CoV-2 infection may bind to receptors in neutrophils and macrophages causing activation and secretion of pro-inflammatory cytokines that results in development of MIS-C [9,28]. Children with MIS-C have higher SARS-CoV-2 IgG titers than those with severe COVID-19 [29], however, this trend is transient in MIS-C [30]. We speculate that the spike protein IgG antibodies are protective innocent bystanders, are a marker of prior infection and do not have a pathogenic role in MIS-C. On the other hand, autoantibodies against endothelial, gastrointestinal, and immune cells are also produced and may potentially play a role in MIS-C [31]. Patients with MIS-C have high levels of certain antibodies against autoantigens (anti-SSB, anti-Jo-1), lending credence to the hypothesis that MIS-C is mediated by a persistent autoimmune response to the original infection [31]. As such, and analogous to neonatal lupus, where anti-SSA and anti-SSB antibodies cross the placenta to cause manifestations such as rash and congenital heart block in newborns, it is plausible that similar antibodies against autoantigens crossed the placenta after a SARS CoV-2 infection and initiated MIS-N disease in these neonates. In our case series, atrioventricular conduction abnormalities were common (Figure 2) potentially secondary to transplacental transfer of similar antibodies.

We would like to differentiate MIS-C in the neonatal period due to early-onset SARS-CoV-2 infection in the neonate from "MIS-N" where the infection occurs in the mother and the neonates present early as shown in this case series (Figure 1). We acknowledge that the CDC has not labelled or described this condition and nomenclature may change in the future.

That maternal antibodies pass transplacentally is a known fact, and maternal infection with SARS-CoV-2 is no different. Multiple studies have reported the transplacental transfer of anti-SARS-CoV-2 IgG antibodies to neonates [32–34]. The majority (87%) infants born to seropositive mothers had detectable IgG antibody at birth, transfer ratios were more than 1.0, and there was a positive correlation between maternal and infant antibody titers, regardless of the presence of symptoms in the mother or the severity of disease [33].

None of the mothers in our case series had received vaccination against COVID-19 (vaccines were only administered to >45 years age strata in India during the study period). Although COVID-19 vaccines were not tested in pregnant mothers, many pregnant health care workers have received the Pfizer and Moderna vaccines in the US [35]. These mothers have a robust IgG and IgA response in their sera and breast milk respectively [27]. Umbilical cord sera were positive for IgG antibodies. We speculate that these vaccine induced antibodies against SARS CoV-2 spike protein are protective and do not pose a risk of MIS-C in babies because they are not directed towards autoantigens. Approximately 4500 pregnant mothers have registered in the V-safe COVID-19 vaccine pregnancy registry. Limited data from this registry have not reported any neonatal deaths to date [9,36].

The majority of infants in our case series were delivered at late preterm gestation. The NICHD Maternal Fetal Medicine Units (MFMU) network has reported a higher incidence of preterm labor and delivery in symptomatic pregnant mothers with COVID-19 (severe symptoms—42%; mild to moderate symptoms—15%; asymptomatic—12%) [37]. Therapy for MIS-N is mainly supportive. All patients in our case series received immunomodulatory therapies (intravenous immunoglobulin-IVIG and steroids), anti-platelet agents (aspirin), and anticoagulants (unfractionated heparin or LMWH). Further studies are required to evaluate the benefits and risks of these therapies in MIS-N [23,25]. While some cases, especially those with cardiac conduction abnormalities responded well to IVIG and steroid therapy, we need randomized trials to evaluate efficacy of these therapies in MIS-C. Overuse of these agents should be avoided. We admit that there was probably overtreatment with steroids, LMWH and IVIG among our patients and many of these patients might have improved without these therapies. More targeted therapy with these agents based on further research is prudent as IVIG use among neonates carries the potential risk of necrotizing enterocolitis [24].

5. Conclusions

We conclude that maternal history of SARS-CoV-2 infection or exposure to COVID-19 may potentially be associated with multisystem inflammation, thrombosis, and AV conduction abnormalities in the early neonatal period. However, neonatal MIS-C and MIS-N are relatively rare. More common causes for cardiac dysfunction and elevated troponin or BNP such as perinatal asphyxia and sepsis should be considered. Based on our case series, we recommend that among neonatal patients born to mothers with a history of COVID-19, neonatal MIS-C or MIS-N be considered in the differential diagnosis to explain unusual signs of multisystem inflammation, after excluding common causes.

Author Contributions: Conceptualization, R.P.; methodology, R.P., V.G., N.P., V.M., A.G., S.L. (Sanjog Loya) and R.S.; validation, R.P., V.G., A.C., V.T., U.P. and N.N.; formal analysis, R.P. and S.L. (Satyan Lakshminrusimha); investigation, V.G., V.M., A.G., S.L. (Sanjog Loya) and A.C.; data curation, R.P., V.G., U.P. and N.P.; writing—original draft preparation, R.P.; writing—review and editing, R.P., N.N. and S.L. (Satyan Lakshminrusimha) All authors have read and agreed to the published version of the manuscript.

Funding: This research received no external funding.

Institutional Review Board Statement: The study was conducted according to the guidelines of the Declaration of Helsinki, and approved by the Institutional Ethics Committee of D. Y. Patil Medical College Kolhapur (438/2021/IEC, on 15 May 2021).

Informed Consent Statement: Informed consent was obtained from parents/guardians of all subjects involved in the study.

Acknowledgments: We thank Rupali Patil, Amar Naik, and all post graduate residents in Pediatrics from all the included NICUs for their contribution in patient management. Also, thanks to R. S. Patil and Akshata Pawar (Pathologists), for laboratory tests and their interpretations in neonates. Special thanks to Shimpa Sharma, Pro-Vice Chancellor, D. Y. Patil Education Society (Institution deemed to be University), Kolhapur, R. K. Sharma, Dean and Anil Kurane, Head of Department of Pediatrics, Dr. D. Y. Patil Medical College Hospital and Research Institute, Kolhapur, for their guidance. We thank Ananya Nrusimha for her critical editing of the manuscript.

Conflicts of Interest: The authors declare no conflict of interest.

References

1. WHO COVID-19 Dashboard. Available online: https://covid19.who.int/ (accessed on 24 June 2021).
2. Gupta, S.; Malhotra, N.; Gupta, N.; Agrawal, S.; Ish, P. The curious case of coronavirus disease 2019 (COVID-19) in children. *J. Pediatr.* **2020**, *222*, 258–259. [CrossRef]
3. Brodin, P. Why is COVID-19 so mild in children? *Acta Paediatr.* **2020**, *109*, 1082–1083. [CrossRef]
4. Rawat, M.; Chandrasekharan, P.; Hicar, M.D.; Lakshminrusimha, S. COVID-19 in Newborns and Infants-Low Risk of Severe Disease: Silver Lining or Dark Cloud? *Am. J. Perinatol.* **2020**, *37*, 845–849. [CrossRef]
5. Whittaker, E.; Bamford, A.; Kenny, J.; Kaforou, M.; Jones, C.E.; Shah, P.; Ramnarayan, P.; Fraisse, A.; Miller, O.; Davies, P.; et al. Clinical Characteristics of 58 Children With a Pediatric Inflammatory Multisystem Syndrome Temporally Associated With SARS-CoV-2. *JAMA J. Am. Med. Assoc.* **2020**, *324*, 259–269. [CrossRef]
6. Verdoni, L.; Mazza, A.; Gervasoni, A.; Martelli, L.; Ruggeri, M.; Ciuffreda, M.; Bonanomi, E.; D'Antiga, L. An outbreak of severe Kawasaki-like disease at the Italian epicentre of the SARS-CoV-2 epidemic: An observational cohort study. *Lancet* **2020**, *395*, 1771–1778. [CrossRef]

7. Belhadjer, Z.; Meot, M.; Bajolle, F.; Khraiche, D.; Legendre, A.; Abakka, S.; Auriau, J.; Grimaud, M.; Oualha, M.; Beghetti, M.; et al. Acute Heart Failure in Multisystem Inflammatory Syndrome in Children in the Context of Global SARS-CoV-2 Pandemic. *Circulation* **2020**, *142*, 429–436. [CrossRef]
8. Davies, P.; Evans, C.; Kanthimathinathan, H.K.; Lillie, J.; Brierley, J.; Waters, G.; Johnson, M.; Griffiths, B.; du Pre, P.; Mohammad, Z.; et al. Intensive care admissions of children with paediatric inflammatory multisystem syndrome temporally associated with SARS-CoV-2 (PIMS-TS) in the UK: A multicentre observational study. *Lancet Child Adolesc. Health* **2020**, *4*, 669–677. [CrossRef]
9. Nakra, N.A.; Blumberg, D.A.; Herrera-Guerra, A.; Lakshminrusimha, S. Multi-System Inflammatory Syndrome in Children (MIS-C) Following SARS-CoV-2 Infection: Review of Clinical Presentation, Hypothetical Pathogenesis, and Proposed Management. *Children* **2020**, *7*, 69. [CrossRef] [PubMed]
10. Consiglio, C.R.; Cotugno, N.; Sardh, F.; Pou, C.; Amodio, D.; Rodriguez, L.; Tan, Z.; Zicari, S.; Ruggiero, A.; Pascucci, G.R.; et al. The Immunology of Multisystem Inflammatory Syndrome in Children with COVID-19. *Cell* **2020**, *183*, 968–981.e7. [CrossRef] [PubMed]
11. Godfred-Cato, S.; Tsang, C.A.; Giovanni, J.; Abrams, J.; Oster, M.E.; Lee, E.H.; Lash, M.K.; Le Marchand, C.; Liu, C.Y.; Newhouse, C.N. Multisystem Inflammatory Syndrome in Infants<12 months of Age, United States, May 2020–January 2021. *Pediatric Infect. Dis. J.* **2021**, *40*, 601–605.
12. Godfred-Cato, S.; Bryant, B.; Leung, J.; Oster, M.E.; Conklin, L.; Abrams, J.; Roguski, K.; Wallace, B.; Prezzato, E.; Koumans, E.H.; et al. COVID-19-Associated Multisystem Inflammatory Syndrome in Children—United States, March–July 2020. *MMWR Morb. Mortal. Wkly. Rep.* **2020**, *69*, 1074–1080. [CrossRef]
13. McCarty, K.L.; Tucker, M.; Lee, G.; Pandey, V. Fetal Inflammatory Response Syndrome Associated With Maternal SARS-CoV-2 Infection. *Pediatrics* **2020**. [CrossRef] [PubMed]
14. Divekar, A.A.; Patamasucon, P.; Benjamin, J.S. Presumptive Neonatal Multisystem Inflammatory Syndrome in Children Associated with Coronavirus Disease 2019. *Am. J. Perinatol.* **2021**. [CrossRef]
15. Khaund Borkotoky, R.; Banerjee Barua, P.; Paul, S.P.; Heaton, P.A. COVID-19-Related Potential Multisystem Inflammatory Syndrome in Childhood in a Neonate Presenting as Persistent Pulmonary Hypertension of the Newborn. *Pediatric Infect. Dis. J.* **2021**, *40*, e162–e164. [CrossRef] [PubMed]
16. Kappanayil, M.; Balan, S.; Alawani, S.; Mohanty, S.; Leeladharan, S.P.; Gangadharan, S.; Jayashankar, J.P.; Jagadeesan, S.; Kumar, A.; Gupta, A.; et al. Multisystem inflammatory syndrome in a neonate, temporally associated with prenatal exposure to SARS-CoV-2: A case report. *Lancet Child Adolesc. Health* **2021**, *5*, 304–308. [CrossRef]
17. Shaiba, L.A.; Hadid, A.; Altirkawi, K.A.; Bakheet, H.M.; Alherz, A.M.; Hussain, S.A.; Sobaih, B.H.; Alnemri, A.M.; Almaghrabi, R.; Ahmed, M.; et al. Case Report: Neonatal Multi-System Inflammatory Syndrome Associated With SARS-CoV-2 Exposure in Two Cases From Saudi Arabia. *Front. Pediatr.* **2021**, *9*, 652857. [CrossRef] [PubMed]
18. Clark, B.C.; Sanchez-de-Toledo, J.; Bautista-Rodriguez, C.; Choueiter, N.; Lara, D.; Kang, H.; Mohsin, S.; Fraisse, A.; Cesar, S.; Sattar Shaikh, A.; et al. Cardiac Abnormalities Seen in Pediatric Patients During the SARS-CoV2 Pandemic: An International Experience. *J. Am. Heart Assoc.* **2020**, *9*, e018007. [CrossRef]
19. CDC. Information for Healthcare Providers about Multisystem Inflammatory Syndrome in Children (MIS-C). Available online: https://www.cdc.gov/mis-c/hcp/ (accessed on 25 June 2021).
20. AAP. Multisystem Inflammatory Syndrome in Children (MIS-C) Interim Guidance. Available online: https://services.aap.org/en/pages/2019-novel-coronavirus-covid-19-infections/clinical-guidance/multisystem-inflammatory-syndrome-in-children-mis-c-interim-guidance/ (accessed on 25 June 2021).
21. Chawla, D.; Chirla, D.; Dalwai, S.; Deorari, A.K.; Ganatra, A.; Gandhi, A.; Kabra, N.S.; Kumar, P.; Mittal, P.; Parekh, B.J.; et al. Perinatal-Neonatal Management of COVID-19 Infection—Guidelines of the Federation of Obstetric and Gynaecological Societies of India (FOGSI), National Neonatology Forum of India (NNF), and Indian Academy of Pediatrics (IAP). *Indian Pediatr.* **2020**, *57*, 536–548. [CrossRef] [PubMed]
22. Kobayashi, T.; Fuse, S.; Sakamoto, N.; Mikami, M.; Ogawa, S.; Hamaoka, K.; Arakaki, Y.; Nakamura, T.; Nagasawa, H.; Kato, T.; et al. A New Z Score Curve of the Coronary Arterial Internal Diameter Using the Lambda-Mu-Sigma Method in a Pediatric Population. *J. Am. Soc. Echocardiogr. Off. Publ. Am. Soc. Echocardiogr.* **2016**, *29*, 794–801.e29. [CrossRef]
23. Alsaleem, M. Intravenous Immune Globulin Uses in the Fetus and Neonate: A Review. *Antibodies* **2020**, *9*, 60. [CrossRef]
24. Navarro, M.; Negre, S.; Matoses, M.L.; Golombek, S.G.; Vento, M. Necrotizing enterocolitis following the use of intravenous immunoglobulin for haemolytic disease of the newborn. *Acta Paediatr.* **2009**, *98*, 1214–1217. [CrossRef] [PubMed]
25. Whitworth, H.B.; Sartain, S.E.; Kumar, R.; Armstrong, K.; Ballester, L.; Betensky, M.; Cohen, C.; Diaz, R.; Diorio, C.; Goldenberg, N.A.; et al. Rate of thrombosis in children and adolescents hospitalized with COVID-19 or MIS-C. *Blood* **2021**. [CrossRef]
26. Lakshminrusimha, S.; Hudak, M.; Dimitriades, V.; Higgins, R.D. Multisystem Inflammatory Syndrome (MIS-C) in Neonates (MIS-N) Following Maternal SARS CoV-2 COVID-19 Infection. *Am. J. Perinatol.* **2021**. (editorial under review).
27. Gray, K.J.; Bordt, E.A.; Atyeo, C.; Deriso, E.; Akinwunmi, B.; Young, N.; Medina Baez, A.; Shook, L.L.; Cvrk, D.; James, K.; et al. COVID-19 vaccine response in pregnant and lactating women: A cohort study. *Am. J. Obstet. Gynecol.* **2021**. [CrossRef]

28. Kabeerdoss, J.; Pilania, R.K.; Karkhele, R.; Kumar, T.S.; Danda, D.; Singh, S. Severe COVID-19, multisystem inflammatory syndrome in children, and Kawasaki disease: Immunological mechanisms, clinical manifestations and management. *Rheumatol. Int.* **2021**, *41*, 19–32. [CrossRef]
29. Anderson, E.M.; Diorio, C.; Goodwin, E.C.; McNerney, K.O.; Weirick, M.E.; Gouma, S.; Bolton, M.J.; Arevalo, C.P.; Chase, J.; Hicks, P.; et al. SARS-CoV-2 antibody responses in children with MIS-C and mild and severe COVID-19. *J. Pediatric. Infect. Dis. Soc.* **2020**. [CrossRef]
30. Vella, L.A.; Giles, J.R.; Baxter, A.E.; Oldridge, D.A.; Diorio, C.; Kuri-Cervantes, L.; Alanio, C.; Pampena, M.B.; Wu, J.E.; Chen, Z.; et al. Deep immune profiling of MIS-C demonstrates marked but transient immune activation compared to adult and pediatric COVID-19. *Sci. Immunol.* **2021**, *6*. [CrossRef]
31. Gruber, C.N.; Patel, R.S.; Trachtman, R.; Lepow, L.; Amanat, F.; Krammer, F.; Wilson, K.M.; Onel, K.; Geanon, D.; Tuballes, K.; et al. Mapping Systemic Inflammation and Antibody Responses in Multisystem Inflammatory Syndrome in Children (MIS-C). *Cell* **2020**, *183*, 982–995.14. [CrossRef]
32. Zeng, H.; Xu, C.; Fan, J.; Tang, Y.; Deng, Q.; Zhang, W.; Long, X. Antibodies in Infants Born to Mothers With COVID-19 Pneumonia. *JAMA J. Am. Med. Assoc.* **2020**. [CrossRef]
33. Flannery, D.D.; Gouma, S.; Dhudasia, M.B.; Mukhopadhyay, S.; Pfeifer, M.R.; Woodford, E.C.; Triebwasser, J.E.; Gerber, J.S.; Morris, J.S.; Weirick, M.E.; et al. Assessment of Maternal and Neonatal Cord Blood SARS-CoV-2 Antibodies and Placental Transfer Ratios. *JAMA Pediatr.* **2021**. [CrossRef]
34. Atyeo, C.; Pullen, K.M.; Bordt, E.A.; Fischinger, S.; Burke, J.; Michell, A.; Slein, M.D.; Loos, C.; Shook, L.L.; Boatin, A.A.; et al. Compromised SARS-CoV-2-specific placental antibody transfer. *Cell* **2021**, *184*, 628–642.e10. [CrossRef]
35. Blumberg, D.; Sridhar, A.; Lakshminrusimha, S.; Higgins, R.D.; Saade, G. COVID-19 Vaccine Considerations during Pregnancy and Lactation. *Am. J. Perinatol.* **2021**, *38*, 523–528. [CrossRef] [PubMed]
36. Shimabukuro, T.T.; Kim, S.Y.; Myers, T.R.; Moro, P.L.; Oduyebo, T.; Panagiotakopoulos, L.; Marquez, P.L.; Olson, C.K.; Liu, R.; Chang, K.T.; et al. Preliminary Findings of mRNA Covid-19 Vaccine Safety in Pregnant Persons. *N. Engl. J. Med.* **2021**. [CrossRef] [PubMed]
37. Metz, T.D.; Clifton, R.G.; Hughes, B.L.; Sandoval, G.; Saade, G.R.; Grobman, W.A.; Manuck, T.A.; Miodovnik, M.; Sowles, A.; Clark, K.; et al. Disease Severity and Perinatal Outcomes of Pregnant Patients With Coronavirus Disease 2019 (COVID-19). *Obstet. Gynecol.* **2021**, *137*, 571–580. [CrossRef] [PubMed]

MDPI
St. Alban-Anlage 66
4052 Basel
Switzerland
Tel. +41 61 683 77 34
Fax +41 61 302 89 18
www.mdpi.com

Children Editorial Office
E-mail: children@mdpi.com
www.mdpi.com/journal/children

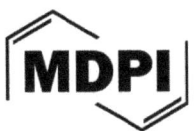